D1567454

Jensen's history
and trends
of
professional nursing

Gerald Joseph Griffin, B.S., M.A., R.N.

Former Head, Department of Nursing, Bronx Community College of the City University of New York, Bronx, N. Y.

and

Joanne King Griffin, B.S., M.A., R.N.

Instructor, Division of Nurse Education, New York University, New York, N. Y.

With a special unit on Legal Aspects by

Elwyn L. Cady, Jr., J.D., B.S.Med.

Medicolegal Consultant, Kansas City, Mo.

and a

Special unit on Nursing in Canada by

Mary B. Millman, B.A., R.N.

Professor Emeritus, University of Toronto, Toronto, Ontario, Canada

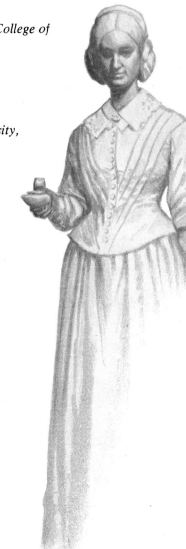

Jensen's history and trends of professional nursing *Sixth edition*

Deborah Jensen

Gerald Joseph Griffin

Joanne King Griffin

Illustrated

Saint Louis

The C. V. Mosby Company

1969

Sixth edition

Copyright © 1969 by
The C. V. Mosby Company

Previous editions copyrighted 1943, 1950,
1955, 1959, 1965

Printed in the United States of America

Standard Book Number 8016-1976-9

Library of Congress Catalog Card Number
69-18835

Distributed in Great Britain by Henry Kimp-
ton, London

To The "Cinders" Three:

Mary Hope, Jerilyn, and Maura

Preface

The revision and updating of any written history about today's nursing world is an all but impossible assignment for anyone who is more than an onlooker in nursing's mainstream. The process of change, usually slow and erosive, has speeded up to a point near visibility. One cannot help but feel that this era in nursing has the potential to effect changes as significant as those we attribute to Florence Nightingale and her time. How it will happen, and where? Who will the leaders be? What changes will occur? Who can really answer these questions? The history we have recorded here should be of some predictive value, at least in comprehending our past, and hopefully, in planning for our future. One cannot but feel that even greater things are in store.

It seems imperative to acknowledge once again our admiration of Deborah MacLurg Jensen who still exemplifies some of the best attributes of the twentieth century nursing educator. In addition, we must express our sincere gratitude to the many generous people who were kind enough to submit thoughtful critiques of the fifth edition. Many of their suggestions have been incorporated into this edition.

Gerald Joseph Griffin
Joanne King Griffin

Preface to first edition

The modern approach to the study of history is sociological, as emphasized by the *Curriculum Guide for Schools of Nursing.** Only thus is it possible fully to appreciate the significance of the broad current of events which out of the past flow into the future, and which will profoundly affect the lives of every one of us, both individually and as a profession. Approaching the subject from this angle, the nurse will reach a fuller understanding of her place in the society of the future. She must, however, learn it against the background of the past, and of those other currents of our social structure by which her own profession has been influenced and moulded.

To clarify the lines of her study these other currents have been traced separately to weave a background, the first part of this book, against which the rise and evolution of modern nursing may be better appreciated. In the second part of the book, an endeavor has been made to give due emphasis first to the pioneer British efforts, then to modern American leadership, and finally to the beginning of international cooperation, to the future of which we all look with such great expectations. At the same time, an attempt has been made to stress the human element by rendering as vivid as possible the sketches of the great leaders of our profession, and by gathering the best available collection of illustrations, including portraits.

The *Curriculum Guide* places the history of nursing with psychology, sociology, social problems in nursing service, and professional adjustments in Group II of the program of nursing education, the section dealing with the nurse's social and professional adjustments. It is recommended that thirty hours be given to the study of the history.

The material for this book has been collected from various sources over a period of many years and it is impossible to mention all those who have, directly or indirectly, contributed to it. I shall always keep in inspiring memory the fascinating course in the history of nursing, which Miss Isabel Stewart gave at Columbia University. Mrs. Dorothy Rogers Williams and many other outstanding contemporary leaders contributed much to the final shaping of the manuscript.

Deborah MacLurg Jensen

---

*The Curriculum Guide for Schools of Nursing, published by the National League of Nursing Education, 1937.

Contents

Chapter 2

Nursing in antiquity

Very little mention is to be found in ancient history of nursing as a separate occupation. Certain activities must be performed, and specific needs must be met by society. Reference is made to the midwife and occasionally to women who looked after children. Of course, in the study of many ancient religions, priestesses are described who often performed functions now recognized as belonging to the nurse. The temple or place of worship in ancient days was also the health center; people who were ill went there for the treatment of disease as well as to worship. In fact, many of the health instructions were intermingled with concepts of religion and magic.

EGYPTIAN MEDICINE

Medicine originated in the practice of magic. In early Egypt certain empirical knowledge regarding sickness slowly accumulated from the witchcraft. The practice of medicine never entirely outgrew the superstitions that surrounded its origin. Today, even the very educated patient looks toward his physician for something more than the logical application of a technical science. Medicine in Egypt reached a surprisingly advanced stage of knowledge. The custom of embalming enabled the Egyptians to become well acquainted with the organs of the human body. From clinical observa-

tions they learned to recognize some 250 different diseases; to treat these they developed a great number of drugs and procedures, including surgery. At the time of Herodotus, about 484-425 B.C., neurosurgery was advanced to a point beyond the imagination of the visiting Greeks. However, their ignorance of normal and pathological physiology and of experimental investigation limited their theories.

Egyptian medical practice was centered in the personage of Imhotep, chief physician to Pharaoh Zoser of the Third Dynasty about 3000 B.C.

Imhotep was not only chief physician but also by far the most trusted advisor to King Zoser. One of his major contributions was in architecture, which affected the beauty of the projects of the dynasty for generations; another major contribution was in the care of the sick. This remarkable man also left behind much wisdom in the formulation of his wise proverbs. The common people sang these proverbs for centuries after his death. His fame was such that he became a demigod almost immediately upon death and was raised to the honor of full diety centuries later. On the Isle of Philae a temple was erected to Imhotep, and actual worship to him continued into the sixth century of the Christian era.

With the decline of Egyptian civilization,

medicine came under Greek influence. Although the Greeks brought their own ideas regarding medicine, they undoubtedly absorbed much of the knowledge found in Egypt, thus becoming bearers of some of the ancient truth to our own time.

GREEK MEDICINE AND HOSPITALS

Hippocrates (about 460 to 370 B.C.) stands out as a real person in the mythology surrounding early Greek medicine. The chief contribution of his school was to change the magic of medicine into science of medicine. Hippocrates taught physicians to use their eyes and ears and to reason from facts rather than from gratuitous assumptions. His writings on fractures and dislocations remained unexcelled until the discovery of the x-ray. The Oath of Hippocrates possesses such a vitality that even today many are admitted to the practice of medicine with it, and the Hippocratian school has perhaps erroneously been given credit for the first ethical guide on medical conduct.

In ancient Greece we distinguish between two refuges for the sick: the secular and the religious. Physicians directed the secular, which corresponded roughly to spas or health resorts of today. Some were endowed and had outpatient departments, and

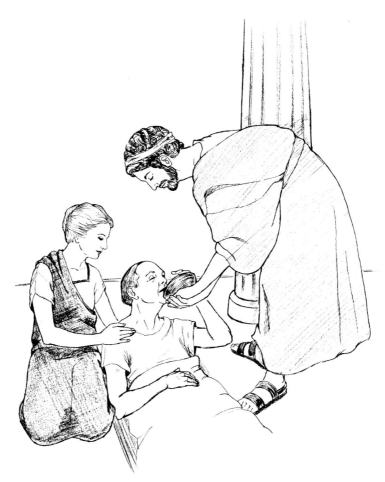

Specially trained care of the sick has been a characteristic of highly civilized peoples. The ancient Greeks had several centers for such care—among them the Temple of Hygeia, named for the goddess of Health, the daughter of Aesculapius.

some were used for the instruction of medical students. The secular places of healing and the sanctuaries of the gods, especially Aesculapius, were closely associated; of these, the one at Epidaurus, his birthplace, is the most famous. Most important here was the play upon the patient's emotions by a complicated ritual. Other practices that may have been more effective in bringing about cure were rest, wholesome food, physiotherapy, and fresh air and sunshine on porches overlooking the blue Mediterranean while the patient awaited the appearance of the god in his dreams. There were more than eighty such sanctuaries throughout ancient Greece. One of the most famous is the Temple of Cos, the birthplace and later seat of activity of Hippocrates.

The first suggestion of women being associated with the healing arts is found in Greek mythology. Aesculapius, who eventually became deified as the God of Healing, had five children; one daughter, Hygeia, became the Goddess of Health, and another, Panacea (our word for "cure-all") the Restorer of Health. Aesculapius is represented by the familiar caduceus. Later most Greek healing centered around shrines in which many patients congregated. Among the attendants were the so-called "basket bearers" and those who were supposed to look after the sick somewhat in the manner of nurses. In the writings of Hippocrates there are many references to procedures that would be undertaken in modern hospitals by nurses but no reference to a nursing vocation as such. In ancient Greece and Rome the nursing of the sick and wounded was probably an incidental household duty, since there is no reference to any organized nursing group.

EARLY CHRISTIAN CHURCH

The great element of altruism contained in the Jewish religion later bcame further emphasized by Jesus Christ. Love is the fundamental element of His teaching. Its practical expression appeared in the early Christian Church in the form of succor to the orphans, the poor, the travelers far from home, and above all, the sick. The deaconesses of the early church visited the sick, much like modern visiting nurses. They were lay women appointed by the bishops. These appointments were highly esteemed and were given to women of good social standing. The women were often sent on distant and varied missions to accomplish

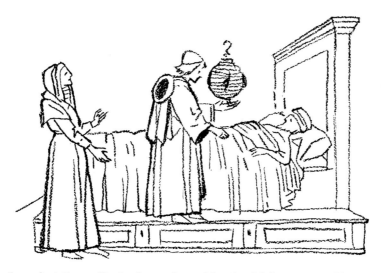

In ancient Greece "basket bearers" cared for the sick in a manner like nurses.

their appointed tasks. Gradually their work was assumed by the various orders, and their activities declined. One of the best known deaconesses of the early Christian Church was Phoebe, a Greek lady who is also remembered as the bearer of St. Paul's epistle to the Romans. Visiting nursing soon became an important part of the work of these early deaconesses, and Phoebe is often referred to as the first visiting nurse as well as the first deaconess. During the fourth and fifth centuries the names of three Christian matrons of patrician Rome, Fabiola, Paula, and Marcella, were associated with charitable work. These matrons were particularly interested in the care of the sick.

In the early days of the Christian era the Roman Empire was at its peak. At the height of its splendor Claudius Galen (A.D. 130-201) was physician to the Emperor Servetus. He worked with incredible industry observing, experimenting, and gathering information. Unfortunately, many of his conclusions were based on speculation. Although his anatomical and physiological observations were admirable, his later dominance over medieval and Renaissance medicine came about largely by the force of obscure and erroneous notions that retarded medical progress for centuries.

However, Galen's voluminous writings contained virtually all of the medical knowledge of his day—knowledge that only through his industry survived the destruction of the Roman Empire. The translation of his writings into the Arabic chiefly accounted for their preservation; therefore, until the time of the Crusades, Arabian physicians became the standard bearers of medical knowledge.

EARLY CHRISTIAN HOSPITALS

Although early Christendom at first encouraged women to visit the sick and to nurse them, refuges for the sick made an early appearance. Patients were sheltered in the bishop's houses, but when this proved impractical, special institutions were estab-

lished by endowments throughout the Roman Empire. In Rome the first large hospital was established by Fabiola, a beautiful, worldly woman, who thereby did penitence for her second marriage. She administered this hospital so well that her death was mourned by all Rome.

In the Eastern Roman Empire several large hospitals were established; the Emperor Constantine founded one at Constantinople, A.D. 330; but the largest of them all was the one that St. Basil of Athens built on land granted him by the Emperor Valerian near the city of Caesarea in Asia Minor. It was tremendous, constituting a town all of its own, with separate hospitals for lepers, children, the aged, and strangers. These hospitals, however much contemporaries may have been impressed by them, did not continue into the later centuries.

A few centuries later in the Western world the first hospitals immediately under the auspices of the Roman Catholic Church were founded; these still exist. In Lyons, the Hôtel Dieu was established in A.D. 542 by Childebert; it is now the hospital with the longest record of continuous service. Detailed records were kept of the Hôtel Dieu in Paris, which was founded about A.D. 650-651 by St. Landry, Bishop of Paris. It was greatly enlarged in the thirteenth century by St. Louis and was the prototype of the medieval hospital. The records of this hospital constitute a principal source of information regarding nursing in those days.

MOSLEM HOSPITALS

During the eighth to the tenth centuries magnificent hospitals were erected throughout the Moslem world. For the times they had excellent endowments. One in Bagdad received about $1,200 a month, and the physician-in-chief served gratuitously. In addition these hospitals had a great advantage over their European contemporaries, for they were staffed by physicians superior to any in the world. Greek knowledge had been preserved by the Moslems.

One large hospital in Bagdad had a staff of twenty-four physicians. In 869 its superintendent published the first known pharmacopeia. By 1160 there were some sixty medical institutions in that city. Best known to Western lands, however, were the big institutions in Damascus and Cairo. The hospital in Cairo was founded by the Sultan of Egypt in 1276 as a thanks offering for having been cured of the colic.

It was endowed with an income of 25,000 pounds, and contained four great Courts, each with a fountain in the centre, wards for each separate disease, a lecture room, and a department for attending patients at their own homes. Musicians and storytellers were provided for the amusement and benefit of those troubled with sleeplessness, and the convalescent patient received, at his departure, five pieces of gold, about 50 shillings, that he might not be obliged to return to work immediately.*

*British Medical Journal, 1908, p. 1448.

Such was one of the hospitals of the "infidels," whom the Crusaders tried so hard to exterminate. These structures were in marked contrast to the rather gloomy, Gothic Hôtels Dieu in France of a few centuries before.

MOHAMMEDAN MEDICINE

Physiology and hygiene were studied by the Arabian scientists, knowledge in materia medica was expanded, and surgeons used various drugs as anesthetics, but Moslem belief in the uncleanliness of the dead forbade dissection. The following names stand out: Rhazes (860-932), noted for his study of communicable disease, and Avicenna (980-1037), who wrote extensively —his *Canon of Medicine* was used long after his death.

Chapter 3

Medieval medicine and nursing

During the Middle Ages, medicine in Europe was under two influences—the lay medicine that followed what was left of the Roman traditions and the ecclesiastical medicine that existed in the monasteries, around which most of the existing hospitals were built.

For one thousand years after Christ, there were no attempts to organize nursing. As the Middle Ages advanced, three organizations developed that have either persisted in some form to the present day or that had established certain principles still recognized as important. These organizations were the military, regular, and secular orders. All worked under the auspices of the Church, which, as we know, profoundly influenced all activities of the Middle Ages.

The most spectacular product of the feudal system was the Crusader, a man who was supposed to combine a lofty spirit devoted to the service of God with a fierce, belligerent temper, ready to fight the infidel wherever he was to be found, that the holy ground upon which Christ trod might again belong to his followers. He carried the principles and the glory of knighthood to its fullest development as he traveled over the continent of Europe and throughout the Mediterranean basin. When he traveled in the Near East, he learned much from the enemy; the idea of the organized hospital

was originally borrowed from the Arabs. The natural places for the establishment of hospitals were the outposts, particularly Jerusalem itself, in which those wounded in battle sought refuge while they recovered. The hospital had to be staffed by physicians and nurses who were members of the regular orders. The nurses went to battle and then retired to attend the sick. They were called "knight hospitalers." In later years they devoted themselves entirely to nursing. Two great influences shaped nursing practice in the Middle Ages—the religious and the military. Gradually the care of the sick was considered more and more to be a religious duty.

MILITARY ORDERS

Three nursing orders became preeminent: Knights of St. John, Teutonic Knights, and Knights of St. Lazarus. Corresponding with these were three orders for women who tended female patients in special hospitals.

Knights of St. John

About 1050, Italian merchants of Analgi founded two hostels in Jerusalem, one for men and the other for women. The former was dedicated to St. John the Almoner; the latter to St. Mary Magdalene. Some fifty years later the Order of St. John became prominent, and it is generally assumed that this order originated in the nursing staffs of these two hospitals. Peter Gerard, an intensely devout man, was active in the organization of the order on a high religious plane under the Grand Master. The members were divided into three classes: the priests, the knights, and the serving brothers. The women's branch of the order, organized under Agnes of Rome, devoted itself to religion and nursing; they gave up the latter pursuit, however, when the order was driven from Jerusalem.

The Order of St. John proved a huge success; branches were established everywhere, and its extraordinary vitality is shown by the fact that it has persisted to the present day and is active in England. St. John's Ambulance Association and the National Association for the Aid of the Sick and Wounded During War are activities of the order. The order was active in the organization of the International Red Cross, which carries its insignia as its mark.

The order had a long and varied career. At the reconquest of Jerusalem by the infidels it was driven to Cyprus and from there to Rhodes where it established a magnificent hospital that was used as recently as World War I. At this very moment some of the apartments once used by the knight nurses house refugees from other eastern Mediterranean countries.

The order became a prominent, affluent, and important factor in medieval Christendom. Many of the customs that it established have remained the heritage of nursing to the present day. Being military in character the discipline was strict, and modern nursing traces its tradition of obedience to superiors to the Order of St. John. The order also established the organization of rank and the principles of complete and unquestioned devotion to duty. Although extreme subservience does not belong to our day and age, it must still be remembered that in an organization in which exact execution of orders and minute attention to instruction may determine the difference between life and death of patients, strict attention to detail must continue.

Teutonic Knights

The Teutonic Knights made up the German equivalent of the Order of St. John. They date back to a hospital founded by Germans in Jerusalem soon after 1100. They took an active part in the subsequent wars in the Holy Land, especially the siege of Acre in 1190, when they established a tent hospital for wounded crusaders. In consequence they were established as Brothers of the Hospital of St. Mary of Jerusalem. Later they become a separate order under the rule of St. Augustine. Their organization was modeled on the Order of St. John, and they seem to have been, for a while,

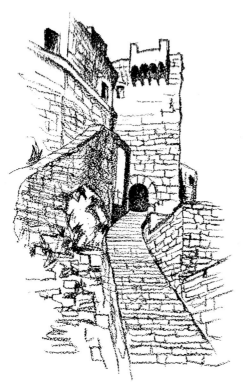

The hospital of the Order of St. John at Rhodes

The Knights of St. John established branches throughout Europe, one of which still exists in England.

under the jurisdiction of that order. Like their model, they gradually came into possession of great property, especially in Sicily. They always remained under German leadership, however, and eventually their main seat was moved to Germany where they became primarily a military order. The nursing of this order was largely done by men; women were not admitted to full membership but retained a secondary position. Sisters of this order were, however, engaged in nursing as late as the end of the fifteenth century.

Knights of St. Lazarus

The Knights of St. Lazarus were established primarily for the nursing of lepers in Jerusalem after this city had been conquered by the Christians. Later, Boigny near Orleans became their main seat, but as leprosy became less prevalent by the end of the fifteenth century, the order was dissolved and its property was absorbed by the Order of St. John.

REGULAR ORDERS

As the early Christian Church developed, those who devoted their lives to the service of God followed the example of Christ, and the very spirit of the Church led it to care for the fatherless, the poor, and the sick. In antiquity, when the Pax Romana prevailed, people could safely travel. The deaconesses could go to people's homes and nurse their sick; later, because of the insecurity of the early Middle Ages, men sought protection behind moats and walls. The men and women of God established monasteries in which they organized hospices to house their charges. In the beginning, travelers, paupers, and patients were housed under the same roof; the modern words of hostel, hotel, and hospital, now with different meanings, all have the same origin—hospice or hospitium, a place of refuge. The early hospital was called a "Hôtel Dieu." Soon, however, it became advisable to care for the sick separately, and with the knowledge the crusaders gained from the Arabs, the hospital, as we

now know it, had its origin. As society again became better organized, and with the growth of cities, hospitals tended to become separate institutions apart from monasteries although many of them continued to be staffed by the regular orders.

Of these, the sisters who took charge of the Hôtel Dieu in Paris are the best known, because their records are the most complete. They began about A.D. 650 as a small group of volunteers who looked after the sick in the hospital. They remained primarily a nursing order called the Augustinian Sisters. For the first 600 years of their existence as a nursing order they were without severe restrictions, but about 1250, Innocent IV caused them to become cloistered under the rigid rules of St. Augustine. The Augustinian nun wore a white robe, and when she become a full Sister, a hood was added to her habit. In Hôtel Dieu she worked very hard, both early and late, with no recreation, and apprenticeship the only method of instruction.

In spite of very inadequate medicine and nursing during the Middle Ages there began to be an increase in the institutions for the care of the sick. Sometimes this was stimulated by epidemics. The number of individuals, mainly volunteers, who devoted themselves to nursing also increased. During the fourteenth century one of the outstanding and devoted women whose activities were linked with the care of the sick was St. Catherine of Siena (1347-1380). At night her lamp represented to the sick of Siena what Miss Nightingale's lamp was to mean in the Crimea. Catherine was not of noble birth; she had been trained in what we would call a middle-class home to help with housework as was the custom of the day. A devout Catholic with a decided bent toward asceticism, she found great happiness in nursing, and in spite of the protest of her parents, she devoted a great deal of her time to working in the hospital in her native town. She taught herself to read and, some years later, to write.

She became a tertiary of the Order of St. Dominic, an organization within the regular order to which she could not be admitted because of her youth. However, the members decided that, because of her great homeliness, it would be safe to allow her to nurse and to visit in the homes of sick patients. In 1372 the plague came to Siena, and Catherine worked day and night at nursing. She became particularly well known about the hospital at La Scala; it stands as a memorial to her today.

St. Hildegarde (1099-1179), a Benedictine abbess in Germany, is associated more with medicine than with nursing, since she actually prescribed cures and was supposed to perform miracles. However, she trained young noblewomen in the care of the sick in her abbey.

In the sixteenth century the Ursulines, an order which emphasized the care of the sick and the education of girls, were founded. It is of great interest to nurses and teachers in the United States, because some of the early schools and hospitals were staffed by Ursuline Sisters.

The nursing provided in the Middle Ages was simple. It consisted mostly of providing for the patient's physiological needs, giving medications and bathing and dressing wounds and ulcers. The ideas concerning cleanliness and ventilation differed considerably from ours: windows were often placed so high that they were difficult to reach, and bathing and the changing of bed linen would not measure up to modern standards. Heating, lighting, and plumbing arrangements were either very primitive or nonexistent. When the Mother Superior made her evening rounds, it was by the light of a torch that she was carrying. Nursing appliances were also primitive. Much equipment that we consider essential such as thermometers and hypodermic syringes were entirely missing; the use of rubber was unknown, and accessories like bed rings were made of leather stuffed with hair; draw sheets were made of leather and later of

oiled cloth. At the Hôtel Dieu there were no washing machines; the nurses carried the dirty linen down to the river on wash days. Many of the activities of the Sisters were limited by prejudices. Because the human body was considered inferior and unclean, it was considered improper for the nurses to undertake certain procedures, such as giving enemas to men or vaginal douches to women. An important duty of the Sisters was to minister to the spiritual needs of the patients; in an age when religious considerations dominated every activity, this took a great deal of time.

The nursing order was definitely organized; the Sisters advanced from the stage of probationer to wearing the white robe to receiving the hood. They were all under a "superintendent of nurses" or director of nursing; in those days she was called a prieuré or maîtresse. In the beginning there was no uniformity of dress; nurses wore their regular clothes when on duty. Clothes became gaudy as the Middle Ages advanced; and because the Church secluded itself from the more worldly aspects of life, there was a tendency to adopt a uniform dress that eventually became entirely standardized. We have thus studied the first organization devoted to nursing; now let us consider its strong and its weak points.

The strength of the nursing order was its organization into an institution under the immediate guidance of the strongest spiritual and secular power of the time, the Church. Absolute devotion to the sick without mundane or selfish motive made the nursing order acceptable to all, and it was thus able to survive for many centuries. The Augustinian Sisters at Hôtel Dieu in Paris can look back upon its record of over twelve centuries of uninterrupted sevice. The nursing order was not firmly associated with the medical profession for two reasons: it was sponsored and dominated by the Church, and the medical profession in the Middle Ages had not developed into a profession capable of exerting leadership over nursing.

However, the strength of the nursing orders was also their weakness. By being so closely attached to the Church, they had to share the vicissitudes of that organization; and because it later suffered censure for practices that were at variance with its professed purpose and ideals, the nursing orders suffered with it. They were sent out of countries in which the Protestant Reformation had gained the upper hand, and their property was confiscated. Those countries then passed into what has been called the "dark age" of nursing. Their close attachment to the Church also sometimes prevented them from enjoying the advantages of the medical progress that did occur. When the interests of Church and medicine conflicted, the Church prevailed, often to the detriment of the patient. As time passed, and as the Catholic Church recovered from weaknesses occurring during the Middle Ages and adopted broader policies of modern days, these difficulties were largely solved. The Catholic nursing orders now seem perfectly capable of serving both Church and patient without detriment to either.

SECULAR ORDERS

Some of the drawbacks of the nursing orders were apparent also to their contemporary observers. Demands for complete and perpetual devotion to God would not always attract those best suited or inclined to care for the sick. Consequently, organizations developed for the primary purpose of nursing. Many of them, it is true, prospered under the auspices of the Church, often as lay branches of the regular holy orders, but some of them remained relatively independent. On the whole, the tendency in the course of time was to make the secular orders approach the regular ones by requiring temporary vows, uniformity in dress, and religious observances. Many of these orders possessed extraordinary vigor and have persisted to the present time. They were very numerous but similar; this description will

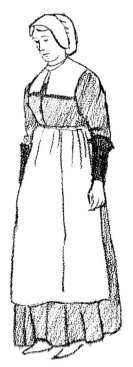

Sixteenth century nurse

Secular nursing groups often had many characteristics in common with regular and religious orders, such as uniformity of dress.

be limited to six of the more interesting ones.

Third Order of St. Francis

About the year 1200 St. Francis was a lively young man in Assisi in northern Italy. He had generally led a carefree life until illness and disagreement with his father brought out the more serious side of his character. At first he retired into the wilderness, but soon he decided to devote his life to the service of God and man. He began by rebuilding a local church, and he attempted to lead a life as similar as possible to that of Jesus. Soon he was joined by friends, all of whom devoted their lives to poverty and service of the poor. When the group numbered twelve, they obtained Papal sanction as an order and dressed in brown or grey woolen hooded robes ("Gray

Friars") with ropes around their waists. They set forth traveling from place to place to spread the Gospel and to teach the better way of life they had learned to live. Eventually their number increased, and they became a great and powerful order with branches throughout the countries of Europe. They were the first Order of St. Francis.

Among those who watched the work of St. Francis was a young girl from his home town. Her name was Clarissa. She was so influenced by his work that one night she ran away from home and joined the small band of Francis and his friends. Francis consecrated her at the altar and cut off her beautiful hair as a sign that she had abandoned vanity and devoted herself to God; she dressed in a simple robe similar to that of the brethren. After having lived in a Benedictine convent for protection, she eventually established an abbey of her own; the Sisters who gathered around her grew into a regular nursing order, "The Poor Clares." These were the second Order of St. Francis.

The work of St. Francis greatly stirred the people of his time; there was a great surge to abandon the temporal for the life of God. St. Francis soon realized that to admit unlimited numbers to his order would not be practical, so he instituted the third or tertiary order, which was secular in the sense that the members did not give up their social relationships or take vows of chastity but devoted their lives to the order in their home town, without neglecting their duties as citizens. These people improved their communities as they served the Order. One of their most important duties was nursing. For centuries male and female nurses belonging to the third Order of St. Francis could be found in hospitals and homes.

Order of St. Vincent de Paul

Nearly 400 years later, about 1600, another inspired priest St. Vincent de Paul, founded with prophetic vision another nursing order that has become very important. St. Vincent lived in Paris, France, where he joined in the care of the sick of a neighboring hospital. Here he discovered that charity was often poorly directed, being bestowed to excess on some, while others equally deserving went without aid; therefore, St. Vincent organized charity wherever he could. He devoted special attention to begging which was rampant at the time, and whenever possible he tried to guide tramps and beggars into useful occupations. His greatest work, however, was done in companionship with Louise de Gras (Saint Louise de Marillac). She was a widow of a noble family who had devoted herself to visiting nursing, and directed a group of volunteer women devoted to this purpose. She was a rare woman, for along with her feeling of social responsibility she was highly educated, being conversant with the Scriptures, Latin, philosophy, and painting. Under the guidance of St. Vincent she studied closely the various lay organizations of charity devoted to the care of the poor and the sick all over France. Finally, on her return to Paris, she organized the "Dames de Charité" (the Ladies of Charity), an institution devoted to social work.

Soon she found that these ladies had difficulty in establishing the right kind of contact with the poor of the slums of Paris; their duties as ladies of charity conflicted too often with their domestic duties. Louise then decided to train her own social workers. In 1633 she opened her home to young peasant girls who as "The Community of the Sisters of Charity" became the foundation of one of the most important of nursing orders. To be accepted the girls must be of good family and of good character; they enter with the consent of a male relative. Each year on March 25 they dedicate and rededicate themselves to their work, but if they do not wish to do so, they are free to resign from the order to marry or to take up some other occupation.

In their training and practice they have made every endeavor to overcome the difficulties that were noted in the discussion of the regular orders, and by working closely with physicians and by assuming all nursing duties they spread all over the world and set a fine example of what a nursing order should be. One of their greatest services was in the Crimean War, for here they not only nursed the French wounded but also, by their example, indirectly stimulated the discontent in the British Army that eventually resulted in Florence Nightingale's great work.

The Beguines

The Beguines are a most interesting group of lay nurses originally organized in Liege, Flanders, about 1170 by the priest Lambert le Begue. The concept of their organization was that it should be liberal but devoted to the service of suffering mankind. Groups of women lived together in little houses, four or five in each. If they occupied a number of houses, these might be surrounded by a wall; however, in small communities this was not the case. These women were available for all kinds of household aid, especially nursing of the sick, but they also sewed, made lace, or taught. They did not beg but supported themselves by their wages and fees for services to those who could pay, as well as by special funds provided for them by the community. They made no vows but accepted certain standards as long as they belonged to the order. For instance, they could not marry and remain Beguines. The adoption of a uniform was optional; when a group designed one for themselves, it was generally in accordance with contemporary dress. They became immensely popular, and the order spread from Flanders into the Netherlands, France, and Germany. At its height about the middle of the fourteenth century it numbered approximately 200,000 members. They staffed hospitals where necessary but generally devoted themselves to work throughout the community; some were found in every community, their number depending upon the need for their services. They always endeavored to live within walking distance of their work. At all times, even to World War II they served their communities, often in a manner comparable to that of the Red Cross.

Similar groups have from time to time come under the domination of the regular orders as tertiaries. Such a fate overcame the entire Order of the Visitation of Mary that was established in Dijon, France, by St. Jane de Chantal with the help of St. Francis de Sales. They began an order of visiting nurses, with activities like those of the Beguines, but because the Church insisted upon cloistered seclusion, they had to change their activities and to restrict themselves to offering succor to those who could come to them.

The Oblates

The Oblates, founded in the twelfth century in Florence, Italy, are another order similar to the Beguines. They gained distinction by the manner in which they staffed the hospitals of Florence and by the broad training that they received for this task. They still remain an established order.

Order of the Holy Ghost (Santo Spirito)

The Order of the Holy Ghost originally had branches for both men and women, although this order is remembered chiefly as a male nursing order. It was founded in Montpellier, France, in the twelfth century by Guy de Montpellier. The numerous "Holy Ghost" hospitals, churches, and streets may be traced back to the activities of this order.

THE MEDIEVAL HOSPITAL

Moslem ideas about hospital construction and administration were adopted by the Crusaders and influenced the great hospitals of the military nursing orders in Jerusalem. Later, as these orders were driven west, the Moslem influence appeared in the hospitals that they constructed in Rhodes and Malta. Inspired by what he had learned in the East, Pope Innocent III about A.D. 1200 decided to build a modern hospital in Rome. He called on Guy de Montpellier of the growing Order of the Holy Ghost to establish this hospital on the bank of the Tiber. Because of its architecture, efficient management, and nursing care, it remained in operation until destroyed by fire in 1922.

When this hospital was finished, the Pope begged the bishops from foreign lands to come and to inspect it and then to go back and to construct similar hospitals in their home dioceses. During the next hundred years literally thousands of such hospitals under the Order of Santo Spirito, Heiligen Geist, or Holy Ghost were spread all over Europe. Street names bear witness to their locations down to the present day. The best of these hospitals were magnificent places, architecturally beautiful with painted Gothic doors, and with window and wall coverings of precious hangings in the manner of the times. The high, wooden ceilings were beautifully carved; privacy of the beds was secured by partitions that could be removed

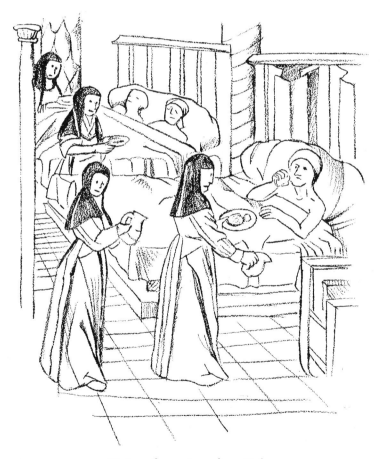

Sixteenth century hospital

Most early hospital architecture was profoundly influenced by Moslem ideas which were adapted by the Crusaders and military nursing orders. Often these hospitals were quite beautiful from an aesthetic point of view.

when mass was said. The greatest artists contributed to these decorations, which made the hospitals beautiful and attractive.

Not until the present day has the wholesome effect that pleasant architectural designs and attractive furnishings have on the patient's morale been appreciated. In fact, some medieval hospitals were so attractive that even well-to-do citizens who were left alone in the world would move into them bag and baggage and turn over all their property to the hospital in return for carefree old age.

In this period a distinction must be made between the two types of hospitals in the medieval towns. There were the city hospitals proper, built within or actually in the walls of the city. There were also the isolation hospitals placed outside the city called "plague" or "leper houses" that served as refuges for those unfortunate outcasts of society. Nursing in them was largely provided by the Order of St. Lazarus. When the Black Death swept Europe in the fourteenth century, it seemed like a fire to consume all who were weak and ailing; following it, leprosy almost disappeared, with consequent neglect and decay of the leper houses.

The better hospitals had resident and visiting physicians who were also often professors of medicine. If they had known a little more medicine, they would have been a setup for fine medical services, for the nursing by religious orders was then at its height, its devotees being enthusiastic servants of Christ.

MEDICAL SCHOOLS AND MEDICINE IN THE LATER MIDDLE AGES

The establishment of the famous medical school in Salerno, Italy, was a great medical event of the ninth century. Until the fourteenth century this school was the center for all medical teaching and was not primarily dominated by the Church. It was abolished by a Neapolitan decree in 1811, but had been in a decline for a long period before

that. In the twelfth and thirteenth centuries, many famous universities were established in Europe. The growth of medieval cities with the corresponding increase in wealth and power influenced this development. The medical school at the University of Montpellier established in the twelfth century was the most famous medical school for several centuries, probably because it was practically independent. The University of Paris had a medical faculty at the same time, but within the department of philosophy. In northern Italy the medical school at the University of Padua was gaining a favorable reputation as was the University of Bologna in France. By the end of the fifteenth century there were well-organized medical schools in many European countries and in Great Britain. Laws governing the practice of medicine were in effect in these same countries. It was to these centers of medical learning that the great medical men of the Renaissance turned for information and inspiration.

Physicians or doctors of medicine at that time considered the practice of surgery inferior and beneath the dignity of scholars. In the fourteenth century the student of medicine in Paris had to swear that he would not do any surgical operations. Surgeons of that period often traveled from place to place performing operations for the stone, hernia, and cataract, as well as blood-letting, pulling teeth, applying cups, and giving enemas. In England the union of surgeons and barbers lasted until 1745, and in 1800 the present Royal College of Surgeons was founded.

By the end of the fifteenth century, the newly invented technic of printing resulted in the rapid increase in both the number and variety of medical books that before then could only be reproduced painstakingly by copyists.

Although names such as Paracelsus (1493-1541) are recorded as outstanding in their time, they do not represent any fundamental advance of physicians of their era generally. What little practice of medicine there was, was so involved in superstitions and erroneous assumptions that it must have done little good. Patients who recovered often did so because their desire to live overcame not only the disease but also the treatment to which they were subjected.

THE RENAISSANCE IN MEDICINE

The well-known name of the forerunner of the great medical developments of this period is that of Leonardo da Vinci whose anatomical studies and sketches remain classic. Vesalius (1514-1564) is remembered as the founder of anatomy as a science and, with Harvey, of a medical science based on fact rather than on tradition. The work of these sixteenth century anatomists enabled the surgeons to work on a more solid basis. Ambroise Paré (1510-1590), a military surgeon, wrote a great book on natural history in general and on surgery in particular in which he emphasized that it was not necessary to dress wounds with boiling oil and that bleeding could be controlled with ligatures as well as by red-hot cautery. He also devised artificial limbs for the victims of war. During this period nursing reached a high level of organization and efficiency in the religious and military orders.

Harvey and his time (1578-1657)

We ordinarily associate William Harvey's name with the discovery of the circulation of the blood, but his contribution to medicine is much greater than the discovery of a single physiological fact, however important, for he established the principle of the physiological experiment. He received his anatomical training at Padua and returned to the St. Bartholomew's Hospital in London where he served as demonstrator of anatomy at the Physicians' College in Amen Street. Here he completed his great discovery, which he communicated in a lecture in 1616. His book was not published until

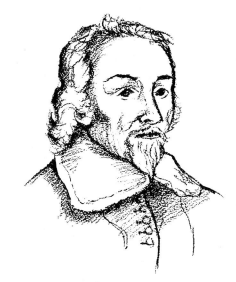

William Harvey

William Harvey is often called the father of modern medicine because he established the principle of the physiological experiment.

twelve years later. In due course, he became attached to the Court of King Charles I, left London with this monarch, and was in Oxford during the siege of that city. While there, his home in London was searched, and all of his manuscripts and notes were destroyed. What loss medicine thereby suffered can only be surmised, for some of the titles were of great promise, including "The Practice of Medicine Conformable to the Thesis of the Circulation of the Blood," and "Anatomy in Its Application to Medicine."

Following these disturbances, Harvey returned to London and became one of the scientific leaders of his day. He donated his library to the College of Physicians and established a lectureship that has continued to this day and to which we owe, among others, Osler's marvelous oration of 1905*

---

*Osler, William: The harveian oration on the growth of truth as illustrated in the discovery of the circulation of the blood, Lancet, October, 1906.

on the founder himself. Harvey exhorted the fellows and members of the college to study out the ways of nature by means of experiment; and, most important, they were urged to continue in love and affection among themselves. These traditions are still highly regarded in the old college.

Thomas Sydenham, 1624-1689

The simple methods taught by Hippocrates were all but forgotten when they were suddenly resurrected by a man who later was called the English Hippocrates, Thomas Sydenham. Sydenham was Puritan by birth and outlook. He took part in both the Cromwellian wars.

Sydenham's great contribution to medicine was that he first set the example of true clinical method. His independent and unprejudiced spirit, combined with great powers of observation, made him the prototype of the clinical investigator. It was he who resurrected the great principles of Hippocrates: to observe phenomena and to let observations logically lead to conclusions. He expounded, "We should not imagine or think out, but find out, what nature does or produces." That this sounds obvious to us is only because Sydenham has succeeded to such an extent that his teaching has become commonplace. In his time medical science carried a superstructure of wanton speculations and theories that made it so complicated and cumbersome that it became deprived of real value. In fact, Sydenham was attacked because he made the practice of medicine too simple and easy. In modern times his name is most commonly associated with his description of chorea, although that of gout was much more of a masterpiece.

Undoubtedly, Sydenham received great support from his friendship with his colleague, the physician-philosopher John Locke, the private physician to Lord Shaftesbury. Locke was a proponent of common sense and straight thinking and the forerunner of Hume and Kant. The essence of his philosophy was to consider the reasonableness of taking probability as our guide in life. In thus eliminating the fantasies and vagaries of the mind, Sydenham met on common ground with Locke; the two must have been great mutual supporters.

It has been stated that Sydenham was considered little better than a quack by his contemporaries. It is true that his views met with great opposition and that he did not participate in the activities of the Royal Society of Medicine. During his lifetime he was considered one of the great physicians of the age although his true magnitude was not appreciated for several generations.

CONCLUSION

At this time London abounded in quackery of all kinds. Quacks, mountebanks, chemists, apothecaries, and even surgeons, who in those days were not supposed to treat internal diseases but nevertheless did, joined in exploiting the healing crafts. Druggists copied prescriptions they were supposed to fill and sold the drugs privately over the counter. One was said to have profited a hundred times as much out of a single prescription as did the doctor who wrote it. Consequently, five sixths of the physicians went with their hands in their pockets all day, the greatest part of the business passing through only a few men's hands (though some of them were more ignorant than the others). It was considered that medicine was overstocked with students graduating from the universities. He who began practice must have had to resolve to be a perpetual slave and servant to the meanest and basest all the days of his life. Upon the physician were imposed taxes, polls, large fees for houses, servants, and entertainments—more in this age than formerly. The main requirements for beginning a practice were to have a good understanding with the druggist and to be seen regularly at church.*

---

*Payne, Joseph Frank: Thomas Sydenham, New York, 1900, Longmans, Green & Co., pp. 165 ff.

Chapter 4

The dark period in nursing and social setting for reform

The dark period in nursing and the social setting for reform dates roughly from the end of the seventeenth to the middle of the nineteenth century. The dark period was characterized by nursing conditions so terrible that some time must be spent on an analysis of how such conditions could come about. It should be noted that during the same period the principles upon which modern medicine was built were established and that remarkable progress in other fields of human endeavor is evident. Medicine developed rapidly during these years. One great man after another made important contributions, not only to detailed medical knowledge but also to its basic principles. There has always been a lag between medical discoveries and their practical adoption. In present times, this is a very short span. One notes, for example, the rapid adoption of insulin or the sulfonamides, but in the old days when postgraduate communication was slow and medical instruction proceeded along primitive lines, physicians persisted tenaciously in old habits.

The general practitioner and most specialists practiced as did their medical predecessors until well into the eighteenth century. During the years that followed, the changes were not great. The doctor of those days simply was not in a position to demand good nursing, for he did not know what comprised good nursing. Good nursing is predicated upon a knowledge of anatomy, physiology, hygiene, and bacteriology; a knowledge that in those days was nonexistent. Assumed knowledge and superstition, the details of which are now practically forgotten because they are worthless, occupied the place of scientific knowledge. Therefore, in the practice of medicine, in spite of the growth of medical knowledge, nothing existed to stimulate the evolution of nursing as a profession. The new knowledge was not to bear practical fruits for many years to come.

The guiding principle of ecclesiastic nursing was charity; there was no concept of medical progress or of medical efficiency. Nursing services, therefore, were as good as the organization within the Church that supported them; some orders continued nursing efficiently until the present time and experienced no "dark age." For the most part, in Catholic countries, nursing remained more or less on the same level, ready to take advantage of progress when it appeared.

The emergence of an organized group such as the nursing profession can be understood only if we understand its back-

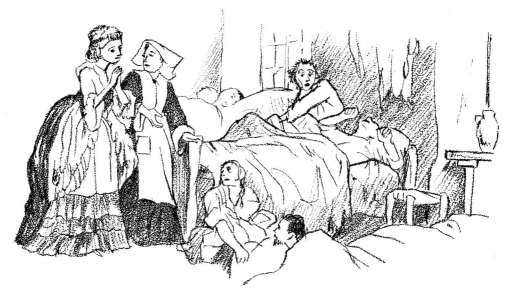

Eighteenth century hospital

Nursing care during the eighteenth century was guided by charity, not by knowledge or principles of safety and hygiene.

ground. Nursing as we know it today was greatly influenced in its professional development by the social and economic change called the Industrial Revolution. By referring to this change as an industrial revolution we do not mean to focus our attention on one element, the mechanical change that occurred in Western Civilization, for it must be realized that the entire process was fostered by economic change. Economy originally meant the rules governing housekeeping; here we use it in the sense of the producing or procuring of the essentials of life. As this activity changed, it altered the entire lives of men, including their environment, their thinking, and their political philosophy and conduct. Out of this setting emerged the world as we know it today. We must look upon the present world as the outcome of the past and the beginning of the future. There is nothing static about it, nor anything hard and fast. Yet to understand nursing we must understand its most important elements of the past as well as those that are likely to dominate its future.

In other words, we must think of nursing as a social function.

INFLUENCE OF THE REFORMATION

Nursing sank to its lowest levels in the countries in which the Catholic organizations were upset by the Reformation. The state closed churches, monasteries, and hospitals. In England alone it was said that over one hundred hospitals were closed, and for a while there was little or no provision for the institutional care of the indigent sick. When the demand became too great to be ignored, lay persons were appointed to run the hospitals. For example, this was done in the case of St. Bartholomew's Hospital in London, in St. Giles in the Fields, and St. Katherine's Hospitals. These hospitals were not run because of the principle of charity but because of a social necessity. There was no honor attached to running a hospital or to being on its staff. At St. George's Hospital a man and his wife were engaged at salaries of £ 8 and £ 10 per annum to be messenger and matron, respectively. The matron remained there in charge of the nurses, and a nurse in charge of a ward or a division was called a "Sister," possibly because it was thought that by retaining the title, some of the devotion and dignity of the old days might be retained also. This, however, was not the case, for when deprived of the dignity of the Church, nursing somehow lost its social standing. Nurses were no longer recruited from the respectable classes of the community but from the distinctly lower classes. The new Protestant Church abhorred cloisters and religious institutions and did not feel the same responsibility to the sick that had characterized the early Catholic Church. Nurses were drawn from among the discharged patients or from the lower strata of society—women who could no longer eke out a living from gambling or vice often turned to nursing.

Another factor in this situation was the status of woman in the social structure of two or three hundred years ago. From the antiquity of Rome to the Middle Ages, the Catholic Church had assigned to woman a place in society that afforded her much freedom and opportunity to move about in the world. Thus women of ability could carve out careers for themselves, and the lay nursing orders especially offered them great opportunities to contribute to the life of the times.

The Protestant Church, although it stood for religious freedom and freedom of thought, did not think much of freedom for women. In the seventeenth and eighteenth centuries and into the Victorian era the place of the average respectable woman was in the home—a "career woman" would have been next to unthinkable around the year 1700. All teaching, secretarial work, and literary endeavors were confined to men, and work then unsuitable for men, such as nursing, was entirely out of the reach of the average woman, even if she had wanted to do it. Housework demanded infinitely more effort than nowadays, and those women who had enough servants to free themselves from domestic tasks gave their efforts entirely to the shallow and superficial life of society. The only profession open to women was acting, and that was not very respectable. So women faced with the necessity of earning their own living were practically forced to enter domestic service; nursing was considered a type, although not a very desirable type, of domestic service. After all, the chief duties of a nurse in those days were to take care of the physical needs of the patient, and to make sure that he was reasonably clean, although this was not considered very essential in the early municipal hospitals. Dressings were applied by dressers or by surgeons; the dispensing of medicines was the responsibility of the doctors and the apothecary.

It is possible to understand the low and dismal state of nursing. It existed without organization and without social standing. No one who could possibly earn a living in some other way performed this service; and those who did lost caste thereby, for, as you are judged partly by the company you keep, a woman who began to practice nursing was almost certain to become corrupted if she was not so already. Most nurses were venal, drunken, and given to even worse vices than these. They expected and took bribes wherever they could be obtained, and liquor was their chief solace.

There were reasons why the nurse should fall a victim to these vices. Her pay was poor; if she had to provide only for herself, she could perhaps eke out a miserable living; but if she had children or other dependents to support, her pay was entirely insufficient, and she was forced to supplement it by any means available in order to survive. Her hours were so long and her work so strenuous that she had no opportunity to supplement her income by additional work. Her work was cheerless and depressing if she thought about it. If she worked in the hospitals, she was dealing with riffraff and the scum of creation; if she were lucky enough to be admitted to nurse respectable persons, she was considered the most menial of servants. As well as the long hours (sometimes nurses worked twenty-four or forty-eight hours at a stretch) they received poor food and sometimes none at all during the long night shift. There was no future toward which these women could look; this was the end of the road. They should, therefore, not be judged too harshly if they turned to the only source of comfort that was open to them—the bottle.

Seen with our eyes, nursing was a blotch on seventeenth and eighteenth century society, but the contemporary attitude was one of inertia and complacency. The high ideals of the Middle Ages were gone, and a demand for adequate nursing had not yet risen. However, when men with the inquisitive spirit of the eighteenth century began to look into social evils, nursing was examined along with the rest of them. Hogarth's cartoons and later Dickens' description of Sairey Gamp were caricatures that had their effect. In a more serious vein the writings of John Howard (1727-1789) have become famous.

INDUSTRIAL REVOLUTION

The Industrial Revolution emerged from a social state called feudalism. Feudalism was stationary, and if it had not been for the Reformation, which really was a product of the Renaissance, and the great scientific discoveries, it might have gone on for centuries. In almost every respect it differed from our world; it was essentially static with fixed concepts of class relationships defined by insurmountable barriers. Life was strictly localized; it centered around the manor, which offered a measure of protection and exercised a crude but effective form of law and justice in return for hard work by the individual to obtain the bare necessities of life. So much work was required to obtain food, clothes, and shelter for the present that there was very little chance of obtaining reserves for the future or for barter. There was little time for education or

for leisure, and freedom to pursue them became, of necessity, restricted; and limitations became further imposed by the social order on the right of movement as well as upon political and religious thinking. It was a conservative, patriarchal state of society, offering few of what we today consider the amenities of life; the individual lived in continuous fear of famine, pestilence, and the figments of his own imagination, such as witchcraft and other superstitions.

The Crusades, acting as a catalyst, began to change all this. Knights returning from the Middle East yearned for the knowledge, pleasures, gracious living, and comforts they had enjoyed so briefly. Out of the ferment came the sixteenth century with its great changes. New, rich lands were discovered beyond the seas, and men began to emigrate and to bring back treasures to the old centers of population. The immediate effects of this were tremendous: the treasures from the new lands made for a richer life, a "surplus economy" was being created, transportation was encouraged, and the center of gravity was shifted from the Mediterranean to the Atlantic seaboard, a change that was to chiefly benefit England. During the time that followed, there was progress in domestic agriculture. Under the feudal system it had been, to a certain extent, communal; it now became more individualistic, and methods were improved. This led to a better yield, fewer men were required to till the ground, and with better food more men survived to a productive age. This agricultural surplus population moved to the cities in which industries had begun to develop in response to the growing wealth. These industries did not offer attractive careers; at first, they had few, if any, machines and it was long before they utilized power other than that of man and beast. There were the guilds, but their range was narrow, and the early industrial worker was limited by fixed wages, inability to move, and many social customs. Essentially the feudal outlook was carried into the early industrial community.

It is questionable whether this Industrial Revolution would have extended very far had it not been stimulated by the new thought.

NEW THOUGHT

The origin of the new thought may immediately be traced to the Reformation. Although the religious aspects of this movement are most spectacular, more important than these fundamental elements is the new stimulus to thought provided by the freedom that generated from the Reformation and eventually transformed our ideas of government, politics, business and philosophy. The right of private judgment was established, which later led to individualism in politics and business and to the concept of the free contract and the right of property. In the feudal order the right of property, by custom, was vested in the sovereign who could, in all ways, abrogate the rights of the individual to hold and to utilize the individual's property. The thinking of Locke, especially, established individual prerogative: the individual's right of property antedates that of the state, and he cannot be deprived of it without his consent (or "due process of law"). With the right of free contract it follows inevitably that the individual is also privileged to acquire and to hold as much property as he can within the limits of the law. This is the fundamental philosophy of capitalism, and it is essential that we grasp it, for without it the Machine Age of the nineteenth century would be unthinkable. Unless we understand it we cannot understand the modifications that it later undergoes and that have profoundly influenced the development of nursing.

Natural sciences

Free thought extended also into the realm of natural science; men began to ask questions to which they expected to find rational answers based on facts alone. The scientific method of inquiry was born. This method of reasoning led to objective observation and to the physical and physiological experiments that form the basis for the modern natural sciences. The writings of Locke, Bacon, and Hobbs guided men's thoughts. Suffice it to mention that Gilbert of Rochester assembled all knowledge pertaining to magnetism and introduced the word electricity; Newton invented calculus and discovered laws governing optics and the law of gravity; Boyle introduced the atomic theory. Thus, through hundreds of observations and discoveries, which often in the most unexpected way gained practical importance, the foundations for sciences were established. It was the scientific attitude that led to the discovery of steam power and the construction of the steam engine and somewhat later to the discovery of electromagnetism and the construction of the electric motor. Without it the modern engines would hardly have come into being, and the Industrial Revolution would have remained unborn. In the course of time, the scientific attitude also laid the foundations for modern medicine, for, as we have seen in Chapter 3, Harvey's and Sydenham's fundamental work was its direct outgrowth. Thus, clearing the air for straight thinking eventually led to the construction of the engine by which our entire lives were to be altered.

Political Philosophy—Mercantilism

Along with studying the laws of nature the philosophers of two and three hundred years ago began to ask questions regarding the conduct and the rights of man. The right of contract to which we have referred was but one of their conclusions. They studied the laws that seemed to govern the growth of population: thus, Petty founded the science of vital statistics and Graunt showed that the population increased in a geometric ratio but that this increase was checked by various factors which in turn were studied by Davenant and de Mandeville; these studies eventually led to the sciences concerning trends in population that are now so essential in grasping the fundamentals of public health. Although purely scientific in their beginning, they were to lead to knowledge of the greatest importance to the modern public health nurse.

The study of the laws of population growth is but a short step to the study of economics, and soon this field was under scrutiny. Gresham founded the science of public finance, and soon the men who guided the new thinking arrived at certain conclusions that by their general acceptance were to exert a fundamental influence on the growth of the state. Their views on the right of property and on national ambition led them to an economic and political philosophy that has been called mercantilism. Property was the watchword, especially property represented by holdings of precious metals or bullion. To obtain these metals foreign trade had to be encouraged, even at the cost of domestic trade. Because trade flourishes when a country has a product to sell, preferably a manufactured product, the importance of manufacturing was stressed. To be able to produce finished goods came to be considered preferable to producing the raw materials from which these goods were manufactured, because the profit was greater.

This was in the days when machines had to be tended laboriously by men and were not the labor-saving devices of today. The chief motor power was man power; therefore, the men of mercantilism began to welcome increases in population, because these increases in man power would eventually mean increases in wealth. We had, at the same time, retained from feudalism the concept of the sovereignty of the head of the state—"L'etat, c'est moi," proclaimed Louis XIV—and that was the view to which most persons acquiesced. It was therefore the monarch or his representative who personified more than anyone else the practical aspects of this philosophy. The common man is the principal asset of the state, and the

personification of the state is the monarch —this is the absolute monarchy. The state became a dynamic entity that, depending chiefly upon the industrial centers of the cities, competed with other states for trade monopolies and far-flung colonies. This was the era in which colonial empires were built.

This political philosophy had one interesting result: since it was realized that the power of the monarch ultimately depended on the number and opulence of his subjects, the monarch became concerned for their welfare. This led to the enlightened monarchy, which was one of the most efficient forms of government ever devised by man. Its defect was the lack of checks and balances that would become effective when the monarch ceased to be benevolent, and that was the cause of its ultimate doom. However, while the enlighted monarchy lasted, the concern of the state for the health and welfare of its citizens resulted in formulation of our first notions of public health. Although factory towns of the eighteenth century may have appeared dingy to us, they were, nevertheless, far in advance of the dirty, smelly cities of the century before. Wealth accumulated, and many strata of the population improved their living conditions. It was also this outlook, which, together with the rapid growth of the cities, was responsible for the rapid increase in hospital construction of this era. Here we have the beginning of public health in the setting of the society that produced it.

Beginnings of revolutionary thought

There were other currents of thought that were to influence men in the future. The philosophers of the seventeenth century who had accepted the right of property and of free contract soon began to ask by what right the sovereign owned the state and by what right he collected tax moneys to be spent on his own personal ambitions rather than on the common good. The answer soon was found to be—by the acquiescence of his subjects. This doctrine of consent of the governed led directly to the political philosophy of the eighteenth century engendered by Rousseau, Voltaire, and Hume.

These political philosophies led to a revaluation of human rights and to the new concept of political liberty. Once the people understood that concept, the Boston tea party was inevitable, leading as it must to the American Revolution and then to the French Revolution. The citizen is no longer the chattel of the sovereign; he is the state, and "citizen" became in France an appellation of honor. The French Revolution and the American Revolution were not revolutions in the sense that the proletariat was placed in power, as occurred in the Russian Revolution a century later; the absolute power of the head of the state was abolished and replaced with a constitutional form of government—immediately in America and eventually in Europe—in which the real power was placed in the hands of the bourgeoisie, the propertied classes.

MACHINE AGE—THE RISE OF ENGLAND

During this same eighteenth century, industrialism, which so far had been very primitive, developed into the Machine Age; the steam engine had now been invented, it multiplied man's power in the factory, and eventually the railroad and the steamship revolutionized transportation. Now factories could be placed near the chief source of their raw materials. All during the eighteenth century and at an accentuated pace during the nineteenth century, England forged ahead of the industrial states. There were many reasons for this: her capitalists had apparently been more awakened by the new philosophies than her Continental confreres, she understood first what production for the masses really implied, her isolated position had largely protected her against the devastation of wars, she was traditionally a nation of sailors, and when it came to getting colonies, she got the lion's share, including the plum of them all—India. The

greatness of the British Empire was to a large extent built upon the riches of India. So we come to look to England as the leader of the Machine Age and consequently as the source of many of the movements that were direct products of this age.

Evils of the Machine Age

England became the first great nation of factories, but certain elements that were part of that development later had to be discarded. We learned that the value of a certain measure of public health was appreciated by the proponents of mercantilism, but these concepts of public health were limited by restricted medical knowledge and furthermore were partly ignored when the absolute monarch disappeared; in fact, they were largely squeezed out by the aggressiveness of the new capitalist. As a type he was so impressed with the right of free contract and the right to acquire and hold property that he forgot that when a man has only the choice between absolute starvation and starvation wages he is not really a free agent. The result was the early dark years of the Machine Age when the capitalist was protected by law in his exploitation of the worker under the guise of free contract. The result was child labor, sweatshops, unhygenic factories, and hours of labor fixed only by the limits of human endurance. This led to the gin shop and all the social evils that soon were to be so graphically described by their reformers. Not the least of these evils were the hospitals. The advances in medicine were so far largely theoretical and had not yet borne practical fruits, so that while medicine definitely was advancing, it was still proceeding slowly and without the dramatic developments that were to mark the end of the nineteenth century. The hospitals were large and crowded, and the conditions of nursing, which were brought about by the Reformation when the Catholic institutions had been closed, had been steadily aggravated until they now reached an all-time low.

HOSPITAL REFORM AND CONSTRUCTION

A new development in our social structure in the eighteenth century, and more so in the nineteenth century, influenced the construction and administration of hospitals: the rise and evolution of capitalism and industrialism. Wealth was created by the manufacture of natural resources brought to the industrial countries from faraway colonies. Manufacture demanded factories, factories required workers, and the profits from individual enterprises went into relatively few pockets; therefore, large numbers of people congregated in the new cities, and the gulf between the new-rich industrial employers, on the one hand, and the laborers, on the other, grew even wider. The result was that extensive sections in industrial cities were inhabited almost entirely by laborers. In sickness, these individuals required ever larger hospitals, and as a direct result of the Industrial Revolution, the demand grew for bigger, but not always better, hospitals. So we see during this period the foundation of the great city hospitals. The London Hospital in the East End of London, the Grosse Charité in Berlin, and the Allgemeines Krankenhaus of Vienna all originated during the eighteenth century, and the development continued through the nineteenth century with the growth of the great cities.

The following notes, taken from the catalogue of the London Hospital, give an interesting account of its progress.

The first course of lectures on surgery was delivered in 1749. In 1772 iron bedsteads were first introduced. In 1780 surgeons were henceforth to be members of the company of surgeons in London. In 1781, Mr. Blizard was granted permission to deliver courses of lectures on anatomy and surgery. In 1791 a thermometer was purchased. In 1820 feather beds were bought for special cases. In 1833 gas was installed in the corridors, though not in the wards. In 1838 an ordinance was passed that medicine was to be administered only by nurses who could read and write. In 1842 special wards were set aside for Jewish patients. In 1849 a microscope was bought. In 1852 the committee held that the apothecary was not the fit person to administer chloroform. In 1856 Miss Florence Nightingale was elected life governor. In 1896 x-rays were introduced.

The evolution during these two centuries cannot compare with the developments of the last fifty years, neither in regard to number of beds nor in regard to technical improvements. Some changes of the nineteenth century must, however, be recorded.

The pavilion system of hospital construction was introduced in the French Academy of Sciences in 1788. It became generally accepted both in Europe and in this country. Its outstanding expression is in the beautiful Bispebjerg Hospital in Copenhagen, which probably is the most expensive hospital to heat yet designed, and also the one which, in proportion to its size, provides the most extensive walking exercises for all who work there, because of the distances between its divisions. As implied in the name, the hospital consists of pavilions and is not built in large blocks as was hitherto the case. In this country the first buildings of the Johns Hopkins Hospital were built by the pavilion system.

Originally as a result of the writings of John Howard, who had severely criticized the hospitals of the eighteenth century, this period also saw the introduction of better hygiene throughout the hospitals, from the nursing service to the plumbing and heating, because the old hospitals had been very cold and unsanitary places. Florence Nightingale, although she failed to appreciate the significance of bacteriology, thoroughly understood the value of fresh air, soap and water, and sunshine. This all preceded the antiseptic and aseptic operating room. We shall learn more later on about the nursing reforms.

During the nineteenth century there was also a tendency to develop hospitals for various specialties. This reached its height in London where the start was made with the Royal London Ophthalmic Hospital, which was founded in 1804 and which was followed by many others: the Royal Free

Hospital run for women by women doctors, St. John's Hospital for diseases of the skin, the Royal Victoria Hospital for diseases of the chest, and many, many others. For a while this tendency also appeared in this country, until the disadvantages of thus emphasizing specialties appeared. The tendency has now been modified so that separate departments are developed within the same hospital, easily accessible to each other.

Outpatient department

With the development of the hospital idea it also became apparent that the hospital's responsibility toward the patient did not always end with his discharge. He may require aftercare while he is ambulatory, or poor patients may wish to avail themselves of the experience of the hospital staff although they are not sick enough to gain admittance to the wards. It thus became logical to establish outpatient departments in connection with the hospitals. Although dispensaries, that is, clinics in which poor patients could be seen gratis and could obtain medicine at cost or free, had been organized in the beginning of the eighteenth century, the outpatient department idea was not thoroughly developed until near the end of the nineteenth century, but when it was developed, the possibilities for medical teaching that it offered were first grasped and best developed in England. In the United States we have been rather slow at appreciating the excellent source of clinical material for nurses as well as for doctors, which is found in the outpatient department.

Early English hospitals

The early movement to construct fine hospitals also reached England. The first one was built at York in 937. This one, however, did not influence further development. For hospitals of enduring importance, we must turn to London, where following the Conquest, three important hospitals were founded—St. Bartholomew's Hospital by Prior Rahere in 1123, St. Thomas' Hospital in 1213, and the Hospital of St. Mary of Bethlehem in 1247. All three of these have so importantly influenced British hospital history that a brief sketch of each is in order.

At the beginning of the twelfth century, a cleric of humble birth became ill while on a pilgrimage to the Holy Land. In his misery, he vowed that, should he be spared, he would on his return to London build there a hospital dedicated to the glorification of God. In answer to his prayer, St. Bartholomew appeared to him in a vision and instructed him to erect a church in Smithfields, London, and name it after him, the Saint. In obedience to his vow, Rahere, who was a courtier as well as a cleric, obtained a grant of land from the King and erected a church and hospital on the chosen site, where it has since remained. The church could still be seen before World War II, but the original hospital had long since been replaced by more recent, if far from modern, structures. St. Bartholomew's Hospital was closed by Henry VIII along with other similar institutions from the Reformation that had ushered in the dark period of hospitals and nursing, but after a few years it was reopened at the request of the Lord Mayor of London. It had then a capacity of 100 beds. During the next century it expanded, and medical teaching was organized there. Since that time "St. Bart's" has been in the heart of British medicine, and some of the most prominent medical men of English history have been on its staff. Outstanding among them is Dr. William Harvey, whose work was discussed in Chapter 3. Although the medical past and present of St. Bartholomew's Hospital has always been outstanding, it shared in the general decay of nursing during the post-Reformation period, and much of our information on how bad nursing became was obtained from the records of that hospital.

St. Thomas' Hospital was founded, south of the Thames, by the Prior of Bermondsey in 1213. It was rebuilt on various sites before it was finally moved to its present location on the south side of the river overlooking the Houses of Parliament. This hospital is of special interest to us, because at the time of this last reorganization, Miss Nightingale established her school of nursing there. St. Thomas' Hospital has, throughout the years, remained among the leading London hospitals. It was badly bombed during the "blitz" of 1940.

Finally there is the Hospital of St. Mary of Bethlehem. In 1247 at the feast for the Translation of Edward the Confessor, Simon Fitzmary gave a tract of land for the erection of a monastery for the brethren of Bethlehem, the second monastic order created in 330 in Bethlehem by Constantine. This land was situated in the eastern part of the city of London, around what is now Liverpool Street Station, and is extremely valuable. In those days it was covered with marshes, fields, and gardens; on this the original Hospital of St. Mary of Bethlehem was erected. It was more of a monastery than a hospital at this time. However, it, too, suffered in the Reformation when Henry VIII expropriated it and handed it over to his political friends who managed it badly. The character thus changed from a monastery, doing charity work, to a regular hospital, and gradually it became purely a lunacy asylum. As such it became a place of horror to the patients and of amusement to the visitors. In those days there was no understanding of mental diseases. The patients were treated with cruel restraint, and it was thought proper to exhibit them to spectators for a small fee. So a visit to see the sights of London included a visit to "Bedlam" as the place eventually was called in common parlance. Later the building was wrecked, and in 1676 a new and magnificent structure took its place. It lasted until 1812 when the last and final structure was commenced.

For many years Bedlam played an important part in London life. Fiction writers sent their characters to languish within its walls, and artists painted its terrors; probably Hogarth's final stage of *A Rake's Progress* was as pictorial a representation of lunacy as was ever accomplished. Awe was inspired by a public exhibition, the horrors of which exceeded the imagination. Although Bedlam presented the horrors of maltreatment of mental disease, it was also responsible for the first rays of the new dawn. It was in connection with the tortures sustained by one American, James Norris, that William Tuke, a York tea merchant in 1792, suggested that mental disease be treated along humane lines. His plea was without immediate effect, but it was the next year that the Frenchman, Pinel, introduced the famous reform of the treatment of mental patients. When reform did occur, the Bethlehem Hospital was again in the van and has taken its place among modern hospitals devoted to the treatment of mental disease. Tuke's work did have an important effect in the United States, for when the Bloomingdale Asylum was opened in 1821 in connection with the New York Hospital, it was molded after Tuke's "York Retreat" and emphasized the mild and humane treatment of the patients.

THE STATE OF MEDICINE

It has been noticed that while nursing was in a very bad condition during this period, medicine was advancing rapidly. During the first part of the eighteenth century Hermann Boerhaave (1668-1738) of Leyden, Netherlands, was easily the most famous physician of Europe. Princes and statesmen alike crowded his waiting room. When he appeared after a sickness, the whole town was illuminated, rejoicing in his recovery. A letter from a Chinese mandarin, addressed "To the illustrious Dr. Boerhaave, Physician in Europe," found him without difficulty. His greatest contribution was his pupils. There was hardly a prominent physician in Europe and North America who had not at some time studied under him. He occupied several university chairs at the same time and excelled in wisdom and classical knowledge. He was one of the first great physicians who appreciated music. When he died in 1738, he left a large fortune of about two million florins.

The seventeenth century had seen two great principles established: (1) disease is to be observed like any other natural phenomenon, and (2) the functions of the human body can be investigated by means of physiological experiments. A third great principle was to be added: symptoms and disturbances of function are associated with changes in the organs of the body and this relation is frequently very specific. It is to Giovanni Morgagni (1682-1771) that we owe this contribution.

His principal work, *On the Seats and Causes of Diseases,* appeared in 1761 when he was 79 years old. It is in the form of a series of letters to an unidentified young man. Morgagni excels in his infinite capacity for working diligently and carefully. He insisted on examining every organ, as well as the one that he suspected of being chiefly affected. He marshalled with the utmost care from his own experience and that of his predecessors all instances in which the disease had existed apart from the symptoms of the lesion or the lesion apart from the symptoms. He discussed each of these incidents with severe exactness, and only after exhaustive investigation would he allow the inference that the organ referred to either was or was not the seat of the disease. Thus he created a work of classical importance and beauty, which even today delights the mind of the scholar.

Thus, Morgagni came to reap the highest honors bestowed on living men. He was a friend of popes and princes, honored by all the scientific groups of importance in Europe, sought by every student of medicine; he died beloved by his family in his eighty-ninth year. Twice when hostile armies invaded his town, their commanders gave strict orders that no harm come to Morgagni and that his work be not hampered.

His wife, who could not have been surpassed in judgment or affection, bore him eleven children—eight daughters who all became nuns, one son who died young, one son who became a Jesuit priest, and one son who married and reared a family.

In Delft, Holland, an unlettered man had the honor of first using the microscope systematically and of perfecting its construction. Anton van Leeuwenhoek (1632-1723) lived quietly, pursuing his microscopic studies and communicating most of his observations to the Royal Society.

In spite of the great leaders who had risen in the seventeenth century, British practice and the teaching of medicine and surgery fell to a low ebb by the middle of the eighteenth century. Obstetrics as a science was just being founded through the efforts of William Smellie (1697-1763). But that was about all. Then suddenly anatomy, surgery, and obstetrics received a great impetus through the efforts of the brothers John and William Hunter. Alike in their zeal and industry for the advancement of science, they otherwise differed most strikingly.

William (1718-1783), the elder, was born in 1718 near Glasgow, where he received his early classical and professional education. Still in his youth he, like so many celebrated Scots, gravitated to London. He became associated with Dr. Smellie, the first male-midwife, founder of obstetrics. He was one of those fortunate few who early in life were placed exactly in the situation for which they are best suited by nature and by education. Given the opportunity to teach anatomy, he soon found himself in charge of the most famous school in the country, and turning to obstetrics he advanced rapidly and eventually became obstetrician to the Queen. In spite of his success, he never let financial considerations crowd out his professional ideals. He realized that a man may do infinitely more good for the public by teaching his art than by practicing it, because the influence of the teacher extends over a whole nation and descends to posterity. So Hunter continued to combine in himself the qualities of a polite scholar, an accomplished gentleman, a complete anatomist, a most perfect demonstrator as well as lecturer. *The Pregnant Uterus* is his main work, which to all times will stand as a landmark in medical literature. About his teaching, he said that he aimed at showing not what he knew but what he thought his students ought to know.

Through his professional efforts he accumulated much wealth, most of which he spent on a magnificent collection now in Glasgow. It contains famous paintings, valuable books, a large number of coins, besides medical and zoological specimens all gathered with great taste and discernment. Thus he combined in himself the qualities of a great teacher, investigator, patron of the arts, and scholar. Besides, he earned additional credit as the man who brought his younger brother to London.

In contrast to the polished William, John Hunter (1728-1793), ten years younger, was considered a misfit for the first twenty years of his life. Not until his brother had introduced him to the art and science of anatomy did his native ability assert itself, but from that day John developed into one of the greatest geniuses of all time. His great intellectual powers triumphed over his early defective training, and he marched onward step by step despite vast obstacles to the highest achievements. After serving a term in the army, he became surgeon to St. George's Hospital, and he gradually acquired the leading surgical practice in London of his day. In contrast to his brother, his progress was slow, for he did not possess the charming manners of William but had to advance by sheer ability. In fact, to the end of his days he remained crude in his expressions and highly undiplomatic; for instance, he generally gave precedence to his poorer patients, saying they had no time to spare, whereas the wealthy ones, having nothing to do, could afford to wait.

Although he had never read Bacon, his mode of studying was as strictly Baconian as if he had. Characteristic is his answer to Edward Jenner (1749-1823), his student: "But why think? Why not try the experiment?" Yet he himself was so busy in his search for knowledge and so cautious in his estimate of it that he always delayed to publish what he knew. He was 43 when he published his first work, and at his death he left many valuable manuscripts and notes, which, to the inestimable loss to the world, were destroyed by his brother-in-law.

A wave of enthusiasm was apparent in France after the French Revolution. Young men now advanced by ability and no longer by privilege and nepotism. This also applied to medicine, and in that century medical science advanced as never before. Beginning with Napoleon's own physician, Jean Nicolas Corvisart (1755-1821), the list runs through Francois Xavier Bichat (1771-1802), the pathologist, who unfortunately died young; Réné Laennaec (1781-1826), to whom we owe the stethoscope and our knowledge of diseases of the chest; to Pierre Louis (1787-1872), who first introduced statistical methods into medicine and who, more than the others, attracted young American students, especially the pathetic figure of James Jackson, Jr., whom he considered almost like a son. The famous school of Dublin, which soon was to shine with the names of Robert Graves (1796-1853), William Stokes (1804-1878), Robert Adams (1791-1875), and Dominic Corrigan (1802-1880), had not yet reached its climax; and on the Continent Karl Rokitansky (1804-1878) and Rudolf Virchow (1821-1902) were not yet famous. By the middle of the eighteenth century interest in real clinical medicine was being stimulated; for example, decisions were based on examination of the patient and the diseased organs rather than on the study of classical texts and the use of metaphysical discussion.

One of the most successful clinicians of the century was William Heberden (1710-

1801). Among other things for which he is remembered is the description of angina pectoris, which has been made available to modern students in reprints. He also described the rheumatic nodules on the fingers called "Heberden's nodes."

William Withering (1741-1799) is remembered for the discovery of the use of foxglove (digitalis) in the case of dropsy.

CONCLUSION

Thus we see the stage being set for the social reforms of the late nineteenth and early twentieth centuries. These reforms included nursing which was soon to be looked upon not only as a skilled technic necessary in scientific medicine, but also as a community service essential to the health and welfare of every community.

Chapter 5

Early reforms

The torch of liberation was carried largely by the intellectuals who continued to follow the views on the human rights to happiness that had been championed by the humanitarian liberals of the eighteenth century. Recognizing the deplorable conditions that existed in the eleemosynary institutions, the Poor Laws were reformed in England in 1832, but even this left much to be desired, and when Dickens, Carlisle, and others of their school revealed the social evils of their time, they met with a ready response among their readers. A sense of social responsibility and a desire to give this feeling a practical response developed among the well-to-do classes. Owen's sociological experiments are an example of this movement, but of greatest interest is its expression in the life work of Miss Nightingale, which was entirely devoted to the relief of the classes in society that could not help themselves. One of the most important accomplishments of this era was the entire reform of nursing education, which is the main topic of this book.

The beginning of the evolution of the nursing profession was primarily the private work of philanthropic persons; it was not sponsored by the state. In time the women who had done nursing in religious or military orders and those untrained and uneducated women who did nursing for money were replaced by the new profession. The govern-ment sponsorship of causes that so greatly increase the fields and scope of nursing is of still more recent origin and has developed out of trends, which we have yet to explain.

EMANCIPATION OF WOMEN

The emancipation of women may be traced ultimately to the trend toward personal freedom, which was one of the factors in the Industrial Revolution. It is part of the fight for human rights, which was first audibly expressed in the eighteenth century and which became one of the principles of the French Revolution. It is a step without which nursing might have developed as a craft but never into the profession as we know it today. Therefore, the emancipation of women forms part of the background which we must know to understand the evolution of nursing. Many attitudes of Florence Nightingale appear peculiar to us if we do not appreciate the difference between the social positions of women a hundred years ago and now. Furthermore, the emancipation of women can no more be considered a completed process than can the Industrial Revolution, the evolution of modern medicine, or even the very evolution of nursing with which we are principally concerned.

The word "moral" comes from the Latin *mos, moris,* custom, and if we use the word in its original sense, we may say that the emancipation of women is fundamentally a moral process, its various practical manifestations—suffrage for women, legal rights, and educational and occupational opportunities—are secondary to the moral aspect.

The customary social attitude toward women a few hundred years ago was one that was almost as old as Christendom and that, in fact, had been dictated by the Church—not by Christ, for his attitude toward women was, as far as can be judged, quite liberal—but by the early Church, especially as influenced by Paul. During the sixth to eighth century the stern attitude toward women was relaxed somewhat, but it was generally believed that woman's place was in the home only.

There were practical reasons for this: the work of housekeeping, like that of producing the necessities of life, was so complicated that it left little time for other pursuits. One part of housekeeping was the rearing of children, which because of the high rate of infant mortality was a most inefficient process. It was not uncommon that out of ten or twelve pregnancies, labors, and months spent taking care of infants there resulted but two or three effective citizens for the community. The energy lost in this manner of procreation was appalling, especially when compared with modern marriages. Young couples today are often limited to two to four pregnancies, but nearly all result in effective citizens. By an effective citizen we mean one who grows to productive manhood or womanhood. Thus there was a good physical reason which would have restrained all but a small privileged class of women from enjoying any measure of freedom even if it had been granted them, and even if the Machine Age had reduced the time required for domestic work, the professional woman as a social class still would not have been possible.

Society's attitude toward women

Another fundamental factor in the emancipation of women was the changing attitude of society toward her. When, during the period of the French Revolution, Concordet upheld the rights of women and Mary Wollstonecraft wrote her *Vindication of the Rights of Women,* it is doubtful if many understood that these were the germs of a movement that eventually was to transform society. Few realized that women needed any "rights." In fact the rights that women already had (such as the franchise, which women had in the United States under the first constitution of New Jersey from 1776 and 1807 and in England prior to the Reform Act of 1832) were not used and consequently were abrogated without contest.

Until the middle of the nineteenth century there was no place for women in the professions or in public life; whatever they wished to do had to be accomplished behind the scenes, hence "the little war office" at Burlington Hotel where Florence Nightingale worked out the army reforms with Sir Sidney Herbert and Dr. John Sutherland. As we shall see later, this failure to recognize women in public life may have been the real reason for Miss Nightingale's illness. Those few who bravely broke the bonds of tradition, such as Elizabeth Blackwell, the first woman doctor, or Miss Dorothea Dix, faced a great resistance, purely because they were women.

The real difficulty in securing for women a place of equality with men was the negative attitude of society; its members took refuge in all kinds of rationalizations. The meeting of the argument, therefore, did not change the fundamental attitude of the opponents. The passing of laws or the exercise of previously unused constitutional privileges or rights does not accomplish much as long as these efforts are not in accord with the emotional attitude of the dominant citizenry, for our moral or customary attitudes are fundamentally determined by emotions. This has best been illustrated in our own country by the failure of the Eighteenth Amendment and the partial failure of the Fifteenth Amendment in the South, attributable to this cause. The relative inertia of our emotional attitudes, together with our social structure, is still effective in maintaining certain social handicaps for women long after they have legally and politically been given rights, which practically equal those of men.

In spite of the fact that the professions are open to women, very few enter the medical, legal, and, especially theological schools or attain high executive positions. On the other hand, society expects some professions to be staffed preponderantly by women, for example, those of nursing, elementary school teaching, and social work. In our evaluation of the progress of the movement for the equalization of women with men, these two distinct aspects must be borne in mind. Nevertheless, the fact that women can now enter almost any career open to men on more or less equal terms is an indication of the trend of the times even though the lag is still markedly felt.

The emacipation of women is characterized in four main areas: judicial, political, educational, and occupational.

Judicial emancipation of women

Before women can hope to advance as a group they must be equal with men before the law. The original concept of the family was that of a unit ruled by a head; the change in legal concept has been to recognize the members of the family as equivalent members of society. This change has been wrought by many individual laws, some of which pertain to franchise or occupation, others again to the civil standing of women in the community. Some of these changes may be mentioned: a married woman is now capable of acquiring and holding property, something that she could not do before; prior to 1925 a mother in England did not possess the same rights as the father did of guardianship of her children; divorce laws have all been changed in favor of the wife. In some cases custom has changed ahead of the law.

Thus, although laws placing women at a

disadvantage have gradually been displaced by others giving women the same equality as men, the increasing participation of women in trade and industry has led to the introduction of many laws protecting but at the same time limiting the activities of women. These laws are justified insofar as they take into account the physical difference of women, but not if they limit their rights and privileges, as, for instance, the many laws that allow lower wages or salaries for women performing the same service as men. There are, in this respect, still many inequalities that should be corrected.

Enfranchisement of women

In recent history the vote has proved to be a most powerful weapon when used by an organized group. This was appreciated by the early champions of women's rights. If a woman could vote, she could enforce the correction of many injustices. In spite of Concordet's efforts, suffrage was not extended to women through the French Revolution; and because this movement soon became unpopular in the Anglo-Saxon countries, the cause did not gain impetus until about the middle of the last century.

The agitation for women's vote was more intense in America than in England. This was brought about especially by the antislavery movement in which women took a very active part. It was led by Lucretia Mott and Elizabeth Cady Stanton and supported by the Quakers. As a result of their activity the first Women's Rights Convention met in Seneca Falls, New York, in 1848. During the next few years the movement continued to gain strength. It received wide publicity in the press, and soon other leaders joined in. Most famous among these was Susan B. Anthony who remained actively interested until her death in 1906.

In England the early efforts were made between 1840 and 1850 when suffrage for women was advocated by such men as Cobden, Disraeli, and Hume. The most potent protagonist, however, was John Stuart

Mill, who entered parliament in 1865, having placed women's suffrage in his election address. Later he published his *Subjection of Women,* which had a tremendous influence. Women now began to organize themselves and to present petitions to parliament. When a reform bill was to be introduced in 1884, they thought that they stood a good chance of achieving their goal; however, Gladstone killed the bill through the treason of 104 liberal members. The movement became greatly discouraged although at this time women gained electoral rights in local government.

The women in America had no better luck in obtaining suffrage. Working through state legislatures was found to be futile; therefore, they turned to national organizations. In 1869 the National Women's Suffrage Association was formed in New York under the leadership of Mrs. Stanton and Miss Anthony, and in the fall of the same year the American Women's Suffrage Association was formed in Cleveland under Lucy Stone; in 1890 the two were joined. By annual conventions and by repeated appearances before the legislature in Washington, D. C., they pressed their claim. The movement grew, and in 1888 it assumed an international character. When the older leaders died, new ones took up their tasks, and eventually the states began to yield. By 1920 general suffrage had been obtained by ratification of the Nineteenth Amendment.

The movement had to pass through more troubled waters in England. After the setback in 1884 it grew without any dramatic events until 1897 when a National Union was formed of the various smaller societies. This step strengthened the effort. In 1903 a Women's Social and Political Union was formed; this was the famous organization that for the next decade, under the leadership of Mrs. Pankhurst, was to obtain such notoriety. Offhand the new Union changed tactics. Formerly each candidate for office had been questioned on his views, but this method had achieved nothing. Now the Union applied directly to the government, and as the liberal party came into power in 1906 it was hoped that it would be more favorable than the previous conservative rule. Instead the new government handled the suffragettes roughly, and when they attempted to hold a meeting, they were brutally thrown into the street and eventually into prison. The ensuing notoriety gave a tremendous impetus to the movement; they now began to adopt "militant" tactics with parades, heckling of ministers when they appeared on public platforms, and general disturbances all in the name of propaganda. Their efforts showed the world what determined propaganda could do: everybody all over the world was talking about them, and the papers carried pictures of their activities, with the result that the movement became tremendously popular. New societies sprang up everywhere, and the membership grew by leaps and bounds. In 1907 they organized their first public demonstration, and on a rainy afternoon 3,000 women marched through London; soon one mass meeting followed another, and no one could move anywhere in England without encountering their propaganda.

After a while the suffragettes became so violent that they had to be arrested; in prison they went on hunger strikes and had to be released, and immediately they resumed their tactics. To combat hunger strikes the "cat and mouse" act was passed, whereby prisoners who refused to eat could be rearrested when they had recovered their health. A few efforts on the part of private members to introduce bills failed, and finally in 1910 a committee was organized under Lord Lytton for the purpose of drafting an acceptable bill. Even this effort came up against the unyielding resistance of the government under H. H. Asquith. The struggle reached its climax when the government, in 1911, proposed to introduce a new franchise bill, "for male persons only." New and violent protests followed, but in decisive matters parliament supported the government, and seemingly the suffragettes made no progress.

The suffragettes now decided to support the party that would further their course. This happened to be the labor party. By 1913 they believed that they had public opinion behind them, and they had. The government's cause was virtually lost and British women would probably have been enfranchised if World War I had not begun in 1914, when all efforts were turned toward winning the war. The Women's Social and Political Union was dissolved, and the National Union undertook war relief work; the women thus gained even greater favor in public opinion. Finally in 1917 a conference called by the speaker of the House (that is, the government) recommended that vote be given to householders and wives of householders. A bill drafted along these lines was passed in the House of Commons by a majority of 7 to 1 and soon became law. The next year women became eligible to run for parliament, and in 1919 Viscountess Astor was elected. The experience with women's franchise was so entirely favorable during the next ten years that by 1928 women were given voting rights similar to those of men, and the movement came to a successful close.

Women's suffrage apparently has not materially altered the course of Anglo-Saxon civilization, but it has given to women a potential power with which they can support any movement in which they choose to take interest, and although it may never be given any bias as a whole (the women's vote has in general been divided among similar party lines to those of the male vote), it is always extant to protect the rights of women before the law in the professions and in the labor market. A movement such as the state (or national) registration of nurses would always receive a more favorable treatment in the hands of legislators if it were to be backed by nurses as voters rather than by a disfranchised profession.

This whole movement, therefore, now successfully completed, has been of the greatest value and may be of still greater potential value in the progress of American nursing.

Education of women

The placing of women on an equal footing with men, before the law, had politically enabled them to seek careers comparable to those of men, but to do so it became further necessary to give them educational facilities equal to those that were offered to men. Early in the nineteenth century it was very difficult for a young woman to obtain an education except through private tutoring, which was very expensive and therefore limited to a privileged few. Thus, Miss Nightingale received much of her education from her father and by travel and social contact. There was no "college" to which she could have been sent. If there had been, the evolution of nursing might have developed quite differently. As it is, the growth of colleges and universities for women has profoundly affected nursing education; therefore a short review of this is in order.

Before 1800, occasional schools in America had been open to girls, but educational opportunities for women were practically nonexistent until 1821, when Emma Willard opened a Female Seminary at Troy, New York. "Academies" and "seminaries" soon followed in various parts of the East, and about the middle of the century the public high schools, which were coeducational, had been extensively established. Higher education for women, however, lagged somewhat behind; the first colleges open to women were Oberlin in Ohio (1833) and Wheaton at Norton, Massachusetts (1835). Mount Holyoke also dates from this early period, having been established in 1857. A number of other colleges were established during the next thirty or forty years. Outstanding among them was Vassar, which opened in Poughkeepsie, New York, in 1865; it is remarkable for its high educational standards, which have been maintained from the first.

During the latter part of the century, when higher education for women became more generally recognized, large numbers of institutions all over the country admitted women. Some of them were separate colleges for women; others were established within already existing universities, some of these being coeducational. Among colleges for women established during this period, Smith, Wellesley, and Bryn Mawr became outstanding. Mount Holyoke also obtained a college charter (1888). Simmons College in Boston was established in 1899 for the specific purpose of preparing women for independent professional careers. Tulane University in New Orleans and Western Reserve in Cleveland were the first universities to open their doors to women (1887 and 1888) and soon others followed their example. The University of Chicago was established in 1893 on the basis that it should be open in equal measure to men and women. To mention them all would be tedious; in general, not only did the number of women admitted to college increase but the educational standards of institutions admitting them advanced rapidly during this period.

These schools and colleges have maintained very high standards. All the good ones have had their pick of students, with the result that their material to start with was superior; they have been led by educators of vision who have emphasized the liberal arts education as applied to the individual, with the result that more and more of their graduates have sought and qualified for distinguished professional careers. The American Association of University Women has been active in creating opportunities, often by establishing fellowships for the advanced education of women, with the result that an increasing number of women Ph.D.'s have been added to the rosters of that degree. Most of these women enter advanced teaching or research in the physical sciences, where they are beginning to occupy an increasing number of the important posts.

The participation of the nursing profession as a whole in the development of the education of women will be extensively discussed later; in addition we may note that an increasing number of women seeking professional education go into nursing.

Thus it will be clear that the advances made in the education of women form an important integral part of the professional evolution of nursing.

Occupational emancipation of women

Perhaps some of the early emancipators of women visualized a world in which woman took a place in society in all respects similar to that of man. Obviously that dream has not been and is not likely to be realized. As long as the family remains the unit of Western Civilization, the larger proportion of women's efforts will be concerned with homemaking and child rearing. Therefore, although the growing freedom of women has resulted in their admission to most occupations, this movement has encountered certain countercurrents of considerable power.

Experience has shown that, physically and temperamentally, women are less suited than men for certain pursuits although they are eminently fitted for others. In certain professions women still constitute a small percentage, and it is of great significance that this percentage in some instances tends to decrease; thus, there are fewer women doctors, both absolutely and proportionately, than there were a few decades ago. It has also been found necessary to protect women in the labor market by limiting their participation in certain activities by law; for instance in England women may not be employed in mines below ground, and they are protected by special hour and wage regulations. On the other hand, in some professions, preeminently nursing, the superiority of women except for certain special tasks has been generally recognized; this profession is unique in that all its positions, even to the highest national offices, are occupied by women.

Thus, as far as the participation of women in occupations and professions is concerned, the movement is finding a level consistent with the compatibility of women for the various tasks.

Another important countercurrent is survival of the old attitude toward women—"prejudice" it is often called—although it is not strictly so, but rather survival of a view that formerly was both justifiable and proper. This, however, is waning steadily, and it is slowly being realized that women should be admitted to any place or career in society for which they are constitutionally and educationally fitted without the handicap of old custom.

RISE OF SOCIALISM

The social reformers of the early part of the nineteenth century were promoting ideas of philanthropic enterprises on the part of those who were privileged to be in a position in which they could carry them out. The power of the organized lower classes was not prominent in the reforms that they suggested, although an awareness of the powers of the French Revolution existed, as is evidenced in the writings of both Carlisle and Dickens. The impulse that eventually was to stimulate action by the workers themselves was to come from another source. About the middle of the century Karl Marx wrote *Das Kapital,* and he and Engel founded the socialistic movement that was directly or indirectly to influence so much political thinking and action. The socialistic way of thinking shifted the center of gravity in society. The industrial system, so far, had acknowledged individual freedom to act and to extract from one's fellowmen whatever one could within the law. The state was for the protection of the individual, but it had no obligation to him. According to the socialistic doctrine it is the duty of the individual to give his work to the state; in return this state will see that he receives his

full share of the proceeds of his labors. In the socialistic state all are politically equal. As this aimed at abolition of political and economic privilege, the masses had but one means to enforce their demands: to organize.

Organized labor movements began to develop in Europe during the second half of the nineteenth century, slowly at first, but gradually gaining momentum. Organized labor advanced in Europe much more quickly than in America where the labor unions are of relatively recent origin. Consequently the by-products of labor organization, with which we are particularly concerned, are of more gradual development in America than in Europe. The chief enemies of the laboring man are old age, sickness, exploitation, and unemployment from the shutdown of factories. It is, therefore, reasonable that requests for protection from these enemies should soon be added to the demands for improved working conditions and that they should become important objects of social legislation.

Social legislation

The first moves for sickness and unemployment legislation were not initiated by the labor movement itself but by Bismarck in Germany, who thought that by anticipating the demands of labor he could control its development. The passing of legislation in Germany protecting labor against sickness and unemployment has progressed even during the more recent periods when the electorate was relatively impotent. Another effect of Bismarck's reform, one that he perhaps did not anticipate, was that it established a precedent and acknowledgment of the obligation of the state to the underprivileged. From this time the revaluation of the rights of man which had been going on throughout the century became rapidly accentuated. The right to life, liberty, and the pursuit of happiness was given an even more liberal interpretation, except perhaps as far as liberty was concerned. The modern era has seen industry regulated to an increasing extent: hours have been shortened, health and safety requirements regarding workshops have been steadily improved and better enforced, and there has been a steady trend in wage increase. Altogether, the present age has been one of social and industrial reform foreshadowed in the preceding century; these reforms are still far from completed.

Extension of medical care

The general trend had embodied an ever-increasing demand for hospitals and medical and nursing services. This demand has had an economic aspect: there has been an increasing interest in the cost of medical care in its broadest sense. Studies have been and are being made of means by which it could be distributed in such a manner that families would not be crippled financially in case of severe sickness and whereby those in society who cannot afford medical care can receive it in a properly organized manner and not as a more or less accidental charity. The attempts to distribute the cost of medical care have led to the developments of numerous schemes; the Krankenkasse system in Germany, the panel system in England, group hospitalization and sickness insurance by private insurance companies in the United States are but examples of a field so vast that it requires a special study to be understood in its entirety.

These developments have been met with resistance, the chief and general argument being that they have led to "socialization" of medicine, by which in general was meant that they would interfere with the professional freedom and initiative of those engaged in the healing art. This social conflict has many aspects that, however, are beyond our scope. We can merely note that in Western Civilization as a whole such schemes have progressed at an accelerated pace. For our purpose, suffice it to say that this evolution of the healing arts is of the greatest significance for nursing, for it con-

tinuously widens its scope: we continue to build new and larger hospitals, public health activities continue to expand, and new industrial positions continue to become available. We shall consider all of these developments in their proper places, but when we do, we should remember to study them against the background we have just described.

Benefits of industry

Social reforms within the society of the United States are premised upon the ability of the industrial system to carry its share of the burden. Now let us consider how industrialism has become so prosperous. When we described feudalism, we noted that most people were occupied fulltime simply in obtaining food and other basic commodities. When we described the advent of the machine, we pointed out how it essentially led to the saving of time that could be used for other work or for leisure (by "leisure" we mean here any activity other than productive labor, such as education, and engagement in the luxury trade). As our machines became increasingly efficient this saving of time became increased at an almost incredible rate. As an example of this we quote A. J. Todd:

It has been calculated that to copy by hand a volume of 100,000 words would require 14 days and cost approximately $54.40; to write 1,000 copies would require 44 years, 45 weeks and 2 days and cost $54,400. To do the same work with a modern power press would require some preliminary work which the author estimates would occupy 96 days and cost some $1,780, but once that was done, 1,000, and as many additional thousands of copies could be run off at less than a cent a copy in less than 10 hours. This example could be amplified by thousands more all showing how the machines increase our efficiency and save us time.*

This tremendous advance applies not only to the production of goods but also to their

---

*Todd, A. J.: Industry and society, New York, 1933, Henry Holt & Co., Inc., p. 109.

transportation. To transport a ton of coal on the backs of coolies in China is far more expensive than to transport a ton of coal in an American freight car the same distance, notwithstanding the fact that the coolies are paid such insignificant wages that they can never become consumers to a significant extent of the goods they help transport.

Modern transport renders it more profitable to carry letters at six cents apiece than it was to carry them at a dollar apiece when mail service was first established.

A further study of this subject will make it clear that there is a striking difference between poverty of feudalism and poverty of the modern Machine Age. Feudal poverty was inevitable, for the work of all the people could produce commodities barely above subsistence level, while the productive power of the modern industrial structure is such that it can produce ample commodities for all the people living under Western Civilization if they will turn it to productive purposes at full capacity. In modern society there are two causes for poverty: either society fails to provide an adequate distribution of its commodities or the citizens at the bottom of the economic scale lack the capacity or education to acquire a reasonable share of the communal wealth.

Public health

Defective distribution of commodities, however intriguing, is too complicated a subject to fall within our scope, but the second cause of poverty is definitely our concern. There is now general agreement that failure to achieve a reasonable standard of living can be traced in many cases to an unhygienic environment with resulting disease that is preventable or curable. The whole subject of hookworm anemia and the deficiency diseases as causes of chronic illness is pertinent. The prevalence of venereal diseases and tuberculosis among the less-favored classes is another illustration. For generations these social evils have been brought to public knowledge by social reformers, and

gradually, though slowly, society has accepted an ever-increasing responsibility for their existence. The acceptance has been furthered by enlightened self-interest, for we are to an increasing extent realizing the truth of the mercantilistic axiom that the wealth of a state depends primarily on the number and opulence (including health) of its citizens. This became particularly evident in the examinations of recruits for World War II. The practical realization of this truth has led the state, be it local or federal government, to assume an increasing burden in the prevention and treatment of preventable diseases. Consequently, governmental medical care in city institutions, veterans' hospitals, or other institutions has greatly increased and is still increasing both in the number of beds being made available and in the quality of services offered.

The field of public health sponsored by public or semipublic bodies is ever expanding. As this view is being accepted the great corporations are following suit either because of pressure of public opinion, ever the severest taskmaster, or because they find that it is to their advantage to maintain a high standard of health and safety measures on their premises and thus avoid damages and compensations that had to be paid in the past. As public good will is becoming increasingly important, many corporations and governmental bodies take pride in making known the health measures that they sponsor. Organized health measures require more and better nursing; it will now be seen how the Industrial Revolution with its collateral economic, political, and philosophical developments may be considered the soil which nurtured the growth of all of the healing arts.

MEDICINE DURING THE NINETEENTH CENTURY

The vigorous intellectual, political, and social activity of the nineteenth century affected medicine and resulted in a remarkable development in America as well as in all of the European countries. Some of the outstanding men and their contributions will be outlined briefly, but the reader is referred to books on the history of medicine for the complete discussion of this fascinating period. During this period the tendency to specialize in a single clinical field had its beginning. General physicians practicing in all brances of medicine became proportionately fewer in number; this trend was encouraged.

Ignatz Philipp Semmelweis, 1818-1865

One of the most tragic figures of medicine —Semmelweis—was the genius who banished childbirth fever from maternity hospitals. Hungarian by birth, he was assistant at the second Vienna clinic about 1845 when the death rate from puerperal sepsis had reached the appalling figure of 10% of all of those delivered. At the same time it was only about 3% at the first clinic. Medical students were taught at the second clinic, pupil midwives at the first. Semmelweis proved that the high rate of death at the

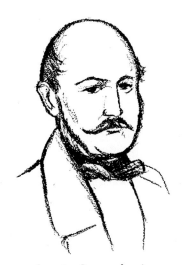

Ignatz Semmelweis

Ignatz Semmelweis had a share in the "emancipation of women" by helping to free them from the spectre of puerperal fever.

second clinic was caused by the filthy habits of the students. They were dissecting and doing postmortem work at the same time that they took their obstetrical work. Often they walked directly from the postmortem room and proceeded to examine a woman in labor without washing their hands. Rubber gloves were not used in those days. Semmelweis showed that this practice was the cause of the appalling mortality; the fever was caused by decomposing organic matter that had gained access to the mother's system through the wounded generative organs. He also showed that other sources could cause it—the examining hand could carry the infection from woman to woman and from infections occurring elsewhere in the body of other patients. Most important, he demonstrated that the infection could be prevented by cleaning the hands with a solution of chlorinated lime before examinations. This work was done before Pasteur began his great task.

Semmelweis died young, at the age of 47 years. His biography is the story of the fight to gain recognition of an idea. In having to wait long years for the victory of his discovery, Semmelweis shared the fate of Harvey, Jenner, and many others. Semmelweis was met by his contemporaries not only with antagonism but also with derision—he was called "The fool from Pesth."

In America, Oliver Wendell Holmes has been extolled as the hero who with Semmelweis conquered the scourge. In fact, the contagiousness of puerperal fever had been suggested by him, before Semmelweis published his papers, in a paper *On the Contagiousness of Puerperal Fever* (1843). Holmes was agreeable to his friends and clever with his pen whereas Semmelweis was difficult to get along with and an awkward writer. Although Holmes held the professorship of anatomy at Harvard, he is now remembered mainly for his wit and clever pen. His work on puerperal sepsis was his most important contribution to medicine.

Another person with whom it is tempting

to compare Semmelweis is Lord Lister (1827-1912), who in 1883 visited Pesth where he learned of the fate of this unfortunate man. Studying the lives of these two men offers a good opportunity to learn the effect of circumstance on the association of fame and genius. Why should Semmelweis' life have been such a tragedy while Lister's was a triumph? The work of Semmelweis was advanced for his time; he died in 1865 before Pasteur's great work was accepted, the year Lister began his researches. Semmelweis had a small and unimportant promoter. Lister's promoter was his father-in-law, the master surgeon of his day in Great Britain, Mr. James Syme (1799-1870). "There are few things more encouraging to aspiring youth than a strong and triumphant master; few things more discouraging than an unpretentious or timorous one." Semmelweis died at the age of 47 years; Lister did not experience his final triumph until 1879 when he was 52 years old. Semmelweis had difficulty with his environment; Lister was never known to speak a sharp word to a house surgeon, dresser, or anyone in his employ. Lister was fortunate in finding prompt support. If circumstances had been different, Semmelweis might have attained a fame as great as that of Lister.

Joseph Lister, 1827-1912

Joseph Lister, the father of modern surgery, was born in 1827, the son of a well-to-do Quaker merchant. He received his early medical training in London, after which he went to Edinburgh and became the house surgeon of Syme, whose daughter he afterward married. In due course, partly through Syme's influence, he became professor of surgery in Edinburgh. In 1877 he came to London where he worked until his retirement.

When Lister entered the surgical wards he found a condition as bad as that found by Semmelweis in the obstetrical wards. Particularly, he was impressed by the huge

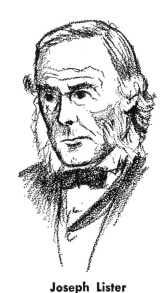

Joseph Lister

Joseph Lister, the father of modern antiseptic surgery, applied the principles of Pasteur's germ theory to the care of wounds.

mortality from sepsis following compound fracture and amputation. After much thought and experimentation, he discovered that if wounds were cleansed with carbolic acid and were kept clean, sepsis did not occur. Out of these observations he developed his antiseptic surgical technique. Although his results were conclusive, his methods were accepted slowly, for it not only takes a great man to make an important discovery but it also takes a great man to be the next to adopt it. Saxtorph of Copenhagen was, in this case, the first to adopt Lister's method, and soon it spread to Germany, France, and elsewhere. England and America were very slow to appreciate Lister's methods. However, by 1879 the evidence in Lister's favor was so overwhelming that it enforced the acceptance of Lister's principles, which since then have guided all surgical work.

Lister, on every occasion, recognized his debt to the genius of Louis Pasteur (1822-1895), whose germ theory supplied the missing link in his reasoning. The assumption of pathogenic bacteria made everything clear. If this effect of great minds upon each other could have happened a few years earlier, another of the greatest catastrophes of history could have been avoided, that is, the casualties from wound infections during the Franco-German war when for the first time the modern war machine was unleashed.

Rudolf Virchow, 1821-1902

In 1881 an international medical congress was held in London under the presidency of Sir James Paget. Among the many thousands attending were some already famous and many destined to become so later. Among them were these four, each of a different national heritage: the Latin Pasteur, the Teuton Virchow, the Anglo-Saxon Lister, and the young and relatively unknown Celt, Osler, who had come from Montreal with his chief, Palmer Howard.

Eldest of these was Virchow. Born in 1821, he soon displayed an interest in natural history which, as so often happens, became supplanted by the love of medicine. He combined a brilliant mind with great industry, and in his twenties the young professor occupied the chair of pathology at the University of Berlin. With the exception of a few years spent at Würzburg, largely for political reasons, he remained in this position until his death at the age of 81. The mind of this intellectual giant was enormous. His fame is founded in his many different contributions to medicine, but he is famous in his own right in many different sciences. He is possibly the greatest pathologist who ever lived. His conception of the cellular changes of disease transformed the entire outlook of the scientific world. Besides his fundamental contribution, he founded or contributed to our knowledge of leukemia, thrombus formation, tumors, septicemia, and much else. Under his direction about fifty thousand postmortem examinations were performed. He founded and personally edited the first 170 volumes of his

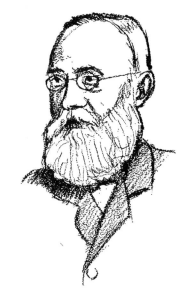

Rudolf Virchow

Rudolf Virchow is justly famed for his many contributions to medical knowledge. His greatest work was probably as a pathologist.

Archives. He was also active in politics; he became associated with the liberal movement of 1848 and suffered for his views.

After the age of 50, at the time when most men willingly slow down, Virchow became active and famous in the fields of anthropology and archeology. His knowledge and contributions were so great that people wondered how he could do this work and still remain a leader in pathology. He contributed to the science of public health; he studied the epidemics of typhus and did much to stamp them out. He helped plan the system of sewage disposal of Berlin. It is partly a result of his efforts that Germany for a while was leading the world in public health research. Virchow was active in the sanitation of the German army in the war of 1870, in the heating and lighting of schools, in the organizing of the duties of school physicians, in the training of nurses, and in the organization of the medical profession into national and local associations. In short, his mind was encyclopedic.

Louis Pasteur, 1822-1895

Then there was Pasteur. The son of a country tanner in moderate circumstances, he did not show any promise of genius at first. His father was one of Napoleon's veterans and instilled into his son a wholesome respect for truth and industry, love of family, and appreciation of the glory of his beloved Fance. Pasteur traveled one road from his youth to his death, but it was a mountainous one leading him, like the youth in Excelsior, to ever greater achievements. He began by solving the molecular structure of racemic acid. He then discovered the true nature of the fermentation of wine and of vinegar and of the production of beer. The relation of these substances to infectious processes and certain fortuitous circumstances led him to the study and eventual conquest of silkworm disease, anthrax, "swine fever," chicken cholera, and finally to the greatest of all his achievements—the preventive treatment of hydrophobia. Each of these conquests would have assured him immortal fame.

He gave all of his attention to his work; thus his wife wrote: "Your father is ab-

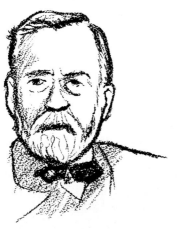

Louis Pasteur

Pasteur's entire life was dedicated to his work in the laboratory where he virtually founded the science of bacteriology.

sorbed in his thoughts, he talks little, sleeps little, rises at dawn, and in one word continues the life I began with him 35 years ago." But with it all, Pasteur upheld the highest ideals. As he himself expressed it: "Blessed is he who carries within himself a God, an ideal, and who obeys this ideal of art, ideal of science, or ideal of gospel virtues; therein lie the springs of great thoughts and great actions. They all reflect light from the infinite." This was the man who established the science of bacteriology —and yet he never possessed a physician's diploma.

Other medical advances in Europe

In 1847 James Simpson in Scotland discovered the use of chloroform, which was the leading anesthetic for many years until its place was taken by newer and safer drugs.

Psychiatry was first considered a separate branch of medicine toward the end of the eighteenth century. The most famous doctor associated with modern reform in the treatment of patients with mental illnesses was Philippe Pinel (1745-1826).

Concern for community hygiene and public health began to emerge during the eighteenth century. At that time there were no city sanitation departments, and open sewers ran through the streets into which people dumped all their garbage and waste. English doctors and medical societies became interested in trying to control communicable diseases as well as in treating them.

The discovery by Edward Jenner (1749-1823) of vaccination against smallpox not only was an important scientific discovery but also was one of the first steps in scientific prevention of disease and has been followed by many other more modern discoveries.

At about the same time that Dr. Jenner was working in England, Johann Peter Frank (1745-1821), an Austrian physician, was outlining the whole structure of modern systematic hygiene. He described the principles of state hygiene and maintained that the government should be responsible for the public health not only during periods when threatened by serious epidemics or disaster but at all times. The theory of Frank was supported in the writings and activities of many nineteenth century social reformers.

Antituberculosis legislation was begun in Italy toward the end of the seventeenth century. Important in the dissemination of medical knowledge among practitioners was the development of medical journals, which began to appear in all countries during the eighteenth and nineteenth centuries. No longer were physicians attached only to the courts of princes, they also began to practice in towns and to appear in localities all over the civilized world.

EARLY REFORMS IN NURSING

Partly as a result of Howard's writings and partly as a manifestation of the general change in attitude toward the penal and eleemosynary institutions, it was realized that nursing, in and out of hospitals, was thoroughly unsatisfactory both in England and on the Protestant continent. At the same time, as we have seen, development for the social liberation of women moved slowly. Because of the great loss of men in the frequent wars, many women could not find husbands and were naturally looking for careers for themselves.

Mrs. Elizabeth Gurney Fry (1780-1845) was an outstanding social reformer in England, particularly concerning conditions in prisons. While she was engaged in this work, she was visited by Fliedner, the father of the deaconess movement. Later she became interested in nursing and established the order that inspired the Fliedners.

Nursing Sisters

In the British Isles, the first efforts at systematic lay nursing institutions were made in Ireland by the Irish Sisters of Charity and the Sisters of Mercy. They antedate the modern deaconesses and orders sponsored by the Anglican Church by a number of years and are more closely related to the Sisters of Charity of de Paul than to the later English orders.

The Irish Sisters of Charity were started by Mary Aikenhead (Sister Mary Augustine). In 1812 she and a friend went to the Convent of the Blessed Virgin Mary at York where they studied the work of nuns who practiced visiting among the poor, and in 1815 they began similar work in Dublin. Some years later they sent three Sisters to study nursing at the Hospital de la Pitié in Paris, and when they came back, the Sisters got their own house and hospital in Dublin. This hospital, which was begun with twelve beds, later expanded into St. Vincent's Hospital, the name of which suggests its relationship to the French order of Sisters of Charity.

The Sisters of Mercy was a similar order founded by Catherine M'Auley. It began as a home for destitute girls but soon included visitation of the sick. In 1830 it was made a presentation order with increasing emphasis on nursing. This order also sent branches to different parts of the world, and from the branch in Bermondsey near London some Sisters went with Miss Nightingale to the Crimea. The order came to the United States in 1843 when Mother Warde brought some Sisters across the ocean. Among their outstanding hospitals in this country are the Mercy Hospitals in Chicago and in Pittsburgh.

These orders are important as being the first modern nursing orders in the British Isles; they are, however, Catholic and derived from the French orders. They did not in their original conception embody the modern training school for nurses. This idea was first propounded by Dr. Robert Gooch, who around 1825 suggested that lay nursing orders should be established for women. The applicants should first be entered as pupil nurses in the big hospitals in London and Edinburgh, should be supplied with regular textbooks adapted to their needs, and should be regularly examined so that their progress could be checked. After graduation they should, after the manner of the Beguines go into the country or districts where they should live together in small houses. This plan, excellent as it was, did not materialize for many years. But Dr. Gooch was a friend of Mrs. Fry's, and it is not impossible that some of these ideas were conveyed to Mr. Fliedner and thus first materialized in Germany.

Deaconesses at Kaiserswerth

The need for better nursing was also acknowledged in Germany. In Hamburg, Amelie Sieveking had organized "The Friends of the Poor," who did home visiting and nursing. Efforts were being made in many towns to improve nursing in the hospitals. Nursing manuals were being written. Still, it all lacked the spark of genius that was eventually to overshadow all similar efforts in Europe.

This spark was contributed by Theodor Fliedner and his wife, Fredericke (nee Münster). As a young minister Mr. Fliedner was called to Kaiserswerth near Düsseldorf. He found a community in the throes of an economic depression and little prospect of earning even a modest livelihood. However, in spite of tempting offers elsewhere, he decided to remain at his post and to travel abroad to raise the funds necessary to work where he was.

In 1822 he traveled through Holland and England, and because he had introductions to all sorts of influential people, he was soon able to solve his financial problem. He also had the opportunity to study firsthand many efforts at relieving shame and suffering; in Holland he observed the work of the deaconesses, and in England he formed a close friendship with Elizabeth Fry, who allowed him to study her work in the prisons. He investigated schools, hospitals, almshouses, and other eleemosynary institutions, so that he returned to Kaiserswerth one of the best-informed men in his field.

It took his wife and him many years to

materialize their plans, and not until 1833 were they able to open their first refuge for discharged prisoners. However, the problem of the deaconesses lay closest to their hearts. They had seen what the Sisters of Mercy were able to do, and they appreciated the intrinsic value of the deaconesses. They also realized that a nursing organization, such as they had in mind, must be modernized to meet the demands of the times. The training had to be more systematic than it had been in the past, and the organization had to be more closely knit although elastic enough to meet the most varied demands.

In 1836 they bought the biggest house they could find in Kaiserswerth, hoping somehow to pay for it later—which they did. Soon afterward their first patient, a servant girl, arrived, and Mrs. Fliedner persuaded her friend, Gertrude Reichardt, to enter as the first deaconess. Mrs. Reichardt was a doctor's daughter, middle-aged, who had already had extensive experience dealing with sick people in assisting her father with his practice. She arrived at the Kaiserswerth Hospital expecting little in the way of equipment, but even that was not there. Four bare walls and a patient were about all the new institution had to offer, and Gertrude Reichardt was just about ready to give up and go home when the first load of equipment unexpectedly arrived, and somehow the young hospital got started. By the end of that year there were six more deaconesses; eventually there were one hundred and twenty deaconesses and, by 1842 the hospital had two hundred beds.

Fredericke Fliedner had a marvelous talent for organizing and soon each girl found herself in charge of her own department with no one else's interfering. Furthermore, to complete their training, the deaconesses rotated from service to service, all the while receiving systematic instruction. Mr. Fliedner instructed them in ethics and religious principles, and Mrs. Fliedner instructed them in the principles of practical nursing.

A physician gave them theoretical training and bedside instruction in the care of the sick, and they learned enough pharmacology to pass the state examinations for pharmacists.

Thus, the fully trained deaconess could nurse sick and convalescent patients, manage children, and dispense medicines; she was familiar with occupational therapy, parish or district visiting, and religious theory and instructions.

The organization that accomplished so much was managed very strictly. No student could assume a privileged position; all were equal before their instructors. In this way they differed markedly from the later English and American orders. To be admitted to the course a girl had to be at least 18 years of age and had to present letters from a clergyman and a physician certifying both her moral standing and her health. She would then be admitted for three months' probation; later this probation was replaced by required attendance at a preparatory school, sometimes for as long as a year. She received a regular, small allowance of pocket money. Rotating through the various services, she in turn became a junior, senior, and finally head sister. Through the course she received, besides practical instruction, regular theoretical classroom instruction. The course took three years, and she was required to wear a uniform. For the first time in history we observe, complete with all the essentials, the modern training school for nurses.

The modern training school was a huge success and it grew rapidly. The Fliedners already had a normal school for the preparation of deaconesses, and soon there was added to the hospital a lunatic asylum for female patients and in 1842 an orphanage for Protestant girls. They also organized an infant school and a day school for girls. Finally, they organized an asylum for released female prisoners and for wayward girls, in an attempt to readjust them to society.

When the hospital was fully developed, its facilities included, besides wards for male and female patients and children, a unit for communicable diseases, one for convalescents (this is remarkable, for many modern hospitals still have no such department), and one for sick deaconesses. There were also an apothecary shop, the administrative offices, the chapel that took care of burials, and the garden that furnished vegetables.

Not only did the institution prosper in Kaiserswerth but there were also calls for branches from all over Europe and from America. As early as 1846 Fliedner went to London with four deaconesses to begin the nursing in the German Hospital there. In 1850 he took a group to Pastor Passavant in Pittsburgh, and at the same time a deaconess home and hospital were founded in Milwaukee. Branches were established throughout the Near East in such cities as Jerusalem, Smyrna, Constantinople, and Alexandria, and by the time Fliedner died in 1864 there were about 1,600 deaconesses working in 400 different fields, and they had thirty mother houses. Since that time the organization has continued to grow, so that there is now hardly a community, excluding the strictly Catholic countries, without its group of deaconesses.

The growth of the organization was a result of the urgent need for such an organization and the incessant industry of the Fliedners. Along with her enormous task Fredericke Fliedner found time to bring into the world five children before she died in 1842. Theodor Fliedner was fortunate in marrying Caroline Bertheau, a former pupil of Amelie Sieveking, one year later. She had been in charge of the nursing of the female surgical department of the Hamburg Hospital. She was able to carry the mantle of Fredericke, and she did not neglect the domestic side of life, for she made her husband a good wife —they had eight children before he died in 1864. After his death she continued to direct Kaiserswerth until 1882.

There remains but a brief evaluation of the order. It was primarily religious, it was modern, and it was practical and democratic. If the directions and the spirit of Theodor Fliedner had always been followed, there would have been no difficulties. However, not all clergymen possessed his wide vision, and sometimes interference by the clergy would hamper its efficiency in spite of the principle that doctor's orders should prevail. Exaggerated idealism on the part of the girls would occasionally lead to excessive self-negation, and sometimes they were exploited by unscrupulous leaders. Some opposition to the order resulted, manifest in the appearance of "free sisters" who later became organized, but, on the whole, deaconesses have weathered all storms and are now the outstanding Protestant religious nursing organization. The security of the mother house, which means so much to the European girl, has been somewhat modified in America. They have offered and still offer a unique opportunity for serious-minded young women to do good in the world. They require no vows; a deaconess may retire or marry, but in return for a life of faithful service a deaconess can look forward to an old age secure from want.

BRITISH NURSING ORDERS
Protestant Sisters of Mercy (the Nursing Sisters)

Fliedner's work made a great impression on interested person especially in England and on the European continent. As we shall see, Florence Nightingale received much inspiration from his work, visited the institution repeatedly, and for a while even participated in the Fliedner's activities. Mrs. Fry also followed the work closely, and finally in 1840, largely under the inducement of Dr. Gooch and the poet Robert Southey, she organized the first Protestant nursing order in England, the Protestant Sisters of Mercy or the Nursing Sisters, as they were later called. These women received some training in their preparation for the care of the sick; they visited Guy's Hospital in London for several hours each day where they received some instruction from the doctors and the ward nurses. However, these doctors and nurses were uneducated and could not be expected to be very valuable instructors. These pupils received neither classroom nor theoretical instruction; they were trained entirely for practical home nursing. The order is still in existence.

Anglican nursing orders

The Church of England sponsored the most important early nursing organizations in England. As a result these organizations were dominated by the cleryman's conception of nursing as primarily an act of mercy and of religious devotion. It was thought that such service must be free to the patient. It took a considerable amount of time before the idea could be accepted that nursing by good, devoted women could be a profession with services rendered for remuneration and that these women should be trained as carefully and thoroughly for this as for any other profession. There was an obvious need for a profession for women, and consequently refined and capable women were attracted to this work. More and more nursing activities were sponsored by the upper classes and recruited from the middle classes of the country.

The Park Village Community, established in 1845 by Pusey, was the first of the Anglican nursing orders. The emphasis here was largely upon friendly visiting of the sick in their homes; there was no emphasis on systematic training or care of patients. About the same time, Miss Sellon organized a similar group, the "Sisters of Mercy" in Devonport. These orders were established for the purpose of home nursing and did not participate in the reform of hospital nursing that took place in the next few years.

A primary factor in this reform was St. John's House, established by the Church of England in 1848. Its purpose was to establish systematic training of nurses in the hospitals and to attract young tladies of the middle classes into nursing. Like the nurses of the Hôtel Dieu they were to advance through three stages. For the first two years they were to be probationers, after which they were to qualify as "nurses," when they would receive board, lodging, and a salary besides. After having worked for five years as nurses, they could advance to become "Sisters," who had the privilege of living at home with their families. Women of the better classes could enter as "nurses." Training in obstetrics was not included until 1861. St. John's House became identified with nursing activities in most of the important London hospitals at one time or another. At first the probationers were trained at Middlesex and Westminster Hospitals, and then, from 1849, at Kings College Hospital where in 1856 they took over the entire nursing service until the hospital established a school of nursing of its own in 1885. The order also nursed in Charing Cross Hospital and was finally taken over in 1919 by St. Thomas' Hospital. The order is now known as the St. John's and St. Thomas' House and is maintained on a cooperative basis as an institution for private nurses. The order contributed twenty-six nurses to Miss Nightingale's expedition.

A similar order, the Sisterhood of All Saints, was founded in 1851 by Miss Byron. This order also concerned itself with the training of nurses in hospitals. It was especially connected with University College Hospital; from 1857 it was responsible for the nursing of a few wards, and from 1862 to 1899, for nursing in the entire hospital. The order assumed direction also of St. John's House from 1883 to 1893.

Finally, St. Margaret's order, established by the Reverend Dr. Neele in East Grimstead in 1854, should be mentioned, Although this order emphasized nursing, the training that it offered its members was not outstanding.

In the United States, the Protestant Episcopal Church established similar nursing orders, patterned after the English. A branch of the English order, the Sisterhood of St. Margaret, nursed at the Children's Hospital in Boston from 1872 to 1912. The Sisterhood of the Holy Communion has nursed in St. Luke's Hospital in New York since 1854, and the Sisterhood of St. Mary has nursed in St. Mary's Free Hospital for Children in New York since 1870.

ON THE CONTINENT
La Source

One Continental development should also be mentioned. In 1859 Comtesse Agenor de Gasperin and her husband established L'école normale evangelique de gardes-malades independents, briefly called "La Source," in Lausanne, Switzerland. They endowed this school of nursing and provided it with a building. The students received instruction for six months during a preliminary course, after which they nursed in the homes of the poor. Since 1891 the institution has had its own hospital. The order, if it may be called that, is based upon the principle of personal liberty. The nurses are salaried and make no vows. The quality of the nurses issuing from this institution has sometimes been questioned, but about its importance as a new departure in the form of an endowed school for nursing, there can be no argument.

Chapter 6

Pioneer days in America

The time of the great discoveries in medicine and the early immigration to America was also the time of the Reformation, which split the European nations into either Catholic or Protestant states. The early Spanish explorers and the French were Catholic and brought with them as missionaries Dominicans, Franciscans, and Jesuits and, later, the nursing orders. The care of the sick and the wounded among friend and foe in the missions and in the wilderness was largely their task. The old term for quinine, "Jesuits' bark," is reminiscent of those days when medical knowledge was in the hands of the clergy. In the Spanish civilization nursing continued to be the responsibility of the monks, and, any high degree of efficiency was never reached. During the eighteenth century, when the great European hospitals began to develop, American hospitals were also beginning to be established. Mexico City can justly claim the first American hospital to be built by the white man—established by Cortez in 1524;—and the early French immigrants built hospitals in Quebec, New Orleans, and St. Louis.

BEGINNINGS OF HOSPITALS AND ORGANIZED NURSING SERVICE

The Charity Hospital of New Orleans established in 1737 is considered by many authorities to be the oldest hospital still existing in America for the care of the sick. In 1737 a sailor, Jean Louis, died in New Orleans and left a bequest of 10,000 liras "to serve in perpetuity and the founding of a hospital for the sick of the City of New Orleans and to secure the things necessary to succor of the sick."* The contract for this hospital gives the following description: "A hall measuring 45 feet in length, by 24 feet in breadth, and 14 feet in height including the foundation, the whole in walls of well conditioned brick."*

This building was completed in 1737 and named St. John's Hospital. In official records it is mentioned as "L'hopital des pauvres de la charite," and it is considered the original Charity Hospital of New Orleans. The institution served both as a hospital and as an asylum, but most of the early hospitals performed both functions. The school for nurses, however, was not established until 1894.

The Ursuline Sisters came to Canada from France in 1639 to teach, accompanied by three Augustinian nuns who were to nurse in a hospital in the new land. However, nursing care was needed so badly that they all did nursing at first until the new Hôtel Dieu was built in 1658. These early settlements

---

*Sister Henrietta: A famous New Orleans hospital, American Journal of Nursing **39**:249, March, 1939.

of New Orleans and farther up the Mississippi at Quebec were to have great influence on American nursing. The early Ursuline Sisters in France had done nursing as well as teaching, and in 1727 a small group of them came to New Orleans where colonial life with certain standards of luxury and with civilization based on slavery were even then achieved. However, the people living in the settlement were ravished by epidemic diseases most important were yellow fever and smallpox; all the scourges of a seaport town were encountered. During the nineteenth century, the Ursuline Sisters were active throughout the entire territory of Louisiana. They opened many hospitals and performed many heroic deeds, which were climaxed in the nursing done during the Battle of New Orleans. Soon after this, they practically gave up nursing and restricted themselves to teaching.

As the growth of settlements in the new country proceeded, the need for nursing became urgent; the various Catholic nursing orders responded to the call. The Sisters of

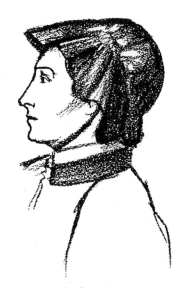

Mother Seton

Mother Elizabeth Bayley Seton founded the American branch of the Sisters of Charity of St. Vincent de Paul.

Charity were among the first; in 1809 Mother Elizabeth Bayley Seton in Emmitsburg, Maryland, established the Sisterhood of St. Joseph as a branch of the Sisters of Charity. In 1849 the Sisters of Charity became affiliated with the Order of St. Vincent de Paul. In 1830 the Sisters of Charity established the first hospital west of the Mississippi River—a log cabin in St. Louis. Almost at once it proved insufficient for the demands made upon it, and in 1831 a larger hospital was built on Spruce and Fourth Streets. This came to be known as the Mullanphy Hospital; in 1874 it moved to bigger quarters, and in 1930, during its centenary, it was replaced by the DePaul Hospital, then one of the most modern and certainly one of the most beautiful hospitals in St. Louis at that time. The Sisters contributed some of the best nursing during the Civil War. Sister Anthony O'Connell, a Sister of Charity from Cincinnati, is remembered in the history of this period as the "Angel of the Battlefield."

The Sisters of Mercy, the Sisters of the Holy Cross, and also the Irish Sisters of Mercy who came to America in 1843 extended their orders throughout the new country, establishing hospitals everywhere and practicing the highest standards of nursing of the times.

EARLY NURSING IN PROTESTANT HOSPITALS

Protestant settlements did not fare as well. We have previously seen the havoc that was wrought during the Reformation to the Catholic nursing orders and to all for which they stood. The result was that wherever Protestant pioneers advanced, there was no organized effort to take care of the sick and wounded. The task was done by persons who felt inclined thereto; although these persons apparently performed their task with kindness, their skill was limited by their inherent ability. As the colonies grew and as settlements became better established, they followed the pattern of their homeland

and organized institutions for the care of the sick and the poor, not so much out of Christian charity as for social convenience —something had to be done with the unfortunate ones. The result, according to the descriptions that have reached us of these early refuges of poverty, sickness, and immorality, was a fair match for what Mrs. Fry found in British workhouses and hospitals during the same era. For in those early days the poorhouse and hospital were under a common roof, and no one who could possibly be nursed elsewhere would go to a hospital. Consequently, the public developed a fear of hospitals, remnants of which survive even today, long after hospitals have ceased to be dens of horror and torment.

The most accurate information about nursing in American hospitals before the reform movement is found in the records of the investigation of 1837 and later of the Bellevue Hospital Visiting Committee. This was an agency of the New York State Charities Aid Association.

Dirt and squalor were predominant factors, no money was available with which to accomplish anything, and everybody lived, or died, close to a subsistence minimum. There was neither ventilation nor hygiene;

plumbing was defective. The "nurses" were ill-paid individuals from the lower strata of the community; they were venal to a degree and tempted to supplement their meager pay with bribes and extortions from the patients. They could be trusted with nothing: neither with administration of medicine nor with gifts of food for the patients. Often they were so deficient in number or health that the sicker patients had to receive most of their nursing from other patients who could move about or from prisoners or inmates of the workhouse. No proper provisions were made for the maintenance of the nurses. Their food was poor, and there is record that they even had to sleep in the barns on bundles of straw. Now we realize that "hospital" and "nursing" had a different connotation in those days than they have today. Only the utterly destitute went to the hospital. Any others who had a home or place to stay remained there when they were sick, and nursing was provided by the mother of the home, or the grandmother, or in well-to-do homes by trusted servants. The "Mrs. Gamp" of English life does not seem to be quite as prevalent in early American days. In many neighborhoods, certain women gained reputation in being especially good in nursing and were sought out for

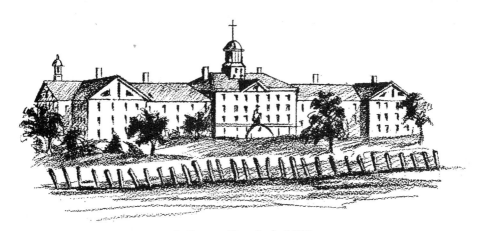

Bellevue Hospital, 1848

Originally Bellevue Hospital was established as the New York Public Workhouse. The name was taken from its second site, Belle View on Kip's Farm, where it still stands.

cases of sickness and confinement. These were called monthly nurses. Most of them were respectable women; many had a great deal of experience and, considering the limitation of medical experience of the period, were fully a match for the family doctors. Thus, considering the general state of medical knowledge and practice a hundred or more years ago, nursing of the sick in the middle and upper classes was not bad.

In order to present a few definite landmarks, we may remember that the Pennsylvania General Hospital was established in 1751, the New York Hospital in 1781, and the Massachusetts General Hospital in 1821. Two other institutions, the Philadelphia General Hospital and the Bellevue Hospital in New York, had their early beginnings before these came into being.

In 1713 the Quakers of Philadelphia established an almshouse for Quakers only. It demonstrated the value of such an institution as well as the need for one that was not restricted to Quakers. Accordingly, in 1731, the town established a general almshouse and, in connection with this, a hospital ward. After this institution had repeatedly outgrown its quarters, new buildings were constructed outside of the city in Blockley Township, and in 1834 it was transferred and, henceforth, assumed the name Blockley, later "Old Blockley." During this period it had become less and less of an almshouse and more and more of a hospital, and an increasing amount of instruction of medical students took place within its walls. Many famous medical teachers, the best known of whom is Dr. Osler, walked its wards. But all that did not prevent the standards of Old Blockley from sinking to a very low level of medical and nursing care, until attempts were made to improve conditions during the early period of nursing reforms. Eventually Old Blockley developed into what is now known as Philadelphia General Hospital, one of the leading Hospitals in the country. Its early origin can probably be traced back farther than any of the other early American hospitals.

About the same time as Philadelphia General Hospital emerged, Bellevue Hospital originated as the New York Public Workhouse. When the New York Workhouse was erected in 1736 where the city hall now stands, one large room in the west end of the building was set aside to be used as an

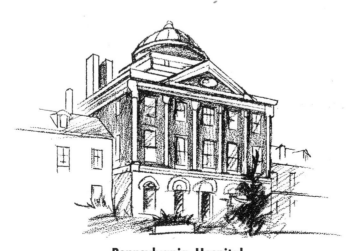

Pennsylvania Hospital

The first hospital to be organized as such in America was Pennsylvania Hospital, whose first administrator was Benjamin Franklin.

infirmary, and a medical officer, Dr. John Van Buren, was employed at a salary of 100 pounds a year to look after the sick inmates. By the end of the century the institution had outgrown its quarters and was moved to Belle Vue on Kip farm. Its name was taken from the place, and it has remained there since then, gradually changing its character from that of a workhouse and almshouse to that of a hospital. By 1825 a fever hospital was added, and from 1836 to 1838 the prisoners were moved to Blackwell's Island, after which it continued as one of the leading American hospitals. The leading part that it took in the development of American schools of nursing will later be discussed.

The first hospital to be organized as such was the Pennsylvania Hospital. It was built in response to a petition presented in 1751 before the Colonial Assembly by a committee of Philadelphia citizens. Prominent men on the committee included Dr. Thomas Bond and Benjamin Franklin. The Governor granted a charter for the hospital and provided 2,000 pounds to be paid in two annual installments toward its construction, provided a like among be raised by private contributions. This was rapidly done, and after some negotiations, a site was acquired and the cornerstone was laid in 1755. The first patients were admitted by the end of the following year. The first president of the organization, Joshua Crosby, died within a month of the laying of the cornerstone. His place was taken by Benjamin Franklin, who remained in the post until he was appointed provincial agent at London in 1757. Among his many other accomplishments, Franklin was thus our first hospital administrator, and his views and organization here as in his other projects were quite progressive. The hospital has since continued its outstanding development.

When the Pennsylvania Hospital was being organized, New York City was still for many years to remain without a regular hospital for its citizens—during a time when all the great cities in Europe were building large institutions for their sick. That the defect was keenly felt was evidenced in the commencement address made by Samuel Bard to medical graduates at King's College in 1769: "It is truly a reproach, that a city like this should want a public hospital." This address immediately stimulated a movement that was heavily backed by Sir Henry Moore, Governor of the Colony. It resulted, in 1771, in the granting of a royal charter to the Society of the Hospital, in the City of New York. A site was acquired on the west side of Broadway, opposite Pearl Street. The necessary funds were procured, and construction was begun on a fine hospital. It was almost finished in 1775 when, accidentally, a fire destroyed the entire inside of the building. However, the men behind the movement, including the new governor, renewed their efforts; new funds were raised, partly by a grant of 4,000 pounds from the Colonial Assembly, and the rebuilding was completed within a year, when the Revolutionary War broke out. With the occupancy of New York by the British, the hospital was used as barracks and occasionally as a military hospital. There followed, after the war, a prolonged period of reconstruction, and not until 1791 was the hospital finally opened for regular medical service.

The Philadelphia Dispensary established in 1786 was the forerunner of our modern outpatient department and clinic for ambulatory patients. It was independent of any hospital and supported by civic-minded citizens in Philadelphia. The Philadelphia Dispensary for Out-Patients was so successful that the idea soon spread to other early American cities.

CONCLUSION

Because of the growth of medical knowledge and of the hospital as a social institution, the deficiencies of nursing became glaringly apparent. As we have pointed out, the growth of modern medicine really began to gain momentum about the year 1800; there were doctors, then, who realized that properly trained nurses would be a great asset. In 1798 Dr. Valentine Seaman, attending surgeon to the New York Hospital, gave regular courses to nurses in anatomy, physiology, obstetrics, and pediatrics. He did not restrict instruction to lectures; he gave practical demonstrations also. He published a synopsis of these lectures, probably one of the earliest attempts at preparing nursing texts.

Questions and study projects for unit one

1. What were the nursing activities of the follow-orders?
   (a) Third Order of St. Francis
   (b) Order of St. Vincent de Paul
   (c) The Beguines
   (d) The Poor Clares
   (e) The Community of the Sisters of Charity
2. Discuss the nursing done by the Sisters of the Hôtel Dieu in Paris during the Middle Ages. Include the real contributions made by them to nursing.
3. Discuss the "Dark Age of Nursing" under the following heads:
   (a) General social conditions in Europe
   (b) Status of medicine
   (c) Status of hospitals
   (d) Status and regulations affecting religious orders
   (e) Status of women
4. Write short sketches of the following persons and show their contributions to nursing and to its development as a profession: Dr. Valentine Seaman, Pastor and Mrs. Fliedner, Mrs. Elizabeth Gurney Fry, Mother Catherine M'Auley.
5. What lasting contributions to medicine were made by Hippocrates, Harvey, Sydenham, Boerhaave, and Morgagni?
6. Write a short paper on early American medicine.
7. Discuss the contributions of Pasteur and Lister to medicine. Show how these discoveries radically changed the nursing care of patients.
8. Show the relation between medical discoveries and the progress of professional nursing.
9. What were the effects of the Crusades on nursing and medicine?
10. What were the contributions of John Howard to the improvement of hospitals?
11. Describe the origin and early history of your hospital.
12. Discuss medieval hospitals and the nursing care given in them.
13. How and why have city, state, and Federal governments in this country become interested in health, medical, and nursing activities.
14. Discuss the development of social legislation and effects on public health during the nineteenth century.
15. Discuss progress of the emancipation of women during the nineteenth and twentieth centuries.
16. Discuss the work of religious orders in hospitals during this period.
17. Describe the development of hospitals and nursing service in pioneer days in America.
18. Make an annotated bibliography of recent articles appearing in *The American Journal of Nursing, Nursing Outlook, Nursing Record,* and any other journals available in your library containing articles relating to the discussion in this unit.

References for unit one

Deutsch, Albert: Dorothea Lynde Dix: Apostle of the insane, American Journal of Nursing **36**: 987-997, October, 1936.

Doyle, Ann: Nursing by religious orders in the United States, American Journal of Nursing, **29**:775, 1929 (Part I, 1809-1840); **29**:959, 1929 (Part II, 1841-1870); **29**:1085, 1929 (Part III, 1871-1928); **29**:1197, 1929 (Part IV, Lutheran Deaconesses, 1849-1928); **29**:1466, 1929 (Part VI, Episcopal Sisterhoods, 1845-1928).

Ferguson, E. D.: The evolution of the trained nurse, American Journal of Nursing **1**:463-468, April, 1901; **1**:535-538, May, 1901; **1**:620-626, June, 1901.

Fishbein, Morris: History of the American Medical Association, Philadelphia, 1947, W. B. Saunders Co.

Gallison, Marie: The Ministry of Women: One hundred years of women's work at Kaiserswerth, 1836-1936, London, England, 1954, The Butterworth Press.

Hamilton, Samuel W.: The history of American mental hospitals. One hundred years of American psychiatry, New York, 1944, Columbia University Press.

Hume, Edgar Erskine: Medical work of the Knights of Hospitalers of Saint John of Jerusalem, Baltimore, 1940, The Johns Hopkins Press.

Jones, Mary Cadwalader: The training of a nurse, November, 1890, Scribner's.

Lady Nurses, Godey's Lady's Book and Magazine **32**:188, 1871.

Levine, Edwin B., and Levine, Myra E.: Hippocrates, father of nursing, too? American Journal of Nursing **65**:86, December, 1965.

Sharp, Ella E.: Nursing during the pre-Christian era, American Journal of Nursing **19**:675-678, June, 1919.

Florence Nightingale—her life and influence on nursing

The Nightingale pledge*

I solemnly pledge myself before God, and in the presence of this assembly,
To pass my life in purity and to practice my profession faithfully
I will abstain from whatever is deleterious and mischievous, and will not take or knowingly administer any harmful drug.
I will do all in my power to maintain and elevate the standard of my profession, and will hold in confidence all personal matters committed to my keeping and all family affairs coming to my knowledge in the practice of my profession.
With loyalty will I endeavor to aid the physician in his work, and devote myself to the welfare of those committed to my care.

---

*This pledge was formulated in 1893 by a committee of which Mrs. Lystra E. Gretter, R.N., was the chairman. It was first administered to the 1893 graduating class of the Farrand Training School, now the Harper Hospital, Detroit, Mich.

Chapter 7

Early life and education

The dominant figure in the development of organized nursing is Florence Nightingale. We have seen in the introductory chapters (1) how the general evolution in medicine was being developed into a scientific practice in which doctors, whether they knew it or not, would soon require more than menial labor from nurses, (2) how the general state of society and the improvement of hospital facilities were amenable to the new profession, and (3) how the Protestant ministers in various countries had begun to realize that in Protestant countries and organization was needed similar to the Catholic nursing orders, but perhaps freer, and how they in various ways had attempted to meet this need.

The training and organization of lay Protestant nurses had begun before Florence Nightingale made her contribution to nursing, but with her powerful personality, her vision, and her practical organizing ability she took the lead in the movement, placed it on a powerful foundation of organization, sound educational principles, and high ethics, and inspired it with an enthusiasm that gave to it an impetus under which it is still progressing. A few years before Miss Nightingale's time there was no such thing as professional nursing. At the time of her death nursing was a profession, administered by women and offering them nursing and educational opportunities, formerly unthinkable.

However, Florence Nightingale devoted only a part of her life to the advancement of nursing; she also contributed greatly to reforms in the army, the Indian Public Health Service, and public health in Great Britain. Her full stature cannot be comprehended unless attention is given also to these accomplishments.

EDUCATION AT HOME AND ABROAD

On May 12, 1820, a daughter was born to Mr. and Mrs. William Edward Nightingale. She was their second girl, and because the family was then staying in Florence, Italy, she was named after the city of her birth. Her family was of considerable wealth, of good social standing, and highly cultured; therefore, they could afford to give their children the best education available. Florence was brought up with a broad outlook and knowledge of French, German, and Italian. Her father took a very active part in her education by personally instructing her in mathematics and the classics.

When the Nightingale family returned to England, they built a new house at Embley Park, Hampshire, and most of their time was spent here or at the old family home

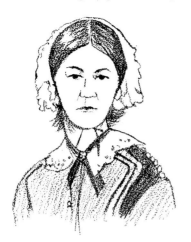

Florence Nightingale

Florence Nightingale is the major personage associated with the development of nursing as an organized occupation.

at Lea Hurst, Derbyshire. Each year during the season an extended visit was made to London, and the young ladies grew up with opportunities to make the best social contacts, which later were to be of the greatest value to Florence.

In 1837 the family again went abroad, touring France, Italy, and Switzerland. In the winter of 1838 they traveled to Paris where Florence was introduced to the salons, in which she made acquaintances that she was to treasure throughout her life. When she returned to London, she was a young lady and was supposed to take her place in society. However, Florence was too serious to be satisfied with such a life. She felt a calling for something greater, although it took some years before her yearnings became articulate. From time to time she made inquiries into the possibilities of becoming a nurse, but knowing what we do of the social status and morals of those creatures, we cannot wonder that Mrs. Nightingale fought such ideas. Nevertheless, Florence had definite plans to become a nurse at the Salisbury Hospital not far from her home. Although these did not materialize, her purpose became even firmer.

In 1844 Miss Nightingale met the American philanthropist and his wife, Dr. and Mrs. Ward Howe (Julia Ward Howe later became known as the author of "The Battle Hymn of the Republic"). They stayed at Embley, the Nightingale home. Miss Nightingale was very much impressed with an institution for the blind that Dr. Ward had founded in New York in which he had worked out a plan to make medical care and nursing available without payment to elderly or ill American citizens. During their stay, Miss Nightingale discussed with them the feasibility of working in English hospitals as Catholic Sisters did. At that time no English women of any social standing would have sought a vocation outside the home, except to enter the Church as a Catholic Sister. During this year, she felt she had reached the turning point of her life, and it was clear to her that her vocation was to be the care of the sick in hospitals. However, her family would not even discuss the possibility of her entering the hospital, so far was it removed from any of their thinking.

Until 1845 she had believed that qualities such as tenderness, sympathy, goodness, and patience were all that a nurse required. After experience in caring for some members of her own family during their illnesses, she recognized that knowledge and skill were also necessary and that acquisition of these required education and training.

It is not surprising that her family was shocked whenever she mentioned going to a hospital, either for training or to nurse, because in the middle of the nineteenth century, hospitals were at a very low level of degradation and squalor. Dirt and lack of sanitation were common. They were crowded, and the patients who were dirty when they came to the hospital were likely to remain that way during their stay.

In 1847 after a busy "social summer" she set out for Rome with Mr. and Mrs. Bracebridge, close friends of the family—a visit that was to result in two important experiences. She went into retreat for ten days in the Convent of the Trinita dei Monti, where she absorbed much of the spirit of the church and where her religious belief greatly matured. Although she was much impressed with the practical endeavors of the Catholic Church, she did not become converted to Catholicism; in fact it could never be said that she strongly preferred any particular branch of the church although she remained deeply religious throughout her life. By tradition she remained within the Church of England.

Her second important experience was the meeting of Mr. and Mrs. Sidney Herbert. Mr.—later Sir—Sidney Herbert was to have the greatest influence on her life; it was through him that she was to go to the Crimea, and with him (and Dr. Sutherland) that she was to form "the little war office." For the present, their contact was largely social, consisting of parties and visits to the galleries. There was some talk of nursing, for there were plans to establish a nursing home when they returned to England. It is interesting to note at this time that Mr. and Mrs. Sidney Herbert and many of their friends were beginning to be interested in hospital reform. Public opinion was being awakened, and Miss Nightingale, who had been collecting facts on public health and hospitals for several years, was able to give this group a great deal of information. Gradually she became known as an expert in hospital reform.

When Miss Nightingale returned to England, she was about 28 years of age, and it was about time for her to marry. In fact, marriage was seriously considered repeatedly but did not materialize. The next year she once more accompanied the Bracebridges abroad to Egypt and Greece. In the meantime she had grown considerably, both emotionally and intellectually, so she studied intently all that she saw; she paid much attention to institutions for the sick and poor. She had learned about the institution at Kaiserswerth. Through some friends she had

received the Yearbook of the Institution of Deaconesses at Kaiserswerth in 1846. She studied it very carefully and realized that here she could receive the training she so keenly wanted. Because the institution was under religious auspices and the character of the deaconesses and pastors above reproach, she could go there without the stigma attached to the English hospitals.

On the return journey she paid it a visit. She was greatly impressed and became very eager to return to participate in the training. Miss Nightingale was so impressed with Kaiserswerth that on her return she issued anonymously a pamphlet called *The Institution of Kaiserswerth on the Rhine for the Practical Training of Deaconesses Under the Direction of the Rev. Pastor Fliedner, Embracing the Support and Care of a Hospital, Infant and Industrial Schools and a Female Penitentiary.* This was a thirty-two page pamphlet and was printed by the Inmates of the London Ragged Colonial Training School at Westminster where Miss Nightingale had taught and in which she had a great deal of interest.

She was well aware that to become a good nurse a thorough training was essential, and when in 1851 her mother and sister went to Carlsbad to "take the cure," she finally contrived to accompany them with the intention of paying an extended visit to Kaiserswerth. She spent three months at the Fliedners' institution and derived from it a great deal of instruction. She participated in the nurses' instruction even to the point of scrubbing floors and left much impressed with the organization and high purpose of the place. Her opinion of the actual training of the nurses was not so high. The experience at Kaiserswerth strengthened her purpose, but as yet she failed to give it practical expression.

In 1851 she met the famous woman doctor, Dr. Elizabeth Blackwell, through the Herberts. Dr. Blackwell visited Miss Nightingale at Embley, and while Miss Nightingale did not approve of woman doctors in general, they had many discussions about hospitals and medical care. In the spring of 1853 she was in Paris again inspecting hospitals and infirmaries; finally she arranged to enter the Maison de la Providence for a course of training with the Sisters of Charity. An attack of the measles, however, promptly forced her to receive nursing care instead of dispensing it. Her illness more or less put an end to this undertaking.

In the meantime she had entered into negotiations with the committee supervising an "Establishment for Gentlewomen During Illness." This was a type of nursing home in London for governesses who became ill, and after appearing before the committee she was appointed superintendent. In 1853 the establishment moved into an empty house at No. 1 Upper Harley Street, and here for the next few years Florence Nightingale found a limited expression for her desire to nurse. She had a number of difficulties with her committee, all of which she negotiated with tact, and she soon had the nursing home running smoothly.

As soon as Miss Nightingale had reorganized the institution, she again began visiting hospitals and collecting facts for reforming conditions for nurses. In the middle of the nineteenth century, social reform was becoming increasingly popular, and people like the Herberts and many of their friends became interested in the reform of medical and social institutions. Miss Nightingale realized that before any nursing reform could be launched, some type of school for the training of reliable and qualified nurses must be organized. At this time, she realized that her first task was to help produce a new type of nurse. Because of her knowledge of hospitals, she was being consulted by social reformers and by many doctors who were beginning to recognize the need for the trained nurse. For example, Dr. Bowman, a well-known surgeon of that day, had performed a difficult operation under chloroform, which was just being used as an anesthetic, and Miss Nightingale had assisted as his nurse. He was very eager for her to accept the position of superintendent of nurses in the King's College Hospital. However, when rumors of this reached her fam-

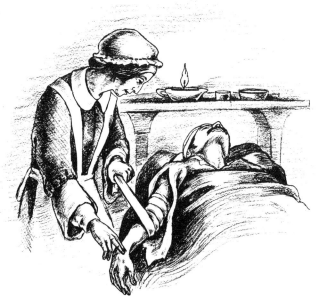

Florence Nightingale's care of the sick at all hours of the day and night during the Crimean War earned for her the grateful title, "Lady with the lamp."

ily, the objections they had always had to Miss Nightingale's going into large hospitals were again brought forward.

She remained in charge of the nursing home at No. 1 Upper Harley Street until her departure for Scutari, with the exception of a vacation to her home and a short leave of absence for the purpose of nursing at the Middlesex Hospital during an epidemic of cholera.

Chapter 8

The Crimean War

In the meantime the Crimean War broke out. The British, the French, and the Turks were fighting the Russians, chiefly near the Black Sea and the Crimean Peninsula. As the war dragged on, it became apparent that there were some serious defects in the organization of the British Army, particularly in the handling of the sick and wounded soldiers. The letters of the war correspondent W. H. Russell to the *Times* stirred up emotion at home. His comparison of nursing in the French Army to that in the British brought things to a climax, which resulted in the letter to the *Times* containing the famous question: "Why have we no Sisters of Charity?"

Many inquiries were made about town in a similar vein, and Miss Nightingale's name was mentioned repeatedly in this connection. Miss Nightingale herself was turning the matter over in her mind and finally wrote to Sir Sidney Herbert, who now was Secretary of War, offering to take a group of nurses into the Crimea. Curiously enough, a letter from Sir Sidney requestion that she do so crossed hers. Her family consented, and she was soon hard at work enlisting thirty-eight nurses. Among these were ten Roman Catholic Sisters, partly from Bermondsey, eight of Miss Sellon's Sisters from Devonport, and six from St. John's House.

These were the best she could obtain at short notice, but several were very inadequate and later had to be returned.

MISS NIGHTINGALE'S ACHIEVEMENTS

On October 21, 1854, the party set out for Scutari on the steamer Vectis. The problems that awaited Miss Nightingale were prodigious. The equipment for the hospital was defective or nonexistent; the staff already there looked upon the expedition as a slur upon their own capability and were not kindly disposed to this arrangement of admitting female nurses into a military hospital. So her job required both organizing ability and tact.

The interested reader may refer to Miss Nightingale's biography for detailed descriptions of the conditions at Scutari. We are concerned with her contribution to organized nursing and may therefore treat the subject in a cursory manner. Plumbing and sewage disposal were next to nonexistent. The simplest means of hygiene and civilized living were lacking. There were no knives and forks, no bedclothes, no scrubbing brushes, no operating room—in fact, hardly anything but a crowded space full of suffering, dying, verminous, undernourished soldiers, attended by inexperienced orderlies and supervised by men who were largely inefficient and who considered the intruders with hostility.

At first Miss Nightingale and her nurses were ignored by the doctors. Although the patients were in great need and Miss Nightingale could get supplies for them, only one doctor would use her nurses and her supplies. She realized that before she could accomplish anything, she must obtain the cooperation and confidence of the medical staff. She was determined to stand by and wait until she was asked for help. This required a great deal of self-control because the need for nursing care and for the supplies that she could get was evident. She was determined that the doctors would ask for her help and was equally determined that no nurse would take care of patients unless she was reliable.

At last, as the fighting increased and the sick and wounded came in ever-increasing numbers, everyone—even visiting representatives from the British government—was pressed into service. At last, the doctors turned to Miss Nightingale and her nurses. It gradually dawned on the medical staff

and the hospital officials that Miss Nightingale was the one person who had money at her disposal and who had contacts with influential people who could help in critical situations.

Miss Nightingale and her nurses set to work at once. They had the authority from the War Office, and they began by requisitioning several hundred scrubbing brushes. Before the war was over, there was a reasonable measure of cleanliness, special diet kitchens had been established, and the rats had been brought under some control. In brief, out of a shambles Miss Nightingale had established a hospital.

The manner in which she handled her staff is also interesting. They were there to cooperate, not to take charge. Miss Nightingale's nurses were strictly instructed not to undertake nursing except when requested by medical officers and to take orders regarding patients from the doctors only. Furthermore, she established herself in the hearts of the men, dividing her time between administration and personal attention to patients. Famous are her nightly rounds when

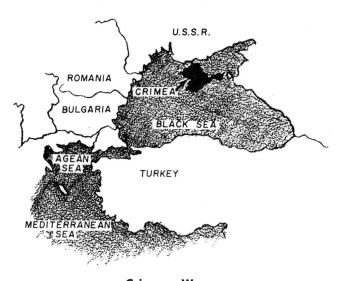

Crimean War

The Crimean War dragged on for many years while the English, French, and Turkish fought the Russians. The English lacked the organization and personnel to care for their wounded until Miss Nightingale came to Scutari.

the day's work supposedly was done. Then with her lantern she made her tour of inspection past the long lines of cots, with a friendly word for some, a smile for others, but in all she inspired a feeling of comfort that someone was sympathizing with them and striving to make their hard lot a little less hard. Of all her activities in Scutari these nightly rounds are perhaps the most famous; they have been immortalized by Longfellow in *The Lady With the Lamp*.

All this was not achieved without difficulties. One of the worst was that she was informed one day that forty-six nurses were on their way to Scutari under the direction of Miss Mary Stanley. It has never been explained who initiated this move or how it was made without consulting Miss Nightingale. They were not sent to assist her but were instructed to report to the Inspector General. Considering the importance of the experiment that Miss Nightingale was performing, her alarm at such an attempt at dual control can easily be imagined. She protested vigorously to Sir Sidney Herbert, and eventually the nurses came into her organization. Other nurses were added from time to time, and at the end of the war she had a staff of 125 nurses.

Miss Nightingale's interest extended beyond nursing. She was in the best sense a social worker. The army in those days had no recreational facilities for the soldiers when they were off duty. The only choice was such entertainment as they might find outside the camp. This entertainment was not of the best and was usually designed to part them from their hard-earned pay with the least possible effort. Many soldiers had brought their wives; these women were painfully neglected, especially during sickness or childbirth. Miss Nightingale did much to relieve the lot of these poor women. She established reading rooms, games, and other entertainments for the soldiers in an attempt to direct their attention away from the dramshop and loose living. She also established in her own office a type of savings bank through which the soldiers might transmit money to relatives in England. She was eminently successful in all of these pursuits.

She gained the sympathy of the medical staff by furnishing them out of her own pocket with a dissecting room and the necessary instruments. In addition to all this she spent the better part of her nights writing: she wrote long official reports and private communications to Sir Sidney Herbert, and did much of the work now incumbent upon the Army Chaplain by writing to the families of sick and dying soldiers.

She had hardly begun to get things into shape when a new and formidable task loomed before her. Her work so far had all been done at Scutari, across the Straits of Bosporus from Constantinople. The war itself was fought across the Black Sea at the Crimean Peninsula, and she felt it incumbent upon her to investigate conditions at the actual theater of war. So in the spring of 1855 she went to Balaklava in the Crimea and worked on the reorganization of the few hospitals there. Here she encountered great obstacles: the roads were dreadful, often nonexistent, and the official attitude of jealous superior officers caused her much grief. However, the Commander of the British forces supported her, and she had done much toward achieving her purpose when she was taken sick with the Crimean fever (probably typhoid or typhus). For a few days her life was in danger. However, her convalescence was slow and she never recovered entirely. She refused a leave of absence to recuperate and returned to work too soon. She stayed until the very end of the war and left with the last contingent of nurses from Scutari.

At the end of the Crimean War, two figures are prominent: the common British soldier and the nurse. At the beginning of the war, most British soldiers were the drunken, immoral dregs of society. The status of the women doing nursing was not very much better. Miss Nightingale, because of her experiment in the Crimea, did much to set the pattern for the improvement of conditions for these two groups.

NIGHTINGALE FUND

The significance of Miss Nightingale's work in Scutari became known and understood far and wide in England: in the future, nurses must be properly trained, and the nursing care of the sick must take its place beside the surgical and medical care. Accordingly, a public meeting was held in London on November 25, 1855, under the presidency of the Commander-in-Chief, the Duke of Cambridge, and it was decided to establish a fund, to be called the "Nightingale Fund," for the purpose of furthering nursing education. Some $220,000, of which $35,000 was subscribed by the army, was collected within a short time in England and in the Dominions. The medical profession, which ultimately was to benefit so greatly from this undertaking, did not enter it wholeheartedly but remained critical.

When Miss Nightingale heard of this fund, she accepted it with the proviso that it would be some time before she could utilize it, and she expressed fear that her health might not suffice for the task. In fact, several years elapsed before she established the first school of nursing.

MISS NIGHTINGALE'S ILLNESS

In August, 1856, she returned from Scutari, six months after the end of the war and began the strangest period of her life. It seemed as if she had spent the strength of her body but not that of her mind. Although there is no record that she was suffering from any organic disease, she was never very well. During the first few months after her return to England she was so weak that she was not expected to live; but when new problems arose in 1857, she rallied to the occasion. For many years she displayed the greatest vigor of mind and undertook the most sustained mental efforts—and yet she was never well enough to see anyone who came to call out of curiosity or on trivial errands. By thus excluding herself from the superficialities of society, she managed to concentrate her energies on the truly great tasks of her life. Much has been written about her "illness." It cannot simply be dismissed as neurasthenia. It could possibly be considered an exhaustion neurosis from which she never recovered because she never afforded herself sufficient rest. It may also be considered an escape through which she, unconsciously perhaps, avoided certain conflicts that would have been inevitable if she had moved about in society hale and hearty. In mid-Victorian England it would have been unthinkable for her to obtain the official position in public life to which she might legitimately aspired. As it was, she was an invalid. Those who wished her advice had to come to her; and by practically living the life of a hermit, she found time and opportunity to gather the tremendous amount of data and information with which she filled the reports that emanated from her rooms.

Chapter 9

Miss Nightingale's postwar activities

Miss Nightingale's first aim was the permanent rectification of the defects that had become glaringly apparent during the Crimean War. This was to be achieved through extensive reforms of the army. She accomplished this by working through a committee, the principal members of which were Sir Sidney Herbert and Dr. Sutherland. This committee, often called "the little war office," sat usually in her rooms, at first at the Burlington Hotel, later in various rented houses. This work was progressing when it was severely upset by the death of Sir Sidney (then Lord Lea) in 1861 and by changes in the government. The reforms were being made slowly; the origins of many reforms carried out years later can still be traced to the activities of Miss Nightingale.

In 1856, the result of Miss Nightingale's conferences and deliberations was published as *Notes in Matters Affecting the Health, Efficiency and Hospital Administration of the British Army.* This was a volume of nearly a thousand printed pages. In 1859 she published a small book called *Notes on Hospitals.* This was so successful that a second edition was published in 1860 and a third, rewritten and with many additions, in 1863. After the publication of this book she was constantly being asked for advice on hospital administration and construction. The plans for many hospitals were submitted to her.

In 1858 she was elected a member of the Statistical Society, and at the Statistical Congress of 1860 she presented a paper for discussion called "Miss Nightingale's Scheme for Uniform Hospital Statistics." Until this time each hospital had used its own method for naming and classifying diseases and keeping other statistics.

While Miss Nightingale's interest in nursing and nursing reform had never diminished, her activities for reforms in the Army had pushed it into the background.

In 1859 her book, *Notes on Nursing,* was published and caused quite a sensation for that day. Habits of personal hygiene taken for granted today were completely foreign to the mid-Victorian days. This book was very widely used, and thousands of copies were distributed to factories and schools. It was also translated into French, German, and Italian.

About 1860 she found time to devote herself to the establishment of a school of nursing to be financed by the Nightingale Fund. St. Thomas' Hospital was finally selected, and for many years Miss Nightingale took a most active part in all details concerning her school. This interest was slackened by only the feebleness of old age.

For the remainder of her life Miss Nightingale's interests were divided among "The Nightingale Nurses," the construction of hospitals, reforms in workhouses, public health measures throughout England (and other countries), and the promotion of public health reforms in India. Because of her powerful personality and her vast knowledge, her advice was sought on most subjects in which she was expert, but she never stood out in official capacity. Somewhat later she was interested in the development of district nursing, and during the Franco-German war she was frequently consulted by both belligerents regarding the care of sick and wounded.

In only two respects was she judged wrong by history. First, she did not appreciate the significance of the bacteriological discoveries that occurred during that period. In spite of her interest in public health and her good judgment regarding hygienic measures, wherever bacteriological facts conflicted with her ideas regarding hygiene, the facts were ignored. Second, she did not appreciate the importance of a central registry for nurses, similar to that for medical men. She thought that the reputation of nurses could be established better through their schools and that a central registry would lead to standardization that would have a detrimental effect on the profession as a whole. Experience, of course, has shown that this was not the case, but she did manage to delay this reform for many years.

In her writings Miss Nightingale dealt with many aspects of the fields in which she was interested. She wrote about the care of the sick in hospitals, workhouses, army camps, city tenements, and rural districts. She also discussed problems in the public health field, such as housing and sanitation, and was interested in health teaching. She wrote extensively on sanitary problems in India, of racial questions, and of the uses of statistics. Her writings appear in books, pamphlets, papers, addresses, articles, and many letters. The Adelaide Nutting Historical Nursing Collection at Teachers College, Columbia University, New York, probably contains the finest collection of her writings

to be found anywhere. Following is a list of some of the writings of Miss Nightingale:

1. The Institution of Kaiserswerth on the Rhine for the Practical Training of Deaconesses under the Direction of the Rev. Pastor Fliedner, Embracing the Support and Care of a Hospital, Infant and Industrial Schools, and a Female Penitentiary. Printed by the Inmates of the London Ragged Colonial Training School, 1851.
2. Letters from Egypt. Privately printed, 1854.
3. Statements Exhibiting the Voluntary Contributions Received by Miss Nightingale for the Use of the British Hospitals in the East, with the Mode of Their Distribution, in 1854, 1855, 1856. Harrison and Sons, 1857.
4. Notes on Matters Affecting the Health, Efficiency, and Hospital Administration of the British Army. Founded Chiefly on the Experience of the Late War. Presented by Request to the Secretary of State for War. Privately printed for Miss Nightingale. Harrison and Sons, 1858.
5. Subsidiary Notes as to the Introduction of Female Nursing into Military Hospitals in Peace and in War. Presented by Request to the Secretary of State for War. Privately printed for Miss Nightingale. Harrison and Sons, 1858.
6. A Contribution to the Sanitary History of the British Army During the Late War With Russia. Harrison and Sons, 1859.
7. Notes on Hospitals. John W. Parker and Sons, 1859. 3rd edition, almost completely rewritten, 1863. Longmans, Green and Co.
8. Suggestions for Thought to the Searchers after Truth Among the Artisians of England. Privately printed for Miss Nightingale. 3 vols. Eyre and Spottiswoode, 1860.
9. Notes on Nursing: What It Is, and What It Is Not. By Florence Nightingale, Harrison and Sons, 1859.
10. Army Sanitary Administration and Its Reform Under the Late Lord Herbert. M'Corquodale and Co., 1862.
11. Observations on the Evidence Contained in the Stational Reports Submitted to the Royal Commission on the Sanitary State of the Army in India. By Florence Nightingale. (Reprinted from the Report of the Royal Commission.) Edward Stanford, 1863. "The Observations."
12. Introductory Notes on Lying-In Institutions. Together With a Proposal for Organising an Institution for Training Midwives and Midwifery Nurses. By Florence Nightingale. Longmans, Green and Co., 1871.

13. Life or Death in India. A paper read at the meeting of the National Association for the Promotion of Social Science, Norwich, 1873. With an Appendix on life or death by irrigation, 1874.
14. The Zemindar, the Sun, and the Watering Pot as Affecting Life or Death in India. Unpublished, proof copies among the Nightingale papers, 1873-1876.
15. On Trained Nursing for the Sick Poor. By Florence Nightingale. The Metropolitan and National Nursing Association, 1876.
16. Miss Florence Nightingale's Addresses to Probationer-Nurses in the "Nightingale Fund" School at St. Thomas's Hospital and Nurses Who Were Formerly Trained There, 1872-1900. Printed for private circulation.
17. Florence Nightingale's Indian Letters. A glimpse into the agitation for tenancy reform. Bengal, 1878-82. Edited by Priyaranja Sen. Calcutta, 1937.*

Thus, for about forty years Miss Nightingale was actively interested in some of the most important reforms of the times, but about the turn of the century her powers waned—she was then nearly 80—and the last ten years of her life she spent in a state of decline until she died quietly in her sleep on August 13, 1910. It was proposed that she be buried in Westminster Abbey, but in accordance with her wish she was interred in the family burying place at Willow, Hampshire.

MISS NIGHTINGALE'S INFLUENCE ON NURSING

Notwithstanding her great contribution in other fields, Miss Nightingale's greatest and most enduring work was done in nursing.

From her youth she believed that her calling was to nurse the sick, and as her purpose in life gradually evolved, she increasingly concentrated her efforts upon the organization of hospitals and the training of nurses. She availed herself of the training that was then available and always deplored that it had not been better. Although she

accepted most of the good aspects of Kaiserswerth, she was keenly aware of the defects in the nurses' training. When she was sick in Paris, she criticized the nursing care that she received. When she was placed in charge of a nursing home, its greatest defect in her opinion was that it gave her no opportunity to train nurses. Again, the lack of trained nurses was at the root of the evils of Scutari and Balaklava, and her greatest single contribution in the Crimean War was the organization of nursing care and such training of nurses as she could effect. The next logical step in her career would have been the administration of the Nightingale Fund, and it was only because of the pressure of the army reforms and her poor state of health that the establishment of a school of nursing under her direction was delayed. However, the time was not wasted, for in 1859 she published two books, *Notes on Hospitals,* which advocated better construction of hospitals and better nursing care, and *Notes on Nursing; What It Is, and What It Is Not.* In the latter book she set forth the fundamental principles of nursing, and it became widely read; it was followed by a "popular edition" in 1861, called *Notes on Nursing for the Laboring Classes,* which included a chapter on infant care. Her *Notes on Nursing* was really one of the first nursing texts and was widely used as such by nurses. It was first published in 1859 and translated into several languages. The first American edition was published in 1860.

Finally, in 1859 a committee was appointed to select a hospital for Miss Nightingale's training school, and, as we noted, St. Thomas' Hospital was selected. The Medical Officer, Mr. R. G. Whitfield, was sympathetic to the plan and the matron, Mrs. Wardroper, was a most capable woman. In 1860 fifteen probationers were admitted for a year's training. Miss Nightingale was consulted on all details of selection of pupil nurses, instruction, and organization. Throughout this chapter emphasis has been placed upon Miss Nightingale's appre-

*Woodham-Smith, Cecil: Florence Nightingale, New York, 1951, McGraw-Hill Book Co., Inc., pp. 368-369.

ciation of the necessity for training of nurses. This is so obvious to us that it is hard to understand that she had to fight to establish this principle. Most people, including many medical men, thought that nursing could be done "by intuition." If that attitude is understood, the magnitude of Miss Nightingale's contribution is better appreciated. Furthermore, she made it clear that she did not advocate a new "nursing order." She wanted to establish a secular career for women, similar to law and medicine for men. And she succeeded. If it had not been for Miss Nightingale, the elevation of nursing from a lowly craft to a respected profession might have been delayed many years, to the detriment of the progress of medicine and hospital administration.

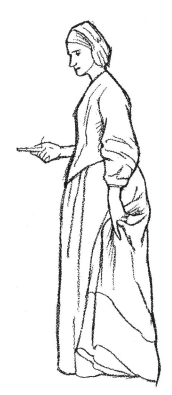

Florence Nightingale from statue

The "Lady with the Lamp," immortalized by Longfellow in commemoration of her nightly rounds at Scutari, left an impact on nursing and hospitals that is felt today.

As it was, Miss Nightingale placed the emphasis on the education of women in an endowed school; in fact she was less concerned with the production, in the first place, of practical nurses than with a group of educated women who could go abroad in the land and establish similar centers of training elsewhere, acting as leaders who would help raise the level of nursing everywhere. Again she succeeded. More nursing pupils were admitted, more instruction was instituted, and gradually the old type nurses were replaced by younger women to whom nursing was a career and not a last resort.

Along with all this she personally kept in touch with her nurses. She rarely went out, but they came to see her in her home at South Street where she lived for many years, and aided by her acute judgment of human character she quickly sized them up and her notes made at the time bear witness to her shrewd and crafty powers of observation. During her lifetime she became an almost legendary figure in English nursing. The growth of her reputation was not hampered by the eventual decline of her frail body. Her name continues to be the beacon light for our profession.

MISS NIGHTINGALE'S INFLUENCE ON NURSING EDUCATION

It is hard for us to realize that recognized preparation for modern nursing and the real beginning of nursing education began with the establishment of the Nightingale School at St. Thomas' Hospital.

The cardinal principles upon which she established that first school were the following:

1. Nurses should be technically trained in hospitals organized for that purpose.
2. Nurses should live in "homes" fit to form their moral lives and discipline.

The direction of her school was largely accomplished through the efforts of others, but she was consulted often about what was being done in the school. She rebuked head nurses who were not giving enough time and thought to teaching students. She also recognized the need for appointing a nurse instructor for classroom teaching. Some of the following points that she made are quite modern.

1. In addition to her salary received from the hospital, the Ward Sister should be paid by the Fund (The Nightingale Endowment Fund) for training these probationers.
2. It was recorded that remuneration was to be paid also to medical instructors.
3. Weekly records of the work of the probationers were to be kept by the head nurses and monthly records by the matron.
4. Diaries (as previously noted) were to be kept by probationers.
5. Miss Nightingale emphasized the need for correlation of theory and practice (although she did not use that phrase).
6. Probationers, she said, must be taught to know symptoms—and the reasons why and they must be given time to learn "the reason why."*

Miss Nightingale established the custom of sending an annual letter to her students. In some respects similar messages are now given at commencement time. Quotations from these letters demonstrate that not only do they contain helpful ideas but also encouragement and inspiration. Many of them are very applicable to students in nursing schools today.

A woman who takes a sentimental view of nursing (which she calls "ministering" as if she were an angel) is, of course, worse than useless. A woman possessed with the idea that she is making a sacrifice will never do; and a woman who thinks that any kind of nursing work is "beneath a nurse" will simply be in the way.

For us who nurse, our nursing is a thing, which, unless in it we are making progress every year, every month, every week, take my word for it we are going back. The more experience we gain the more progress we can make. The progress you make in your year's training with us is as nothing to what you must make each year after your training is over. A woman who thinks of

herself "Now I am a full nurse, a skillful nurse. I have learnt all there is to be learnt," take my word for it, she does not know what a nurse is, and she will never know: she has gone back already. Conceit and nursing cannot exist in the same person.*

The principles upon which this first school of nursing was established exerted great influence as the need for trained nurses increased. These graduates went out to establish schools and to become matrons in hospitals throughout England and her colonies and in the United States of America. Because of inadequate financial arrangements few schools remained separate from the hospitals even if they had been organized as distinct units. They were all soon part of the hospital and controlled by its administration. This important principle of Miss Nightingale's, namely, that the school be considered as an educational and not as a service institution, is being revived today in the recent reorganization of nursing schools.

It was natural that there should have been opposition to Miss Nightingale. There was a growing need for nurses, and many believed that the type of training demanded, the close supervision, and the very strict regulations insisted upon would never produce enough nurses to meet the need. In 1866 a committee of the Hospital Association proposed that an independent body of examiners should be created to set an examination and that when a nurse had passed it, her name would be placed on a register of nurses. Thus, the public would be protected from incompetent or unscrupulous nurses. Miss Nightingale opposed this step because she thought nursing was still too young and too unorganized for such a standard examination and because she did not believe that any examination could test the character of the nurse, which she held to be so very important. She believed that only a certificate from the matron in the nursing

---

*Roberts, Mary: Florence Nightingale as a nurse educator, American Journal of Nursing **37**:775, July, 1937.

*Pavey, Agnes E.: The story of the growth of nursing, London, 1938, Faber & Faber, Ltd., p. 296.

school would be a guarantee that the nurse had the necessary qualities of character as well as the technical skill. An examination conducted by strangers, she thought, could never test this important aspect of the nurse's qualifications. This controversy continued between Miss Nightingale and a few of her royal matrons for some years. Later the British Nursing Association was granted a royal charter but not in the terms they had sought, so that actually neither side won.

In 1893 she prepared a paper on "Sick Nursing and Health Nursing," which was read at the Chicago Exhibition of Women's Work at the World's Fair.

Many memorials have been erected to Miss Nightingale. National Hospital Day is celebrated on her birthday; on the Sunday nearest that date nurses all over America hold memorial services. In 1912 it was proposed at the International Council of Nurses in Cologne that an international memorial be developed; a Florence Nightingale Foundation was set up for this purpose. Before World War II a group of nurses from many countries lived at Florence Nightingale International House in London for one year and acquired a better conception of international understanding while studying together in three courses: (1) public health, (2) nurse administration and teaching, and (3) social work. The courses were given at Bedford College in cooperation with the College of Nursing.

Questions and study projects for unit two

1. In what ways did the Crimean War affect nursing and the development of professional nursing?
2. To what other fields besides nursing did Miss Nightingale contribute? What were some of these contributions?
3. What were the basic principles upon which the Nightingale School was established?
4. Be prepared to discuss the life of Florence Nightingale under the following heads:
   (a) Her early life and education
   (b) Her preparation for nursing
   (c) Her activities during the Crimean War
   (d) Her contributions to the development of professional nursing
   (e) Her contributions to public health
   (f) Her writings
   (g) Her influence on the first schools of nursing established in this country.
5. Make an annotated bibliography of recent articles appearing in *The American Journal of Nursing, Nursing Outlook, Nursing Research,* and any other journals available in your library relating to the discussion in this unit.

References for unit two

Andrews, Mary R.: A lost commander: Florence Nightingale, New York, 1938, Doubleday & Co., Inc.

Banworth, Calista: A living memorial to Florence Nightingale, American Journal of Nursing 40: 491-497 May, 1940.

Cook, Sir Edward: The life of Florence Nightingale (2 vols. in 1), New York, 1942, The Macmillan Co.

Editorial—Dedication of the American Nurses' Memorial, Florence Nightingale School, Bordeaux, France, American Journal of Nursing 22:799-804, July, 1922.

Editorial—The dedication of the Bordeaux School Building, American Journal of Nursing 22:635-636, May, 1922.

Editorial—The imperishable glory of Miss Nightingale, American Journal of Nursing 36:491-492, May, 1936.

Extracts from letters from the Crimea, American Journal of Nursing 32:537-538, 1932.

Florence Nightingale is placed among mankind's benefactors, American Journal of Nursing 50: 265, 1950.

Lee, Eleanor: A Florence Nightingale collection, American Journal of Nursing 38:555-561, May, 1938.

Noyes, Clara D.: American nurses complete fund for Memorial School in France, American Journal of Nursing 29:1189-1191, October, 1929.

Nightingaliana: American Journal of Nursing 49: 288-299, May, 1949.

Pavey, Agnes E.: The story of the growth of nursing, London, 1938, Faber & Faber, Ltd., pp. 267-298.

Roberts, Mary M.: Florence Nightingale as a nurse educator, American Journal of Nursing 37:773-778, July, 1937.

Scovil, Elisabeth R.: Florence Nightingale notes on nursing, American Journal of Nursing 27: 355-357, May, 1927.

Seymer, Lucy: St. Thomas' Hospital and the Nightingale Training School, International Nursing Review 11:340-344, 1937.

Stephen, Barbara: Florence Nightingale's Home, International Nursing Review 11:331-334, 1937.

Strachey, Lytton: Eminent Victorians, New York, 1918, G. P. Putnam's Sons.

Trevelyan, George Macaulay: History of England, London, 1928, Longmans, Green & Co., Ltd.

Whittaker, Elvi W., and Olesen, Virginia L.: Why Florence Nightingale? American Journal of Nursing 67:2338-2341, November, 1967.

Woodham-Smith, Cecil: Florence Nightingale, New York, 1951, McGraw-Hill Book Co., Inc.

Unit three

Early American nursing

The humanitarian impulse that developed at the dawn of the Christian era resulted in many hospitals' being established. The industrialization of the community emphasized the need for hospitals and the training of personnel as a community as well as a religious obligation. The concept of group responsibility for the individual was beginning to develop.

Chapter 10

Medical and social setting

Medical science was confronted by a host of problems. More than a hundred years ago Louis emphasized the importance of the numerical method in medicine, but few doctors properly appreciated the necessity of the suitable application of statistical methods in determining effective treatment and in evaluating data. Tuberculosis, although receding, was still a formidable enemy and required much preventive work and improvement of treatment during its early stages. Venereal disease, especially syphilis, was yet to be conquered; in this field, however, notable beginnings had been made by the discovery of the spirochete, the Wassermann reaction (1906), by further development of the specific drugs, Salvarsan and its derivatives, by the use of the heavy metals, and by the general recognition of venereal disease as a public health problem. Maternal mortality was still too high for the country as a whole. Further advances in surgical technic were expected. (In this connection, however, we may remember that at a Congress in England in 1872, just before Lister's work was generally appreciated, the opinion was expressed that surgery had then almost reached the limits of its achievement.) The greatest advances in the near future were expected in increased knowledge of the endocrine glands and of the vitamins, in the control of cancer, in mental illness, and in preventive medicine.

During the late eighteenth and nineteenth centuries, scientific progress in all phases of diagnosis and treatment of disease had been very great. This increased knowledge had resulted in the beginning of specialization in all health activities. Increased knowledge meant the need for more and better equipment in doctors' offices, in clinics, and in hospitals. All of these changes were beginning to increase the cost of medical care. As the community became educated in health matters and as confidence was created in hospitals, doctors, and nurses, increasing demands were being made on the health program of the entire United States. As health and disease became matters of public concern, we find that communities began to make plans for assuming certain responsibilities in these areas. This was observed particularly in countries in which socialism was advancing. Chancellor Bismarck was instrumental in working out a plan of compulsory insurance against illness in Germany in 1883. The German example of providing social insurance made quite an impression on other European countries. Compulsory health insurance for those of low incomes was adopted in Austria in 1888. Other countries in Europe adopting some type of compulsory health insurance or subsidizing voluntary societies were Sweden in 1891, Denmark in 1892, Belgium in 1894, Italy in 1898, and Switzerland in 1912. In

Russia in 1918 "A People's Commissariat of Public Health" was established, and in line with other developments in the communist state almost complete state medicine developed. All of these developments and their underlying social philosophies, naturally, were studied by and had some influence on other countries. England, although probably more individualistic politically than some of the continental countries, had become highly industrialized during the nineteenth century, and even the poorer classes were becoming better educated. In 1911 a National Insurance Act was adopted by the English Parliament. In England the state as well as employers and employees contributed to the cost. Patients had a free choice of doctors, and what has become known as the "panel system" developed.

EARLY AMERICAN MEDICINE

American medicine was still in its infancy in the eighteenth century. Many doctors came from Europe to settle in America, and many students went from this country to study in the European centers. Benjamin Franklin influenced American medicine not only by inventing bifocal glasses but also by preaching the use of fresh air and by helping in the foundation of the Pennsylvania Hospital.

Too, in America, medical teaching was for the most part at a low ebb. Only Philadelphia had attained any reputation; New York and Boston were still struggling into existence as medical centers. It was therefore simple and logical that American doctors should be divided into two groups: those with the ambition and resources that enabled them to visit Edinburgh, London, and Paris, from which they returned to become leading surgeons and physicians, mostly in the larger cities of the East, and those content with the preceptorship of an older practitioner—by far the majority.

The first medical schools in the United States were organized in the second half of the eighteenth century, the first one being the College of Philadelphia, now the University of Pennsylvania, founded by John Morgan, modeled after the Edinburgh School. The first M.D. degree was conferred in 1771 at the King's College School in New York, now the College of Physicians and Surgeons of Columbia University, founded in 1767. Harvard did not start a medical school until 1773. Other schools founded in this century were Dartmouth College and School and the Transylvania University School in Kentucky.

It is no wonder that with a few exceptions medical practice in the United States a hundred years ago was very bad; it could not be other wise. It is remarkable that in America, largely through the efforts of the American Medical Association, the profession has been raised to the level at which it stands today and that in spite of all handicaps, Americans have been able to make important and fundamental contributions to the science.

One such contribution was McDowell's operations on ovarian tumor. Having had his attention drawn to the problem when he was a student in Edinburgh under John Bell, Ephraim McDowell (1771-1830), when he became a backwoods practitioner in Kentucky, had the courage to perform the operation. He was successful and gained fame by several reptitions of his feat. So incredible was his achievement that when reports first reached Europe, they were simply not believed.

During the early nineteenth century, a physiologist became noted because of his studies of gastric digestion and gastric motility, which formed the basis for all later work on the physiology of gastric digestion —William Beaumont (1785-1853).

On the morning of June 6, 1822, an accident happened on the little Island of Mackinac, north of Michigan, which was destined to bring fame to one man and a great increase of knowledge to the world. A young voyageur, Alexis St. Martin, happened to be in the way of a shotgun that accidentally went off two feet from his body. The entire charge entered his left side, tearing his clothing with it. At first the wound was thought to be fatal, but under the care of a regimental surgeon stationed at the fort the lad recovered. However, a fistula, or opening from the stomach to the surface of the body, remained. The surgeon, whose name was Beaumont, seized this opportunity for study of gastric function and attached the boy to his household for the next few years. He performed a series of experiments which have become fundamental in our knowledge of that organ, and Beaumont's name is now known to every young medical student. His studies were performed under very primitive conditions, and the brilliant results are due to Beaumont's ability for research and not to his equipment. Alexis was an unworthy fellow who repeatedly left him, and at last Beaumont failed to recover him. In 1839 Beaumont was stationed in St. Louis. Later because of a difference with his superiors he retired from the Army and entered private practice there, where his fame and ability soon made him the leading doctor of St. Louis.

Best known of all American doctors of the period was Benjamin Rush (1755-1813). He has been referred to as the "American Sydenham." His influence in furthering the clinical method in America continued long after his death; and his descendants are still practicing medicine in Philadelphia.

Perhaps the greatest medical advance made in America during this period was the use of ether for surgical anesthesia. For this great book to medicine we are indebted to a Boston dentist named William T. G. Morton (1819-1868). Through careful research, Morton chose ether as the drug for his purpose. He demonstrated his discovery to the Boston surgeons, and it was soon broadcast all over the world. Along with the work of Pasteur and of Lister it made possible the great advance of modern surgery. It is a curious and sordid fact that Morton, instead of granting his gift magnanimously to the world as most medical benefactors did, tried to exploit it by patent rights. This soon involved him in litigation, which broke him bodily and financially; so instead of reaping the laurels of fame his last years were spent in ignominious misery.

A historical figure in American medicine during the late nineteenth and early twentieth centuries, one whose influence is still felt today, was Sir William Osler (1849-1919). His activities were shared by three countries—Canada, the United States, and Great Britain. He combined with a thorough training in pathology outstanding clinical abilities, both as a teacher and as a diagnostician. Thus he came to be one of the founders of Johns Hopkins Medical School in Baltimore, and it was here he achieved his greatest fame.

The last years of his life were tragic. All through his life he had given of himself freely for the advancement of knowledge and love of mankind. For himself he had but one thing, a son, and that son was sacrificed in World War I. When Osler received the telegram from the War Office, his spirit died within him, and his body survived but

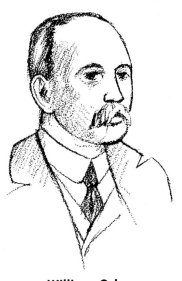

William Osler

a few years. No more direct impression of the futility and bestiality of war could be given than that conveyed by the description of that father's grief for his son.

In 1898 Pierre Curie and his wife, Marie, isolated radium, now used in the treatment of certain types of cancer. In 1910 Paul Ehrlich discovered a cure for syphilis in the form of arsphenamine. Large sums were being appropriated, particularly in America, for scientific investigation. In 1901 John D. Rockefeller endowed the Rockefeller Institute for medical research. Simon Flexner, an outstanding scientist, was director. He gathered about him outstanding scientists in medical and allied fields; many discoveries have come from that Institute.

In 1908 the Carnegie Foundation financed a study of medical schools in the United States and Canada, and on the basis of this report medical schools began to be graded in 1910 and have been graded ever since—a measure that the nursing profession is just beginning to take.

EARLY REFORMS IN NURSING

The first attempt at a regularly organized school of nursing was made in 1839 by the Nurse Society of Philadelphia under Dr. Joseph Warrington. It was inspired by the work of Elizabeth Fry in England. The instruction was very elementary; there were regular courses, with lectures and demonstrations using a mannikin. After a stated period and evidence of proficiency the nurses received a "Certificate of Approbation." Dr. Warrington taught nursing students at the Philadelphia Dispensary together with medical students.

The nurses were called "pupils," and in 1849 they were housed in a home of their own. Another Philadelphian attempt was the school of nursing established in connection with the Women's Hospital of Philadelphia in 1861. The course was supposed to last for six months and was designed to appeal to the better type of young women in order to "train a superior class of nurses." Lectures were given in medical and surgical

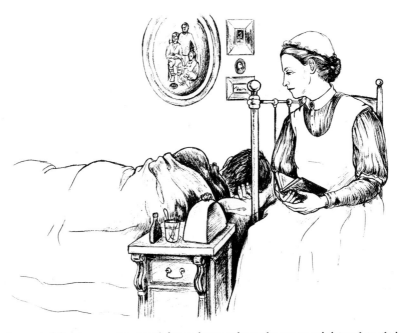

Formerly most sick persons were cared for at home where the nurse ministered to their needs.

nursing, materia medica, and dietetics. These nurses were given a diploma at the successful termination of the course.

Another aspiration to form a nursing school was frustrated by the Civil War. Dr. Elizabeth Blackwell had closely studied Florence Nightingale's ideas and wanted to establish a school for nurses in connection with the New York Infirmary for Women. This school did not materialize.

The realization of the need for nursing reforms remained, but ideas were slow in maturing. The agitation that had been going on in England and the schools that were opened following the leadership of Miss Nightingale had become known in America. American reformers, inspired by visits to England and the continent, began investigating conditions at home. Attention was also paid to the struggling efforts to establish schools for nursing. The cause was not without the support of the medical profession, for in 1869 the American Medical Association accepted a report from its Committee on the Training of Nurses. The chairman was an outstanding Philadelphia surgeon, Dr. Samuel Gross. The committee appreciated the importance of adequate training for nurses and recommended that schools of nursing be established in connection with hospitals all over the United States.

CONCLUSION

In the early nineteenth century a new era began in hospital construction and in medicine, which laid the foundation and emphasized the need for a trained group of nurses to meet the growing complexities of medicine and to staff the growing number of hospitals. One of the important hospitals of this period was the Massachusetts General Hospital. It was established in 1810 as the result of a letter circulated by fifty-six men of Boston who believed that Boston, too, should have a hospital for the poor. The movement was backed by leading Boston doctors and resulted in 1821 in the opening of the Massachusetts General Hospital. Ever since its opening, it has maintained standards often far ahead of its time. The deplorable conditions of nursing that developed in many of the hospitals at this time never existed here. Another hospital that led in nursing reforms was the Johns Hopkins in Baltimore, built in 1889. Many other communities built large hospitals because, with the growing industrialization, cities needed some place in which to house the sick. In America as in Europe, the process was largely a result of urban development occasioned by the growth of the industrial Age. The main purpose of the hospital in the nineteenth century was to serve as a dormitory or a place of sojourn for the sick. It served incidentally as a convenient place for the practical training of the doctors and later of nurses. The events of the Civil War particularly emphasized the urgent need in the United States for adequate hospital facilities and for trained personnel.

Chapter 11

Nursing during early American wars

The need for nurses has always been accelerated in wartime. During the Crusades and the Wars of the Middle Ages, nursing orders such as the Knights of St. John, the Teutonic Knights, and the Maltese Knights were organized to meet the crises. In America the crisis of the Revolutionary War occurred before Miss Nightingale's day, but it is interesting to note that George Washington asked Congress for a matron and for nurses to care for the sick and wounded. However, we know that the number of women with any nursing experience was pitifully small and that many lay women volunteered their services more on a community level than anything else. The Catholic orders were the only organized groups with any actual knowledge of nursing, and they placed their hospitals and personnel at the disposal of the Army. As was the custom of the time, wives, sisters, and mothers followed the men in the Army and took care of them when they were sick and wounded.

REVOLUTIONARY WAR

During the Revolutionary War the Continental Army Medical Corps was not very successful at the beginning, and conditions were not improved until 1781 when Dr. John Cochran was appointed General Director. Anesthesia and modern aseptic technic were unknown, the hospitals were un-

sanitary, and there was a shortage of food, medicine, and trained personnel. Epidemics were common in the Army, and preventive medicine was unknown. It is interesting to note that during the Revolutionary War, chaplains from both the Catholic and Protestant faiths were appointed not only to improve morale but also to "recommend cleanliness as a virtue conducive to health." These conditions were common during all the wars of the nineteenth century and were not brought to the attention of the public in any organized and penetrating way until Miss Nightingale's efforts during the Crimean War.

CIVIL WAR

As was the case in England, the stimulus of a war was necessary to produce an effective demand for modern nursing. Some Americans had begun to hear about the Red Cross and Florence Nightingale's work during the Crimean War, but when the Civil War started, little organized information was available. We find that independently of M. Dunant's efforts at that time, the United States Sanitary Commission was established in April, 1861.

A branch of this commission opened a bureau in New York for the examination and registration of nurses for war service; about a hundred applicants were obtained and offered as nurses to the Federal Army.

When the war finally broke out, this arrangement was totally inadequate, and the Surgeon General agreed to the organization of its own Sanitary Commission as part of the Army. The nurses for this arrangement were supplied largely by the Catholic orders: Sisters of Charity, Sisters of Mercy, and Sisters of St. Vincent. The Holy Cross Sisters, an Anglican Order, also supplied some.

Protestant nursing orders, including the deaconesses, did good work in the war, but all that organized nursing units could do proved insufficient after the big battles when experiences similar to those depicted in *Gone With the Wind* were reenacted all over the war-ridden area. Classical are the descriptions by Louisa May Alcott in her *Hospital Sketches*. She was one of the thousands of women who, anxious to aid the cause, signed up as nurses without other prerequisites than a warm heart and an eager hand. She vividly described her feelings when she

was first faced with the invasions of bloody, filthy, smelly human wrecks, whose wounds were covered by remnants of uniforms matted with filth and clotted blood. Victims came in numbers far exceeding the capacity of the accommodations prepared for them. Somehow everybody had to go to work with soap and brushes and try to clean them up and get them ready for surgical attention. Food had to be provided, and when the confusions of the first rush had subsided there were hundreds of little jobs, apparently trivial, yet important to the patients or those they had left behind: letters to be written and valuables to be received and kept or transmitted to relatives.

Thus, in the American as in other armies, two kinds of nursing developed: a regular Army nursing service, which was placed under the direction of Miss Dorothea Dix, and an organization sponsored by private citizens, at first tolerated, later supported, by the government.

Dorothea Lynde Dix (1803-1887) was

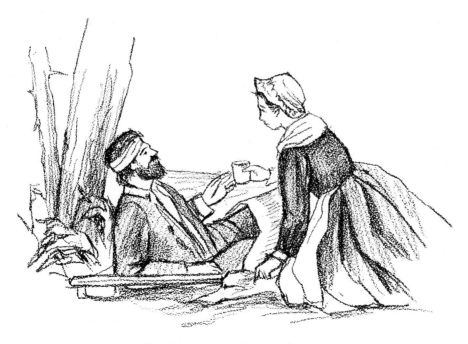

Nursing during the Civil War

known for her interest and activity in the field of reform for the mentally ill. She had studied in England and on the Continent and was a friend of both Elizabeth Fry and Mr. Rathbone. Returning to America, she had worked unceasingly to improve conditions for the care of the mentally ill.

In 1861 a meeting of interested women resulted in the formation of the Women's Central Association of Relief. Out of this activity grew the Sanitary Commission. Influential lay women and physicians became interested because it was necessary that they have some central organization through which supplies could be distributed. The Sanitary Commission attempted to bring together the relief work of many scattered organizations and groups. It was interested in recruiting and in everything associated with the health and welfare of the troops. It studied ways and means of supplementing government appropriations from private funds.

In some ways it might be said that this organization was a forerunner of the Red Cross. The Confederacy had no such type of organization, but as we know from official and unofficial stories, valiant work was done by lay women and religious groups. In 1861, although Dorothea Lynde Dix was not a nurse, she was appointed Superintendent of Female Nurses, and then she proceeded to get together the first Nurse Corps of the United States Army. At this time Miss Dix was about 60 years of age, and by some her standards were considered very rigid and inflexible. She would not have any nurses less than 30 years of age and preferably very homely. Although no uniform was designated, somber colors were insisted upon, black or brown. An allowance of $12 a month was paid these nurses, Miss Dix herself serving without remuneration. Miss Dix found as Miss Nightingale did in the Crimean War that most of her nurses came from religious orders, both Protestant and Catholic.

Although eventually some 2,000 nurses

participated in the Civil War, their number was entirely inadequate. Their equipment was worse than primitive, and hospital facilities were whatever could be found, although in this respect the Civil War contributed one thing: hospital ships were first placed in service at this time. Not only were hospital and nursing facilities insufficient but the hygiene was atrocious; there were in that war about six million medical hospital admissions, mostly from epidemic or contagious diseases, against about 425,000 surgical cases, that is, actual war casualties. It is no exaggeration to state that in those days war claimed more victims from disease than from bullets.

This experience made clear, especially in the light of what Miss Nightingale had done, the desperate need for organized schools of nursing; such schools were accordingly started in New York City, Boston, and New Haven.

SPANISH-AMERICAN WAR

At the turn of the century when trouble between America and Cuba was imminent, Congress authorized employment of nurses under contract. This was necessary, because military nursing had not developed at all since the Civil War and because no mechanism existed by which the Surgeon General could find nurses if needed. However, by 1898 when the Spanish-American War began, schools of nursing had been training young women for this profession for about twenty years. More than 500 schools of nursing had graduated about 10,000 nurses by 1900.

Dr. Anita McGee, at that time vice-president of the Daughters of the American Revolution, had interested the Surgeon General, George M. Sternberg, with a plan for a nurse corps, which was to be organized with the D.A.R. acting as an examining board or a clearinghouse for all applications. Congress gave him authority to employ as many nurses by contract as would be needed. Nurses in the Spanish-American War received $30 a

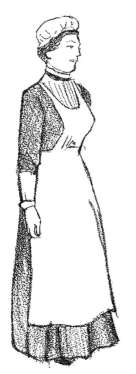

Spanish-American War Nurse

geon General, they gave very satisfactory service, and the Army doctors depended on them more and more. More than 1,500 nurses had been accepted as Army nurses during the Spanish-American War.

The Nurses' Associated Alumnae of the United States and Canada were disturbed with the nursing conditions at the outbreak of the Spanish-American War, and at a meeting, its president, Mrs. Isabel Hampton Robb, suggested that the Association offer its services to the government in an attempt to obtain more and better nurses. When this suggestion was taken to Washington, it was found that Dr. McGee had already been appointed and had set up her own standards. Several prominent superintendents of nursing schools volunteered to help in the organization of Army nursing, among them Anna C. Maxwell, Superintendent of Nurses, Presbyterian Hospital in New York City. Miss Maxwell was appointed Chief Nurse at the hospital at Chickamauga Park, Georgia.

In 1900, 202 nurses remained in the Nurse Corps, and the Army Reorganization Bill presented to Congress in that year provided for a permanent Nurse Corps as part of the Medical Department of the Army. The Army Nurse Corps was created by law on February 2, 1901.

month plus ration allowances. In spite of the great need, not all medical officers were willing to accept Army nurses in the beginning, but since they were carefully selected by Dr. McGee, assistant to the Sur-

Chapter 12

The Red Cross—organization and early development

All over the world the symbol of the Red Cross stands for help in wars or in civilian disasters. What is the history behind such a unique organization?

UN SOUVENIR DE SOLFERINO

In reviewing the life of Florence Nightingale, it was noted that her first great task was to care for the sick and the wounded of the battlefield. That accomplished, her attention turned to the general welfare of the men in the army. They had more coming to them than a cot, three meals a day, and small pay, and she began to organize all those recreational facilities that, as we know today, add greatly to the comforts of army life. Finally, after the war she turned her attention to many activities concerned with the health of the civilian population. In many respects the life of Miss Nightingale after 1854 epitomizes the later development of the Red Cross, which she inspired.

The story of this institution begins on June 24, 1859, near the town of Solferino in Northern Italy. About 300,000 men, Italians and French, were locked in mortal combat, and the carnage was terrific. Yet the work of Florence Nightingale but a few years previously had gone unheeded, and the provisions for taking care of the wounded were

woefully insufficient. Hundreds died from inadequate attention. The appalling horror of the situation struck a tourist who accidentally happened to be there, to the point that he assembled such volunteers as he could gather, mostly women of Solferino, for the work of bringing succor to the wounded. The name of this gentleman was Jean Henri Dunant; he was a Swiss, and he later described his experience in the classic *Un Souvenir de Solferino*.

Inspired by the work of Miss Nightingale in the Crimea, he then decided to devote his life to the prevention of a repetition of the needless horrors of Solferino. He traveled from country to country explaining his scheme to all responsible persons who could help him further it. In France, Napoleon III lent a willing ear, not knowing how badly he himself would need the services of the Red Cross but a few years later. Dunant's idea was to establish bands of volunteer helpers who would seek out and treat the wounded of the battlefield without regard to nationality and in complete neutrality under the protection of all the armed forces. Further, this establishment should be sanctioned by convention and respected by all belligerents. Dunant addressed international congresses, and finally M. Gustave Moynier, president of the Society of Public Utility of Geneva, Switzerland, convened a congress in October, 1863, of thirty-six representatives from fourteen different countries, for the purpose of studying M. Dunant's proposal. At this meeting the fundamental principles of the Red Cross were established, and plans were laid for organizing Red Cross societies in various countries with organization and powers to render aid to wounded soldiers and other victims of war. The congress adjourned and work progressed to secure for the movement the necessary international legal status and to devise an acceptable emblem that would be recognized everywhere.

THE GENEVA CONVENTION OF 1864

Even before it could be further organized, the young organization was put to a test. A short but bloody war broke out in the winter of 1863-1864 between little Denmark and Bismarck's newly organized Prussia. The Danish armaments were hopelessly outmoded, and the war was one long debacle for the Danes. However, it did offer the first opportunity for trying out the Red Cross, and when the Federal Council of Switzerland in August, 1864, convoked an international diplomatic conference, practical experience was available for the organization of what came to be known as the Geneva Convention of 1864. Dunant's original principles were established: the wounded must be respected, military hospitals must be considered neutral, and all persons, equipment, and buildings under the jurisdiction of the institution were to be marked with a red cross on a white background (the reverse of the Swiss flag).

In spite of some infractions, with many more accusations of infractions and very few abuses, these original principles have been accepted and respected by almost all nations. At a conference held in The Hague in 1899, the principles were extended to sea warfare also, and at conventions held in 1906 and 1907, the Geneva and Hague conventions were revised. Curiously, Turkey, by special arrangement, has substituted for the red cross the crescent; and Iran, the lion and the rising sun. Thus, out of the Geneva Convention came the International Red Cross Committee, which is the coordinating agency of all the National Red Cross Committees. Its purpose is to establish Red Cross Committees in countries in which they do not exist, to act as a liaison between the various committees, and to endeavor to have the Geneva Convention accepted by all civilized countries and to ensure that it is observed. In time of war it establishes international agencies for the assistance of war prisoners and other victims of war, and in recent years it has added to this plans for relief during national disasters, such as floods and earthquakes. Thus the International Committee acts in any matter that is beyond the scope of the National Committees. In 1912 the International Committee instituted the Florence Nightingale medal to be given to nurses who had especially distinguished themselves.

The National Red Cross Societies are the component parts of the International Red Cross. They were originally formed purely for war service, but, as we shall see, their scope has been greatly widened. To be accepted by the International Red Cross, a National Society must be recognized as an auxiliary to the army of its country by its government, which, in turn, must have subscribed to the Geneva Convention. It must accept the emblem of the red cross (with the exceptions noted above) and the organization must be open to all citizens of the country irrespective of sex, politics, or religion. It must also cooperate in all required respects with the International organization, which, in return, will recognize only one National Red Cross Society in each sovereign state. Within the country a National Red Cross Society is autonomous and free to develop its own ideas.

It may thus be seen that the Red Cross has a very important official standing. In war it becomes indispensable, and it has assumed so many peacetime activities that it is rapidly becoming one of the most important social agencies of the state, and yet it is entirely independent and supported by voluntary contributions.

FUNCTIONS OF THE RED CROSS

During war, then, the National Red Cross Society assists but does not replace the regular army medical service (which, however, also uses the emblem of the Red Cross in accordance with the Geneva Convention). It mobilizes nurses, nurses' aides, and voluntary helpers and sets up ambulance services, hospitals, hospital ships, canteens, libraries for the soldiers, entertainments, occupational therapy, and many other activities. It renders aid to war refugees and prisoners of war and may assist groups of citizens in devastated countries (for instance, by feeding children). When the war is over, the Red Cross becomes active in the identification and return of prisoners of war, resettlement of refugees, fighting postwar epidemics, reorganization for the next war, and relieving suffering arising from the war. It will see that disabled men get the best treatment and will train them by establishing orthopedic and other special clinics and by establishing trade schools. It may extend direct aid to widows and orphans of soldiers, or it may undertake to house permanently disabled men, as the British Red Cross does in The Star and Garter at Richmond, England.

These, then, are some of the principal activities of the Red Cross in connection with war. It is easily seen how many of these tasks concern nurses or are entirely dependent upon professional nurses. Nurses, therefore, form an important part of the organization, and any properly qualified nurse in good professional standing is encouraged to join the Red Cross reserve, which thus becomes the reserve upon which the military forces largely depend in time of war.

THE AMERICAN RED CROSS

So far we have considered the Red Cross as an international institution. The American Red Cross, however, has its own interesting history.

The Red Cross was organized in many European countries. Clara Barton went aboard and spent years studying the organization in various countries; she established close contact with Miss Nightingale, who later followed American developments with warm interest. Miss Barton's studies were very practical—during the Franco-Prussian War from 1870 to 1871, she actually accompanied one of the Red Cross ambulances into the field. She came back firmly convinced that America must have a Red Cross Society that would adhere to the Geneva Convention. The result of her efforts was the incorporation in 1881 in the District of Columbia of an American Association of the Red Cross with Miss Barton as president. Ratification by the United States was accomplished in 1882.

The young organization was first put to the test in the yellow fever epidemic in Florida in 1888 and in the Johnstown flood in 1889. For the epidemic Miss Barton supplied around thirty volunteer nurses, mostly from New Orleans; they were supposed to be immunized to yellow fever, having had the disease. There was friction with the local board of health, and not without justification, for some of the volunteers were without

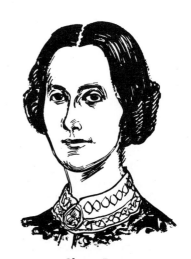

Clara Barton

previous experience in nursing. In the relief of the Johnstown disaster, Red Cross units came out from Philadelphia, and worked under the direction of physicians.

During these years Miss Barton and others interested in the cause worked hard to develop the American Red Cross. An organization evolved with local committees and sections for the purpose of selecting and training volunteer nurses, so that in time of war they could be promptly mobilized and placed in active service. The American National Red Cross was established on a firmer basis in 1893, again with Miss Barton as president. The New York branch opened a hospital for the training of Red Cross nurses. The course was planned to take two years and three months, after which the nurse graduated as a Red Cross sister. This organization adhered to the Geneva Convention, and while on service the nurses devoted their full time to their work; they received no salary but were given the best maintenance obtainable. Gradually the Red Cross School of Nursing failed, because in the meantime the general education of nurses was advancing so fast that the purpose of the school was better fulfilled by some of the new modern training schools, which developed in connection with the larger hospitals.

Toward the end of the century, trouble was brewing in the Caribbean, and the war with Spain was approaching. The Red Cross was enlisting nurses for war service, and in March, 1898, the Cuban Relief Committee chartered the *S.S. State of Texas* as a Red Cross relief ship to sail under the Red Cross flag. Miss Barton was to meet the ship in Florida, but in the meantime war was declared, and the *Texas* sailed with an American convoy to be of aid to American soldiers.

Up until now the American Red Cross had had no official standing, but its work became increasingly important. A special committee was set up to supply nurses, and in New York Mr. William Wardwell organized the American National Red Cross Relief Committee. Now the Red Cross obtained Government sanction as the proper and sole representative of the International Committee in the United States. Its position was thus official.

The Red Cross nurses went to the war in Cuba under the direction of Miss Barton and nursed under her in American hospitals. However, the amount of nursing work increased beyond all expectations, and it became necessary to send for reinforcements. Before these could arrive, the entire staff, including Dr. Lesser, the staff surgeon, came down with yellow fever and, to make matters worse, the hoped-for reinforcements failed to arrive. At the same time the Army organized its own regular nursing service; Dr. Anita Newcomb McGee was placed in charge directly under the Surgeon General.

Following World War I the Red Cross nurses were called upon in much reorganization work and in the fight against the epidemics and the pandemic of influenza which swept the war-torn world. The enlarged scope of the Red Cross was then generally appreciated; it participated in disaster relief and also in public health projects in areas in which local resources proved to be insufficient. This was accomplished particularly through the Delano Red Cross Nursing Service, established by the will of Miss Jane A. Delano, and has provided nursing service for several undeveloped and inaccessible regions.

However, disaster relief remains one of the chief peacetime tasks of the Red Cross Nursing Service, and since World War I there has not been a disaster of any magnitude in which that organization has not taken an important part in the rescue work.

Other activities of the Red Cross were developed about this time. Although instruction in home hygiene and care of the sick had been conducted by the Red Cross branch in the District of Columbia as early as 1908, these programs were not promoted nationally until 1913. The first edition of the Red Cross textbook on home hygiene and care of the sick was also published in 1913.

Public health nursing was first proposed

as a Red Cross program by Lillian D. Wald as early as 1908. It was financed mainly by Jacob H. Schiff, an officer of the New York branch. It was first confined to rural nursing but by 1913 extended to towns having populations as large as 25,000. This activity of the Red Cross was known as Town and Country Nursing Service. In 1915 the first plan for training nurses' aides was proposed. Although it was put into operation that year, it did not really develop fully until World War I. Miss Delano was, in 1917, appointed head of the New Department of Nursing. All phases of nursing service were included in this department: home hygiene and care of the sick, dietetics, public health nursing in rural areas and small towns, disaster nursing, and instruction of nurses' aides.

Miss Delano was succeeded by Clara D. Noyes, who had been her assistant since 1916. Miss Nowes was known internationally as well as nationally. She was twice elected first vice-president of the International Council of Nurses.

The basic international policies under which the Red Cross was first organized have permeated the national programs in all countries recognizing the Red Cross. The American Red Cross Nursing Services assist in various nursing activities all over the world. It cooperates with the director of the Nursing Bureau of the League of Red Cross Societies. It shares knowledge and resources with Red Cross Societies of other countries, including provision for visitors to study in this country.

The American Red Cross method of teaching instructors has been adapted to the needs of many countries and is being used in more than twenty Red Cross Societies. The opportunities for nursing service and nursing education under the banner of the Red Cross are a challenge to all nurses interested in working toward *One World for Nursing*.

The Red Cross Nursing Service no longer assumes responsibility for recruiting nurses for the Army or Navy. Legislation in 1947 establishing a permanent nurse corps for the Armed Forces, including the maintenance of nurse reserves, did away with the need for the Red Cross to maintain a roster of reserve nurses. Since then, local Red Cross chapters have enrolled nurses for community services, including local and national disasters.

Since 1945 Red Cross home nursing instruction has become part of the curriculum in many secondary schools. At first instructors for these courses were nurses, but since 1948 the Red Cross has authorized for this task not only nurses but also teachers and others with teacher-training experience, who complete the instructor's course given by the Red Cross. In 1947 the new blood program was established by the Red Cross, and in 1948 an intensive training program was begun for volunteer registered nurses. By 1956 more than 60,000 registered nurses had been trained in some phase of blood collection activity.

The various services that have developed within the Red Cross since World War II are provided to communities through approximately 3,700 Red Cross Chapters throughout the nation. Each of these local chapters is an administrative unit of the Red Cross, operating within the limits of a charter granted by the national organization. A volunteer board of directors and volunteer committees direct the work of the chapter. One of the important committees in every community is the Nursing Services Committee. This committee is responsible for planning and carrying through the nursing programs within the Red Cross, in accordance with community needs and demands. The nursing programs within the Red Cross are planned in close cooperation with recognized health groups, such as the National League for Nursing, the American Nurses' Association, the Children's Bureau, and the United States Public Health Service.

Contemporary programs of the Red Cross Nursing Service are planned to meet the present-day needs of American communities and include disaster nursing, home nursing, including mother and baby care, the instruction of volunteer nurses' aides, enrollment of graduate nurses in local chapters in community service, the blood program nursing, and educational and technical assistance to nurses in Red Cross societies in other countries. Some very fine educational materials in the form of bulletins describing the work of the Red Cross nurse, to be used in the recruiting of graduate nurses for these activities, have been prepared.

Chapter 13

Early schools and leaders

During the nineteenth century a greater sense of social responsibility for community health and welfare developed. Medical science was advancing more rapidly than ever before in the history of medicine. Traditional concepts of the woman's place in society and of her educational needs were changing. It was time for the development of a formal education for nursing. Close association between Florence Nightingale and early leaders in America resulted in many similarities between the early schools in the United States and those in England.

PRINCIPLES OF THE EARLY SCHOOLS OF NURSING

Finally, in 1873, three important schools appeared, almost simultaneously. All of them were destined to influence the development of modern nursing. These schools were organized more or less in accordance with Miss Nightingale's ideas. Some of these ideas later tended to be forgotten. The main principle was that the school must be considered primarily an educational institution, not a source of cheap labor. The earliest schools of nursing in America were created independently of hospitals by boards or committees with power and freedom to develop the school. However, mainly because of lack of endowment the schools were early absorbed into the hospitals with which they were connected. Therefore, the history of

nursing in America is inextricably bound up with the growth and development of hospitals, and most of the schools were created and conducted by hospitals to serve their needs, while the education of the nurse became a by-product of her service to the hospital.

As schools of nursing developed rapidly during the years that followed, many hospitals, especially the smaller ones, discovered that a school of nursing under the guise of "practical experience" could be made a valuable source of free, or almost free, labor. Consequently formal instruction was often neglected, and it was not until the modern reform movements became effective that this principle again became firmly established. Now it is increasingly realized that Miss Nightingale was right when she said that the education of nurses, like that of doctors, is a public duty and emphasized that a school of nursing must be endowed or supported by public funds—it cannot be self-supporting and remain a good school.

The second principle was that the school of nursing must be administratively independent although closely connected with the hospital. The head of the school, whether she is called "matron" as in England or "director" as in America, should be a nurse, responsible only to the hospital or school of nursing board. This point has been highly disputed. Another school of thought would

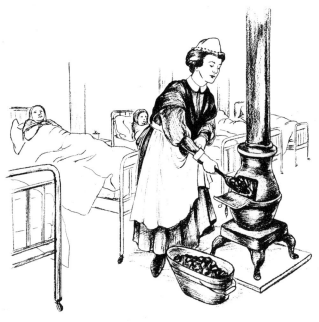

Until recently custodial jobs such as stoking the stove were part of the hospital nurse's regular duties.

have the director of nursing responsible to the hospital superintendent for the nursing care and—under a separate budget—the instruction of nurses. Only through an independent connection with the hospital can the education of nurses be ensured, free of interference by interests that may disrupt orderly planning of the course.

It was generally thought advisable that student nurses live in a nurses' home. Hours of work were often irregular and discipline of necessity was strict. This arrangement was, however, not always considered necessary during preclinical courses or postgraduate work.

The importance of the head nurse, or the "sister" as she is called in England, was also an integral part of Miss Nightingale's scheme. She is a professional nurse responsible for the administration of a ward or a division and for the teaching of the student nurses that come under her care. Much of the clinical instruction is thus her responsibility.

The young schools that came into existence could not fill all of these requirements—in fact many modern schools are still striving to solve these problems—but they were ideals at which they could aim, and during the next few years notable progress was made.

BELLEVUE HOSPITAL SCHOOL OF NURSING

When American women interested in the Sanitary Commission no longer had to worry about the war, they turned their interests to domestic eleemosynary institutions. They formed the New York State Charities Aid Association under which the Bellevue Hospital Visiting Committee operated, directed by Louisa Lee Schuyler. Reference has been made to the shocking revelations of that committee, and it was realized that improvement of the nursing was one of the essential requirements for hospital reform. In all this the committee met the resistance of most of those in authority, but that did not stop it. It publicly appealed for funds; Dr. Gill Wylie, who had been an intern in the hospital and who was sympathetic to the reform movement, was sent abroad to learn what he could directly from Miss Nightingale and from the schools that she had helped to organize. Consequently, the plan for organization of the school of nursing at Bellevue followed closely Miss Nightingale's principles; in America the system became known as the "Bellevue System."

There was some difficulty in finding someone to take charge of the new school. Public announcements were made, in response to which Sister Helen of the Order of the Holy Cross offered her services. She was accepted, and the school was established May 1, 1873.

Sister Helen (Miss Bowden), a member of the Sisterhood of All Saints, had been trained at the University College Hospital in London, when nursing there was in the hands of the Order of the Holy Cross. Later she had had extensive experience in workhouse infirmaries, in epidemics, and during the war between France and Germany in 1870-1871. At the time of her application she was in residence at the Community House in Baltimore. Therefore, she brought to Bellevue Hospital a thorough training, and although she was not a Nightingale nurse, she was fully conversant with the principles of that school. She carried out these principles successfully until the school was well established in 1876, when she went to South Africa to take part in pioneer nursing there. She was a strict, austere woman with profound knowledge of human nature and of politicians, for whom she was always fully a match.

Under her direction, the pupil nurses were housed in a building rented for the purpose. Although many of the old nurses applied for acceptance, they were refused; an attempt was made to recruit the classes with young girls from above the servant class, in order to make nursing attractive as a career. Their training was planned but included no regular classwork or lectures. In the begin-

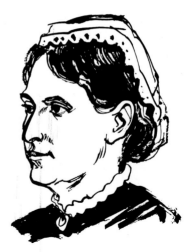

Linda Richards

ning only a few wards were placed at the disposal of the new school for instructional purposes. This proved to be so successful that more were soon added. Although the school did publish a *Manual of Nursing* in 1876, the formal instruction left much to be desired.

In 1874 Miss Linda Richards, America's first "trained nurse," came from Boston to become night superintendent. She instituted the system of keeping written records and orders, which has since become a requirement in all nursing schools. After a while, uniforms were introduced; the nurses were reluctant to wear them until someone had the idea of encouraging one of the pupil nurses from a very good family to wear one. Then a general clamor for uniforms arose. It was readily gratified.

Thus, the school, founded through the efforts of Louisa Lee Schuyler, flourished and became a leading school of nursing. It has had many brilliant alumnae, notably Jane A. Delano, Isabel Hampton, and Lavinia L. Dock. In 1967 it became part of Hunter College of the City University of New York.

EARLY BOSTON SCHOOLS OF NURSING

The New England Hospital for Women and Children attempted to form a school in

1861, but was not successful until it was re-formed in 1872. Dr. Marie Zakrzewska, who studied in Berlin but took her medical degree in Cleveland, Ohio, urged that the New England Hospital be given a school of nursing. A charter for a training school for nurses was included in the hospital charter of 1863. She personally took active part in the training of nurses, but it remained on a rather informal basis until the hospital was rebuilt in 1872 and placed under the charge of Dr. Susan Dimock who, like most good American doctors of the time, had been trained in Europe. She had been to Kaiserswerth, and when the reorganized school opened in 1872, it largely followed that pattern. The course lasted one year and included both practical instruction and lectures. The school achieved its greatest fame because one of its alumnae became one of the leaders of nursing throughout the following generation.

Miss Linda Richards began her nursing career in the Boston City Hospital. Eager for training and advancement she entered in the first class of the New England Hospital and graduated one year later. Following graduation she worked for a while as night superintendent at the Bellevue Hospital, she later returned to Boston and took over the school at the Massachusetts General Hospital. When this school was well organized, she resigned to study English methods. During this period she became personally acquainted with Miss Nightingale. On her return she began a remarkable career reorganizing the nursing services of hospitals throughout the country; in 1885 she was called to Japan where she organized and for five years led the first Japanese School of Nursing at Kyoto. Back in the United States she took up the organization of mental hospitals and spent the remainder of her long and remarkable career moving from one mental hospital to another, improving their nursing services. She has left a record of her experiences in her *Reminiscences,* published by Whitcomb and Barrows.

The nursing instruction at the New Eng-land Hospital as described by Miss Richards was largely practical, hours were long, and time off was limited to an afternoon every two weeks. There were no night nurses. Very sick patients could interfere seriously with the nurses' sleep, for their rooms were between wards. In this early school there was little formal teaching and there were no textbooks. Some bedside instruction was provided by women interns.

As we note from the general tenor of such descriptions, which practically applied to other Boston hospitals as well, they were a far cry from the medieval conditions at Bellevue and many other places. Nursing was to a certain extent systematized, and a measure of cleanliness and acceptable care was extended to the patients. There was still plenty of room for reform.

Perhaps even better conditions obtained at the Massachusetts General Hospital. In fact, according to those times a nursing reform was not urgently needed, both governors and medical staff prided themselves on the care that their patients received. Nevertheless, the spirit of nursing reform, which the Civil War had engendered, extended to Boston where the Women's Educational Union appointed a committee to look into the opportunities that nursing could offer women as a career. We note here the appearance of professional aspiration, for on the committee were ladies of the best families of Boston. They were looking not for hospital reforms but for opportunities for career women. Purely on the strength of the social and intellectual standing of the women on this committee the hospital trustees and doctors accepted the experimental establishment of a school of nursing in the Massachusetts General Hospital. It was opened on November 1, 1873; six pupil nurses enrolled.

The equipment was elementary, but there was an organized attempt at formal instruction closely supervised by the members of the committee, and certain innovations were actually tried. It is to this school that we may trace the first "preliminary course" in America. In spite of all this the young school had difficulties getting started. The early superintendents seemed to lack vision and were unable to break with the old ways. Long hours and menial duties interfered with the efficiency of the students. It was necessary to establish the proper leadership. Miss Richards, then in New York, was selected. She accepted, and within a year conditions were much improved; classes were organized, and the proper emphasis was placed upon the training that was the purpose of the whole undertaking. The more menial tasks were gradually relegated to attendants, and the doctors began to recognize the advantage of having properly trained nurses. After a year's trial under Miss Richards' guidance the school was accepted by the hospital, and it has ever since maintained the highest standards and traditions. This feat was all the more remarkable when we compare Miss Richards' professional training with minimum requirements today. After some preliminary work at Boston City Hospital, she had received such formal training as was possible in the first class of the New England Hospital; her "postgraduate" experience was limited to what she had been able to learn as night superintendent at the newly reorganized Bellevue. She herself realized that she still had much to learn, and after two and one-half years she resigned to visit England and Miss Nightingale and to study the work that was being done overseas.

CONNECTICUT SCHOOL

Among the three early schools of nursing, the Connecticut School was the first to receive its charter but for some time it admitted no pupils. In 1872 the New Haven Hospital appointed a committee to investigate the feasibility of organizing a training school for nurses. In their study they heavily relied upon the report of Dr. Wylie, which had just become available. They were remarkably farseeing in adopting one of Miss Nightingale's principal ideas: they did not want the hospital to start a school, but they wanted a school organized independently of the hospital, which then would serve as a field for the practical training. By such an arrangement they made it difficult for the hospital to use the nurses as cheap labor. After extensive advertising for potential students they finally were able to open on October 1, 1873.

It was an immediate success; the number of pupils rapidly increased, and soon the school was a source of superintendents for other hospitals. In 1879 it published the *New Haven Manual of Nursing,* a textbook created by the committee, which consisted of both nurses and doctors; it was a comprehensive text and soon found wide acceptance among the nursing schools, which by then were being organized all through the country. The New Haven school has retained its leading position. Later, when it became endowed and obtained university affiliation, it made another important contribution to nursing.

All of the more important schools have their history, but because of limited space a detailed description cannot be included here.

EDUCATION IN THE EARLY SCHOOLS TO ABOUT 1900

The period that followed was one of quiet progress in nursing education. To it we trace the early development of many movements that later were to become important, including the Red Cross, Army nursing, and some of the functions of public health nursing, but these will be considered in later chapters.

There was also a steady growth of nursing schools. The growth was closely associated with development of modern surgery and medicine, which as we have seen occurred very rapidly as the result of Pasteur's and Lister's work and the advances in bacteriological knowledge. As it was realized that so much new work could be done if hospital facilities were available, hospitals grew rapidly in number and size all over the country. Now they changed their function from being refuges of the destitute to becoming

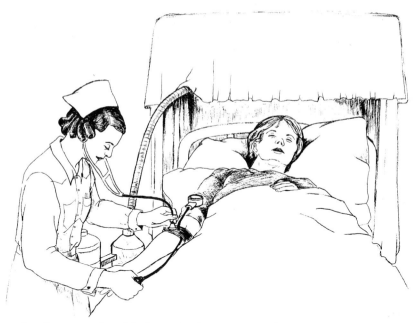

Prior to the discovery of antibiotics and other modern miracle drugs, a large number of patients had to be cared for in croup tents.

the natural work grounds for surgeons and physicians whenever patients demanded more than the most general care. Facilities had to be created and organized to provide for all classes of the population, and part of the original function of the hospital was taken on by the infirmary. With such increase in both the quality and quantity of hospital work the demands for trained nursing care grew accordingly. Nursing developed very largely as an inevitable consequence of these circumstances. It was fortunate that within its membership the necessary leaders existed to carry it through this formative period.

The improvement in educational standards occurred in several areas. Originally one year had been considered sufficient for the training of a nurse; that was Miss Nightingale's idea, and it was the accepted period of training in the early schools. It was probably sufficient for the needs of the times. We must realize that most of the items of a modern nurse's education are necessitated by contributions to medical knowledge and to

public health, which have received practical application since the first schools were opened. So, as more knowledge and more skill became necessary, the course had to be extended, At first it was done by adding a few months for special work. Soon, however, it became necessary to reorganize the courses completely, and courses were planned for two and eventually for three years. The full three-year course was, however, not generally accepted until well into the present century.

The problem was not merely one of lengthening the course; it was also one of the student nurse's understanding. It is not enough that the nurse be told that she must not touch the instruments on the operating table, she must understand why she must not touch them; she must understand why it is dangerous, and not just unpleasant, to have a diphtheria patient or a tuberculous patient cough into her face. She can administer a dietary or drug treatment far better if she knows something about the physiology and pathology of the diseased organs and about the action of the drugs. The nurse's place in the whole structure of the care of the sick is occupied much better if she understands rather than if she slavishly follows directions. To the modern reader this sounds like a statement of the obvious, and yet it was not at all accepted outside of nursing circles. Actually, seventy years ago medications in some hospitals were dispensed by number in order that their contents remain secret to all but the initiated—which did not include the nurses.

As nursing has evolved, there has been a constant struggle against the attitude that modern nurses are being "overtrained." It was argued that by knowing too much the nurses became unfit for the essential nursing task or that we were wasting our time educating a group of "semi-professionals." This attitude among members of the medical profession and among others upon whom the nurses must rely for advancing their standing has been the chief obstacle against which they have had to fight. However, it rather strengthened than weakened their fight, because it made it necessary for every advance to possess the vitality of inherent value to survive. Since 1872 the education of nurses has advanced in spite of this opposition. It still has to show that a nurse is inefficient as a result of education and an understanding of what she is doing. Inadequate nurses are generally so because they are not suited to nursing, not because they are overeducated. Some are inadequate because they have not had a good basic course in nursing.

Thus, we see an increasing demand that promised lectures actually be delivered, that lecture courses be split up and lengthened, and that new subjects be added to the curriculum. In the beginning pupil nurses attended lectures for medical students; later, lectures were prepared especially for them. Better and better choice was made of instructors. Not all nursing lectures were best given by doctors. Specially prepared instructors, themselves nurses, were perferable for many subjects. It was found essential to add courses that were not strictly technical but which dealt with ethical and professional problems and attitudes. In some respects the preparation of nurses has a broader base in the social and behavioral sciences than is required of medical students. The period with which we are dealing was very much concerned with the germination and growth of these trains of thought.

Because of these advances it became necessary to provide the proper equipment. The early pupil nurses often slept in rooms between the wards, where they were readily available for nocturnal emergencies; some were housed in special buildings. The facilities for instruction were meager, and the requirements for equipment were simple: a few mannequins and models of limbs, upon which to learn how to apply bandages, a skeleton, a blackboard, and a few books. As standards rose, demands rose with them, and gradually beds, ward equipment, laboratories, and up-to-date libraries became essential if schools were to meet even minimum standards.

EARLY LEADERS

The early leaders were consistent in their wish to improve the educational program in these schools because of their feeling that the professional nurse could not fulfill her responsibilities to the patient and the community until she was really prepared to do so. Two names stand out in connection with almost every development of professional nursing. One woman was the product of the nineteenth century but was farsighted enough to envision the possibilities and tireless enough to try to improve educational facilities. The name of Isabel Hampton Robb is linked with almost every type of nursing organization, every plan, and every activity at the turn of the century. One of her outstanding students at the Johns Hopkins Hospital was Mary Adelaide Nutting. Miss Nutting complemented Mrs. Robb in many ways and lived long enough to carry out many of the plans and programs that had been the dreams of her teacher. Also important were Lillian Wald, Mary Eliza Mahoney, Mary Sewell Gardner, Annie W. Goodrich, and Isabel Maitland Stewart.

There were other leaders in nursing too numerous to mention. In fact, every school had its leaders during the period of organization, growth, and change which every good school experiences in meeting the changing needs of the nursing profession.

Isabel Adams Hampton (1860-1910)

Miss Isabel Adams Hampton was born in Canada in 1860 and began her career as a schoolteacher. This, however, did not satisfy her, and she applied for nurse's training at Bellevue, from which she was graduated in 1883. In 1886, following two years in Italy, she became superintendent of nurses at the five-year-old Illinois Training School for Nurses. During her three years of office in Chicago she introduced two important reforms. She began a graduated course of clinical experience and classwork, so that nurses advanced step by step, and she arranged for affiliation of her students with other hospitals that possessed advantages, especially in private nursing, not obtainable at Cook County Hospital. When the school of nursing at Johns Hopkins opened in 1889, she was

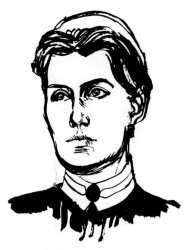

Isabel Hampton Robb

made its "principal" (a term then used for the first time in this connection). Her chief contributions here were in better organization of the work so that the pupil nurse's day could be limited to twelve hours, including two hours off for recreation. Both the hospital and Miss Hampton earned the highest reputation. She was made chairman of the nursing section of the Congress of Hospitals and Dispensaries which was held at Chicago in 1893. She read a paper on nursing at the meeting. When, at the subsequent meeting, the Society of Superintendents was formed, she was one of the leading organizers, and became the first president. The next year she married Dr. Hunter Robb and resigned from active administrative work. Her interest in nursing continued as is evidenced by the two texts that she wrote at this time (*Nursing, Its Principles and Practice for Hospital and Private Use* and *Nursing Ethics*) and by her further organizational activities.

In 1896 she became the first president of the newly formed Nurses Associated Alumnae of the United States and Canada; as such she was active in the scheme of offering the services of that association in the Spanish-American War. Her next important activity was the part she played in the work for establishing university affiliation for nursing education and postgraduate courses. At first courses were offered in Hospital Economics in the Department of Science. Officially, the Department of Nursing and Health began some eleven years later in 1910 at Teachers College, Columbia University. After the turn of the century she again came into prominence as one of the founders and original stockholders of *The American Journal of Nursing.* Her authority and prestige did much to bring the young journal through its first difficult years. When she died in 1910 in a street accident, at the relatively early age of 50, she had in a short career of less than thirty years in nursing done more for American nursing than any other person. It will be noted from studying the subsequent pages that there was no important nursing enterprise during the years when she was active in which she did not take a leading part.

Mary Adelaide Nutting (1858-1947)

When Mrs. Hampton Robb resigned from her post at the Johns Hopkins Hospital, her place was taken by Miss Adelaide Nutting, a graduate of the first class of the school. A warm friendship developed between Miss Nutting, a Canadian by birth, and her teacher Isabel Hampton (later Mrs. Robb). As Superintendent of Nurses and Principal of the School of Nursing at the Johns Hopkins Hospital she carried out many of the reforms initiated by her predecessor. Early in the year of 1896 she established the three-year course and the eight-hour day for student nurses and abolished the monthly allowance to students. In 1901 she initiated a six months' preparatory course, which served as a model for many other schools. A lasting memorial to Miss Nutting is her unique collection of works on the history of nursing. From this interest emerged the four-volume *History of Nursing* written in collaboration with Miss Lavinia Dock.

Miss Nutting was convinced early that progress in nursing education would be slow until two reforms could be brought about:

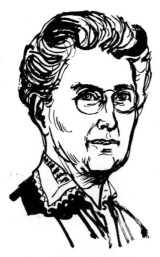

M. Adelaide Nutting

the provision for endowments or other financial support for schools of nursing and the separation of schools of nursing from hospital ownership and control.

Perhaps she is best known for her work in the creation and development of the Department of Nursing and Health at Teachers College, Columbia University. When she resigned her position at Johns Hopkins in 1907 to take the new Chair at Columbia University, she became the first Professor of Nursing in the world. She held that professorship until her resignation in 1925 when she was succeeded by a former student and colleague, Miss Isabel Stewart.

Miss Nutting's interest in all aspects of nursing education and her vital personality have made a deep impression on nursing throughout the world. She took a prominent part in nursing organizations and through her interest in international developments was influential in the formation of the International Council of Nurses.

Lillian Wald (1867-1940)

Lillian D. Wald was graduated from the New York Hospital School of Nursing in 1891. She became interested in the need for nursing among the poor, and in 1893 Miss Wald and a friend, Mary Brewster, rented a tenement in Henry Street, New York. This tenement developed into the famed Henry Street Settlement. These two women soon recognized what many leaders had seen: the need for nursing was just one of the many needs of these people, and so the social aspects of nursing began to develop, and modern nursing in the community began. Miss Wald was one the lecturers at the new Department of Nursing Education at Columbia University and was a leader in most of the activities of public health nursing during her lifetime.

Her activities at Henry Street Settlement are those for which she is most famous, and the story is dramatically told in her two books, *The House on Henry Street* and *Windows on Henry Street*. When the National

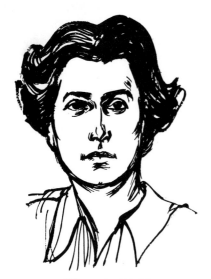

Lillian D. Wald

Organization for Public Health Nursing was organized in 1912, Miss Wald was elected its first president. She was interested in legislative reforms. The result of her interest and suggestions were the organization of the Children's Bureau, the development of the Nursing Service Division of the Metropolitan Life Insurance Company, and the organization of the Town and Country Nursing Service of the American Red Cross.

Mary Eliza Mahoney (1845-1926)

The first professional Negro nurse in the United States entered the New England Hospital for Women and Children in 1878 and completed the course of sixteen months in 1879. Miss Mahoney had a good record at the school and after graduation did private nursing mainly in Boston and its suburbs. Miss Mahoney gave the address of welcome at the first conference of the National Association of Colored Graduate Nurses in 1909. She died in the New England Hospital in January, 1926, 81 years of age. After her death, the Mary Mahoney medal was established by the National Association of Colored Graduate Nurses and was first presented in 1936 to a member of the organization making an outstanding contribution to

nursing. Throughout her more than forty years of professional activity, Miss Mahoney gave devoted service to her patients and the nursing profession and did much to further intergroup relationships so that the Negro nurse could become a vital part of the community.

Mary Sewell Gardner (1871-1961)

Probably one of the most outstanding nurses in the history of public health nursing is Mary Sewell Gardner. She was born in 1871 in Massachusetts and was graduated cum laude in 1905 from the Newport Hospital Training School for Nurses. Soon after her graduation, she became the director of the Provident District Nursing Association, Rhode Island, a post she held until her retirement in 1931.

She is probably best known for her influence on the development of the National Organization for Public Health Nursing. She was one of the nursing leaders who helped to initiate the National Organization for Public Health Nursing in Chicago in 1912. Miss Lillian Wald was the first president, and Miss Gardner was the first secretary. In 1931 she was made honorary president of the organization, which she had done so much to develop.

Miss Gardner was instrumental in the transactions that resulted in the taking over of the *Cleveland Visiting Nurses' Quarterly* when it was offered to the National Organization for Public Health Nursing as an official journal, and as the *Public Health Nurse* it became the monthly magazine of this new public health organization.

Miss Gardner was also responsible for helping to develop public health nursing services in the American Red Cross. In 1912 she was given leave of absence from the Provident District Nursing Association for a year and became temporary director of the Town and Country Nursing Service, the Public Health Nursing Service in the Red Cross. After World War I she visited many European countries as special adviser to the nursing service work being done by the American Red Cross.

Miss Gardner is well known for many articles published in the *Public Health Nurse, The American Journal of Nursing,* and many other magazines. However, in nursing literature she is best known for her book which has become a classic, *Public Health Nursing,* first published in 1916. A second revision of this book was published in 1924 and was translated into French, Chinese, Spanish, and Japanese. A third and last edition of this book was published in 1936. For the lay readers she wrote *So Live We* in 1942, and in 1946 *Catherine Kent* was published, which contained many autobiographical experiences.

Annie W. Goodrich (1876-1955)

Annie Warburton Goodrich was graduated from the New York Hospital Training School for Nurses in 1892. She was one of the pioneer leaders who actively helped nursing develop from an apprenticeship to a profession. She was an outstanding and inspired nurse educator. Her first important position was as superintendent of nurses at the New York Post-Graduate Hospital, a position she held for seven years. Then she was superintendent of nurses at St. Luke's Hospital in New York and then superintendent of nurses at the New York Hospital. She left the New York Hospital in 1907 to become superintendent of Bellevue and Allied Training Schools for Nurses. In 1910 she resigned to become state inspector of nurse training schools in New York. In 1914 she went to Teachers College as assistant professor.

All during these years she had worked with other leaders in nursing organizations, both national and international, to develop the nursing profession. She was president of the International Council of Nurses from 1912 to 1915. She had always been interested in public health and in 1916 became director of the Visiting Nurse Service of the Henry Street Settlement. During these years of great developments in nursing, Miss Nutting, Miss Wald, and Miss Goodrich were often referred to as "The Great Trio." All three were associated with every great idea and movement of the young profession.

In 1918 she was given leave of absence from Henry Street to make a survey of the Military Hospitals with the Nursing Department of the United States Army. When the Army School of Nursing was organized in 1918, she was appointed Dean. At the same time she was instrumental in developing the Vassar Training Camp Program.

After the war she returned to Henry Street and continued her activities in nursing education. She was particularly interested in the Goldmark Study, "Nursing and Nursing Education in the United States." In 1923 she was appointed Dean of the new school of nursing at Yale University, endowed by the Rockefeller Foundation, a position that she held until 1934. Miss Goodrich received many honors and was one of the outstanding nurse educators of this century.

Isabel Maitland Stewart (1878-1963)

The influence of Miss Stewart as an educator, writer, organization worker, and important figure in international nursing affairs for over forty years is just now being recognized. She took her basic training at the Winnipeg General Hospital Training School and, being atracted by an article written by Miss Nutting in *The American Journal of Nursing,* entered the course in hospital economics at Teachers College, Columbia University, in 1908. She was the first nurse to receive a master's degree from Columbia University. She remained at Teachers College for the rest of her professional career, holding the position of assistant instructor, assistant professor, and finally in 1925 succeeding Miss Nutting as the Henry Hartley Foundation Professor of Nursing. She was keenly aware of new concepts in the field of general education and always tried to evaluate new developments in relation to the specialized field of nursing. She was very active on the Education Committee of the National League of

Nursing Education. While she was chairman, the Curriculum Committee first published the original guide to curriculum upgrading in 1917, with revisions published in 1927 and 1937 under her guidance.

She served as chairman of the Vassar Training Camp Program during World War I and wrote a pamphlet for general circulation on this and on other wartime activities. In July, 1940, when the National Nursing Council for National Defense was organized, mainly as the result of Miss Stewart's suggestions, one of the important committees appointed was that on Educational Policies and Resources with Miss Stewart as chairman. She was interested in international affairs and was very active on the Committee on Education of the International Council of Nurses. She prepared a pamphlet called *The Educational Program of the School of Nurs-* *ing,* which was translated into English, Spanish, German, and French by the Nursing Bureau of the League of Red Cross Societies. In 1950 she finished a study of postgraduate education in nursing for the International Council. As author and editor she is well known to nurses all over the world for her books *Education of Nurses* and *A Short History of Nursing,* which she coauthored with Lavinia Dock.

In 1916 she became the first editor of the Department of Nursing Education of *The American Journal of Nursing.* She participated in the founding of the Association of Collegiate Schools of Nursing and in the early developments of the National League of Nursing Education, the International Council of Nurses, and the Florence Nightingale International Foundation.

Questions and study projects for unit three

1. How did the investigations of the New York State Charities Aid Association during the nineteenth century affect the development of nursing?
2. What were the principles upon which the early American schools of nursing were founded?
3. What was the origin of the Red Cross?
4. What are the functions of the Red Cross?
   (a) In times of war?
   (b) In times of peace?
5. Discuss the activities of the Sanitary Commission during the Civil War and compare them with the activities of the American Red Cross during World War I.
6. Discuss the first schools of nursing established in this country following the Nightingale System. What was the effect of the Nightingale System on nursing education and nursing service?
7. Discuss revolutionary changes in medicine of this period and show how these changes and their combination with the development of social conscience in matters of health set the stage, so to speak, for the emergence of nursing at this time.
8. Be prepared to describe the life history of six nursing leaders of this period. Tell why you selected these individuals as the six outstanding nursing leaders and show how their backgrounds and training helped them to take their place in the nursing service.
9. Make an annotated bibliography of recent articles appearing in *The American Journal of Nursing, Nursing Outlook, Nursing Research,* and any other journals available in your library relating to the discussion in this unit.

References for unit three

A century of nursing. Reprints of four historic documents, including Miss Nightingale's letter of Sept. 18, 1872, to the Bellevue School; Foreword by Isabel M. Stewart and Agnes Gelinas, for the National League of Nursing Education, New York, 1950, G. P. Putnam's Sons.

American National Red Cross: The American Red Cross: a brief story, Washington, D. C., 1951, American National Red Cross.

Baker, Nina Brown: Cyclone in Calico, the story of Mary Ann Bickerdyke, Boston, 1952, Little, Brown & Co.

Baker, Rachael: The first woman doctor (Elizabeth Blackwell), New York, 1944, Julian Messner, Inc.

Barton, William E.: The life of Clara Barton—founder of the American Red Cross (two vols.), Boston, 1922, Houghton Mifflin Co.

Blackwell, Elizabeth: Pioneer work for women, New York, 1914, E. P. Dutton and Co., Inc.

Blanchfield, Florence A., and Standlee, Mary W.: Organized nursing and the Army in three wars. Unpublished manuscript on file, Historical Division, Office of the Surgeon General of the Army, Washington, D. C.

Brockett, L. P., and Vaughan, Mary C.: Women's work in the Civil War: a record of heroism, patriotism and patience, Rochester, New York, 1867, R. H. Curran.

DeBarberey, Helen: Elizabeth Seton, New York, 1931, The Macmillan Co.

Dock, Lavinia L., and others: History of American Red Cross Nursing, New York, 1922, The Macmillan Co.

Dubos, Rene J.: Louis Pasteur: free lance of science, Boston, 1950, Little, Brown & Co.

Dulles, Foster R.: The American Red Cross: a history, New York, 1950, Harper & Brothers.

Epler, Percy H.: The life of Clara Barton, New York, 1919, The Macmillan Co.

Gladwin, Mary E.: The Red Cross and Jane Arminda Delano, Philadelphia, and London, 1931, W. B. Saunders Co.

Greenbie, Marjorie Barstow: Lincoln's daughters of mercy, New York, 1944, G. P. Putnam's Sons.

Gumpert, Martin: The Story of the Red Cross, New York, 1938, Oxford Press.

Kernodle, Portia B.: The Red Cross Nurse in action, 1882-1948, New York, 1949, Harper & Brothers.

Livermore, Mary A.: My story of the war, a woman's narrative of four years' experience as a nurse in the Union Army, Hartford, Conn., 1888, A. D. Worthington Co.

Marshall, Helen E.: Dorothea Dix, Chapel Hill, 1937, University of North Carolina Press.

Pickett, Sarah Elizabeth: The American National Red Cross, New York, 1924, Century Co.

Stimson, Julia C.: Earliest known connection of nurses with Army hospitals in the United States, American Journal of Nursing **25**:15, 1925.

Stimson, Julia C.: Medical Department of the United States Army in the World War, vol. 13, part II. The Army Nurse Corps, Washington, D. C., 1927, United States Government Printing Office.

Stimson, Julia C., and associates: History and manual of the Army Nurse Corps, Medical Field Service School, Carlisle Barracks, Pa., 1937.

Stimson, Julia C., and Thompson, Ethel C. S.: Women nurses with the Union Forces in the Civil War, Military Surgeon, January, February, 1928.

The American National Red Cross: Jane A. Delano: a biography, ARC 781, Washington, D. C., 1952.

Tiffany, Francis: Life of Dorothea Lynde Dix, Boston, 1890, Houghton Mifflin Co.

Williams, Blanche Colton: Clara Barton, daughter of destiny, Philadelphia, 1941, J. B. Lippincott Co.

Expansion of nursing

With better hospitals, better medical practice, better education of doctors, nurses, and all health workers, and more effective health teaching throughout the community, the welfare of the group has emerged as a definite concept. Modern medicine is interested in protecting every individual from the hazards of life, particularly disease, by scientific knowledge. In order to do this the health of the individual becomes the concern of many groups in the society. Thus, we have the development of sanitary legislation, city and state public health societies, and the organization and support of many private health organizations, particularly in the fields of tuberculosis, cancer, heart disease, and mental illness. In some countries medicine is being socialized. In other countries, such as the United States, public and private enterprises are working together to control disease and to provide the best care possible for every individual.

Organizational developments and specialization were evident in the professionalization of nursing. Nursing education has become established in universities, and the profession has become vocal through its publications.

Chapter 14

Organizational developments

The period up to 1900 is, in nursing, characterized by the rapid increase in the number of schools, by improvement and extension of the courses, by better equipment, by the early beginnings of libraries and textbooks, and finally, although perhaps it was not so obvious at the time, by the appearance in the nursing world of a group of women who were to bring about the next two great reforms. These reforms, the organization of nursing schools by the universities, and the organization of the nursing profession, culminated in the formation of the American Nurses' Association and the National League of Nursing Education, which definitely established the nursing profession.

Professional societies can be developed in two ways. Someone can decide that it would be well for the members of a certain group to be organized for the purpose of controlling conditions of training, of work, of compensation and of controlling new knowledge concerning the group. On the other hand, persons who have lived closely together during a period of training and education may wish to meet or at least keep in touch with each other when they scatter after graduation. This sentiment is the primary cause for the organization of alumni associations. Both of these purposes can be found in the organizations of the young nursing profession.

It is not possible for professionals to form organizations until certain basic concepts have been accepted by the members. It is not strange to learn that the earliest American nurses' association of which we have knowledge is the Philomena Society formed in New York in 1886. Only its name is known, for it died after a year, leaving no records. Professional nursing organizations did not develop until almost ten years later. Small local groups and alumnae associations began to be organized in the late eighties and early nineties. In a short time these joined together and formed the basis for a national association.

As one studies the purposes and activities of the two major professional nurses' associations, it is evident that from the beginning the members understood the real meaning of professional organization. The function of a professional organization in general is to protect the members and the public it serves. Specifically, this is done by formulating and imposing a code of ethics upon its members and assuring the public of the proficiency of its members by testing their ability before allowing them to practice. The evolvement of educational standards and the licensing of professional nurses developed early and are controlled by the profession. The professional organization is pledged to safeguard its members from unfair competition, to guarantee conditions of employment, and to ensure a fair remuneration. Study the program of the American Nurses' Association throughout the years.

ALUMNAE ASSOCIATIONS

As the nursing schools developed, the alumnae formed associations; the first were those of Bellevue (1889), Illinois Training School (1891), and Johns Hopkins (1892). It may be more than a coincidence that these were the very schools with which Miss Hampton had been connected, for, as we noted, she became their first president when they were consolidated into a national association. These associations must not be looked upon as being primarily social in purpose. In a few years these groups had joined together to become the Nurses' Associated Alumnae of the United States and Canada. The purpose was enlarged and became national in scope to embrace the general betterment of the profession. This occurred especially because the advancement of educational standards was being sponsored by the Superintendents' Society, which also was active in organizing the Associated Alumnae. As soon as the greater scope was considered, incorporation became necessary. For legal reasons Canadian nurses then had to organize a separate society, which, however, continued to cooperate cordially with the sister society south of the border. The aims and purposes of the two societies remained closely similar.

As the society developed as a national organization, it naturally became organized into city, county, and state societies, and it affiliated with similar groups in other countries into an International Association.

AMERICAN NURSES' ASSOCIATION

It became clear that as the Alumnae Association developed it no longer fitted its old name. It was no longer primarily an alumnae association, and besides the old name was rather clumsy. So in 1911 the Association made a new departure under the name the "American Nurses' Association." As such

it has continued to grow and is largely responsible for the reforms that developed during the following periods. In December, 1962, its membership was 168,912. When it was organized in 1897 the purposes of this Association were (1) to establish and to maintain a code of ethics, (2) to elevate the standards of nursing education, and (3) to promote the usefulness and honor, the financial and other interests of the nursing profession.* Throughout the years the association has continued its work. Its program has been altered and shaped by the continuous changes that have taken place in nursing as the profession has developed.

The American Nurses' Association has continued to help the individual nurse. Uniform licensing laws in the states have been developed in order to protect both the nurse and the public. Today professional nurses of every state have to be registered; the registration of practical nurses is also being developed.

The membership in the American Nurses' Association is open to all graduate nurses registered in the state, who join through their local district or who join directly with the State Nurses' Association if the state is not districted.

The platform of the American Nurses' Association, adopted at the biennial in Chicago in 1948, emphasized the expanding role of the American nurse in world affairs, increased participation of the nurse in national affairs, and provided for the rapid expansion in nursing service to meet the health needs of the American people.

NATIONAL LEAGUE OF NURSING EDUCATION

Another nurses' society was organized in order that nurses could work more efficiently. When, in 1893, Chicago decided to celebrate the March of Civilization toward the West with a World's Fair, a Women's Building was in the plans. One exhibit in this

---

*The A.N.A. and you, New York, 1941, American Nurses' Association, p. 2.

building was to be sponsored by British nurses under the direction of Mrs. Bedford-Fenwick. Knowing the difficulties that the British nurses had surmounted when organizing their society, Mrs. Fenwick suggested that a place be provided where American nurses could meet and get acquainted. She visited Miss Hampton, and as a result the superintendents of eighteen training schools for nurses met and formed a section under the chairmanship of Miss Hampton. As could be expected, the heterogeneous nature of nursing education was then revealed. Although most schools had been patterned from the Keiserswerth or Miss Nightingale's ideas, the whole program was still so young that the various courses could not be compared, so much had they been shaped by local circumstances. If a profession were to be created, certain standards had to be universally accepted, and new departures had to be watched and controlled.

For this purpose plans were made toward forming a permanent organization, and in January, 1894, the American Society of Superintendents of Training Schools came into being. In the beginning, membership was limited to the heads of the larger schools, but it gradually became apparent that it would be for the good of the profession to include the smaller schools also. Later it was also decided to extend the membership to others interested in nursing education even though they were not heads of schools. It is this society that has sponsored the reforms in nursing education that have gradually evolved and that are still going on. The work has particularly been along the lines of: (1) higher minimum entrance requirements in order to attract an even better class of student into nursing, (2) improvement of living and working conditions, and (3) increased opportunities for postgraduate and specialized training. In 1952 the National League of Nursing Education, in conjunction with the National Organization of Public Health Nurses and American Association for Collegiate Schools of Nursing joined to become the National League for Nursing.

ORGANIZATION OF PUBLIC HEALTH NURSES

The appearance of a new group of nurses with different interests—the public health nurses—demanded some form of organization. This did not happen, however, until 1911 when a joint committee was appointed by the two national nurses' organizations, the American Nurses' Association and the American Society of Superintendents of Training Schools, for the purpose of standardizing nurses' services outside the hospital. The chairman of the committee was Lillian D. Wald and the Secretary was Mary S. Gardner. After thorough consideration of the problem, it was decided that what was needed was a brand-new organization that in its own right could answer the needs of the new profession. So the committee invited all the 800 agencies, which they knew to be engaged in public health nursing activities, to send delegates to the forthcoming meeting of the two established nursing organizations in Chicago in June, 1912. At the meeting, the interest was great, and a most heated discussion continued for two days. One of the difficulties was to find a suitable name for the new organization. Finally at noon on June 7, the "National Organization for Public Health Nursing" was unanimously voted into existence, with Lillian D. Wald as its first president. That the discussion during the proceedings must have been heated in more than one respect is apparent from Miss Gardner's description, for she refers to the "hot morning of June seventh."

The purpose of the new society was to standardize public health nursing activities on a high level and coordinate all efforts in the field. Although primarily a nurses' organization, membership was not restricted to registered nurses but included all whose work properly concerned this field. The organization was ready to cooperate with all other groups having mutual interests. It soon grew quickly, and it has almost ideally served its purpose, for its growth has intimately reflected the growth of public health nursing in America.

Chapter **15**

Developments in nursing service

Until the time of Florence Nightingale, nursing as a profession had not been sufficiently developed to make worthwhile differentiation between nursing services within and those outside the hospital. She, however, developed the nursing school, with resultant better nursing in the hospital, the opening of hospital careers, and the consequent organization of nursing service and nursing education. As the schools of nursing attracted more and better prepared young women, the nursing service in the early hospitals sponsoring such schools improved.

Not all sick people go to the hospital; in fact, we saw that for many centuries none but the poor went to the hospitals, and even the improvements that followed Miss Nightingale's reforms still left a great field of nursing service outside the hospital among both the rich and the poor.

In "private nursing" the patient bears the entire cost of the nursing. If he cannot do so, the cost is borne partly or entirely by the community either in the form of some private organization or by some public body. This latter form of nursing was at first called visiting nursing. Later, as the emphasis changed, it was called public health nursing.

A hundred years ago people who were ill had nurses in their homes. They were women often with vast practical experience but without formal training because none existed at that time. Naturally, as young women received such training and acquired special skill in attending the sick and carrying out doctors' orders, which were becoming ever more technical in nature, people who could pay for their services would demand them, and nurses trained in hospitals would go into private homes. There was nothing striking or dramatic about such a development, and it leaves no historical landmark. In the early days of many schools, student nurses did private duty in both hospital and home. The hospital usually collected the fee.

About the turn of the century, emphasis on prevention of disease began to emerge as a principle underlying all health care, including nursing service. In many instances, the reason disease is not prevented is not always poverty but often ignorance of the simplest rules of health. The difference in cost between, simple, clean, and healthy living and squalor is not as great as one would think. So it became impressed upon these young professional nurses, as they worked in the slums or in the wilderness, that if people knew a little more, much suffering could be avoided.

This was a period of changing social outlook. The duty of the state to improve and to protect the health of the citizens who cannot do so themselves was just beginning to be emphasized. Furthermore, it is good business to do so, for it is ultimately the state that stands to lose through sickness and premature death of its citizens. It is cheaper to prevent an obstetrical complication than to have the mother of a family a chronic invalid for years; to have a child properly fitted with glasses than to spend money on his education, which he partly misses because he cannot see; to have a tuberculous patient isolated than to lose years of work from others who have become contaminated because the patient was allowed to go about his business when he should have been in a sanatorium; or to treat and to cure early syphilis rather than to have the loss and expense later of keeping the patient for years in a mental hospital or to have him die prematurely from syphilitic heart disease. The age of "rugged individualism" was giving way to a sense of social responsibility.

Thus the obligation of the community was readily recognized once it was pointed out, but who was to bear the expense? Charity (for "free" preventive medicine is a form of charity) to a large extent, has been borne by private organizations. The visiting nurses' societies were private enterprises; the Rockefeller Foundation was promoting public health, and so was the Red Cross. On the other hand, the local communities were establishing health departments. Problems vary so much from locality to locality that prevention of disease is often best handled locally by municipalities or state governments. The United States Public Health Service was developing quickly, and there were many health problems that definitely were nationwide, such as harbor quarantine and maintenance of food and drug standards in interstate commerce. Later, the prevention of spread of certain infectious diseases, such as leprosy and syphilis, was deemed to be a Federal problem. All these arguments had something in their favor, and all classes of agents sponsored health services, so we now have work done by private organizations, by municipal and state governments, and by the Federal Government, all of them needing the aid of nurses. Often they cooperate; sometimes they act independently of each other.

PRIVATE DUTY NURSING

Hospitals a half century ago would retain the private duty nurse on their payroll and collect the fee for services rendered. It was satisfactory to the nurse because it provided her with security and occupation between private cases. As private nursing grew, this arrangement was found to be unsatisfactory. A system of nursing through "registers" or employment offices developed. A certain percentage of the wage was retained as a commission. Sometimes such registers provided not only private cases but permanent appointments, and some of them are still doing well in this respect. Registers for private nursing, however, sometimes fell into unscrupulous hands, and the nurses were exploited. Therefore, they often placed the register in the hands of someone whom they cooperatively employed or with their professional organization. These methods reduce the cost to a minimum and are extensively used now.

Another aspect of private nursing that had become a serious problem was the cost to the individual patient. As the nurse's education and skill became more complicated, her expected financial return naturally had to be greater. With the introduction of the eight-hour day, twenty-four hours of private nursing became quite expensive. Three attempts were made to overcome this difficulty: "hourly nursing," admission to private hospitals in which nursing service could be obtained from general duty nurses, and insurance. This leaves only the more serious cases still requiring full-time private nursing.

In "hourly nursing," the nurse, like the doctor, goes from patient to patient in the home, carrying out the procedures that requires extensive nursing skill, leaving the simpler tasks to an attendant or member of the family. The most common practice today is admission to private hospitals. As well as the nursing service it offers many other advantages, such as the services of laboratories, diet kitchen, and resident physicians. Insurance schemes to pay for the rising cost of nursing are also gaining ground, especially in the form of group insurance, which lowers the overhead cost. In historical perspective, private nursing was at its height during the halcyon days of the twenties. In the subsequent depression many private duty nurses fell into dire need.

NURSING DEVELOPMENTS IN THE COMMUNITY

It is important that the American nurse understand the development of nursing in the community, for although the first organized attempts at visiting nursing began quite early in this country, the movement was slow to gain momentum, and many influences can be traced back to English beginnings.

In 1842 an early Philadelphia institution established a Nurse Society for the purpose of supplying nurses alternately to indigent sick and to those who could pay for them. This service was similar to what we now call visiting nursing. Then in 1877 the Women's Branch of the New York City Mission established a nursing service for the sick poor by graduate nurses. However, their usefulness may have been somewhat impaired by the fact that while nursing they were supposed to actively proselytize for the church. Although the religious motive in nursing always has been and always must be highly respected, it has been the general experience that the cause of God has always been better served by the gentle, loving example than by aggressive agitation. This very factor may have induced the Ethical Society of New York to place four nurses in New York Dispensaries for the purpose of spreading the gospel of healthful living, thus establishing early in New York a service that was not to become general for several years.

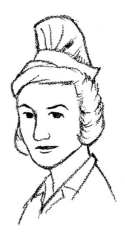

Lenox Hill graduate nurse—New York

During this period visiting nursing in England had passed through its initial stages, had been under scrutiny, and now was developing into a valuable social service. With such an example before them it is not surprising that various American communities established similar societies. During the middle eighties visiting nurses' associations developed in Buffalo, Boston, and Philadelphia. Although the first of these were started under the auspices of the Presbyterian Church, all of them soon became independent societies organized solely for the purpose of maintaining visiting nurses. These societies, inspired partly by those in England and partly by those in New York, have survived to become some of the leading organizations of this kind in our day. The example was soon followed by New Bedford, Chicago, and Kansas City.

THE SETTLEMENT

A new development occurred in the year 1893 that was to have an enormous influence on work among the poor, for much of public health and social service actually stems from the first American settlement. The "settlement" was not a new idea. For years English philanthropists had gone to live among the poor, but this was the first time that an American nurse brought her special training to the task. Miss Lillian D. Wald and her friend, Miss Mary Brewster, settled in Henry Street, one of the poorest neighborhoods in the metropolis, in order to give their lives to the betterment of the conditions of the poor. In other words, their scope extended far beyond nursing their sick; it even extended beyond preventing disease; they aimed at rectifying, so far as it was in their power, those causes that were responsible for poverty and misery. That, in its essence, is social service. The experiment was so successful that Miss Wald became an accepted authority on all subjects within this sphere, and the place itself, Henry Street Settlement, has become the field-ground for training and experience in social work for students from Columbia University and other educational institutions.

The social aims, however, were not pursued to the neglect of nursing or preventive medicine. All of them are considered important, and the institution itself has become the prototype of others of its kind elsewhere in the country. Among the first to follow were the nurses' settlements in Richmond, Virginia (1900), San Francisco, California (1900), and Orange, New Jersey (1903).

SCHOOL NURSING

School nursing has become one of the most important public health functions. In the nineteenth century, when compulsory schooling became general, it was necessary to pass certain health measures that eventually became centered in the periodical medical inspection of premises and pupils. In 1872 in the school of Wild Street, Drury Lane, London, a desire arose to have a nurse look into the method of feeding the school children. A request was made to the Queen's Nurses, and Miss Amy Hughes, then their superintendent, decided to look into the matter herself. Her investigation revealed much unnecessary suffering among school children, and she began at once to place Queen's Nurses in London schools. However, the London school board was very

slow to see the value of this service, and eventually it became necessary for the London County Council itself to appoint a staff of municipal school nurses. This did not happen until 1904. By then, Liverpool had already an eleven-year-old school nursing service financed by voluntary subscription. However, by 1902 when Miss Wald visited in England, school nursing there had reached such a high level of development that she returned, inspired to fight for the institution of a similar service in the New York schools.

In those days children were barred from school if the teacher found reason to do so, but no effort was made to see that such exclusion was on sound medical grounds or that the children excluded received proper care. Miss Wald was able to convince the authorities of the inefficiency of this method. In 1903 she was permitted to place a nurse experimentally in each of the four schools showing the highest incidence of exclusions. The nurses' work was so successful that in the experimental schools the exclusion fell some 90%. Such a result naturally led to the employment of school nurses throughout New York and other large cities, Los Angeles following suit as early as 1904. School nursing is now universal. The nurse supplements the work of the doctor, and she can handle most routine matters. She can follow cases during treatment until recovery, and she can make the necessary contacts and readjustments within the home. This leaves the doctor time to do physical examinations and diagnostic work and to direct treatment. Such activity has since been adopted in many schools other than those of the municipal school system, and it is practically the pattern of the health service of private and special schools as well as colleges and universities. Nowadays an American college would be unthinkable without its health service.

Miss Gardner pointed out that school health service has passed through three stages. At first, it was thought sufficient for the health officer to conduct periodic "inspections" of school children, thereby to discover those who obviously needed medical care. When it was realized how inefficient such a method was, it was supplemented by periodic examinations of the individual children to discover defects not immediately apparent, such as defective vision, poor teeth, or heart murmurs. This was a great step forward but did not realize the full scope of health service, which is essentially the preservation of health, that is, prevention of disease. So now a great emphasis is placed on this phase, by instruction in hygiene and inoculation against preventable communicable diseases. This instruction should not stop in the classroom but should be carried to the very homes of the children when necessary.

Chapter 16

Nursing education is established

In 1896 the maximum hours of theory in the few good schools of nursing were 105. The standard course included 38 hours practical nursing, 36 hours anatomy and physiology, 4 to 6 hours gynecological nursing, 4 hours obstetrical nursing, 1 hour each in eye, ear, nose, and throat, and 2 hours in hygiene. When one compares this with the course suggested in *A Curriculum Guide for Schools of Nursing* and with the course being taught in good schools today, some measure of the progress made in nursing education in over sixty-five years may be appreciated.

The curriculum committee of the National League of Nursing Education made an outstanding and tangible achievement in the compilation of *A Curriculum Guide for Schools of Nursing*. It was originally titled *A Standard Curriculum for Schools of Nursing,* published in 1917. This publication offered concrete suggestions on how standards in schools could be improved, included outlines for courses, mainly in the theoretical subjects, and outlined the classwork for the three-year course.

In 1927 a revision was published under the title *A Curriculum for Schools of Nursing,* embodying the advances in nursing education since the first edition and emphasizing courses in public health, prevention of disease, and sociology, which began to be included in the basic course in the 1920's. The third edition was published in 1937 under the name *A Curriculum Guide for Schools of Nursing.* The revision contained two important changes:

1. It no longer laid down hard and fast rules. Recognizing the varying conditions of different schools, it called itself a "curriculum guide" rather than a "curriculum."
2. To counteract the charge that the many classes would render the nurses' course too theoretical, it was proposed to move the instruction back into the wards as "ward teaching."

The latter suggestion has proved very practical, and much effort is now being expended to develop this practical form of teaching, which compares with some of the most important parts of the training of medical students.

When the schools of nursing developed, as they did toward the end of the century, under the leadership of ambitious and far-seeing women, it was natural that these leaders should strive for the highest standards for their young profession. They were favored by an ever-increasing demand for well-qualified nurses and an ever-increasing number of tasks that nurses could do if they were properly prepared. All this called for

123

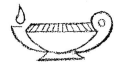

Nursing education lamp

increased basic experience in nursing. On the other hand, there remained the noneducational duties of making beds, giving bed baths to convalescent patients, and many tasks of hospital housekeeping, which required some training for their expert performance. The problem then developed about whether all nurses should receive the highest possible professional education and to an increasing extent relegate simpler tasks to less trained attendants or whether there should be established various degrees of nursing education.

It was soon realized that nurses wishing to prepare for administrative and teaching positions must have certain experiences not offered in the organized courses, to train themselves for such tasks. These principles evolved fairly promptly and have in the course of time obtained general acceptance, but the major problem still remains: how far should the nurse's basic preparation go? The question is to some extent answered by its economic aspects: there must be a certain proportion between the expense involved in obtaining an education and the financial reward that can be anticipated.

The American Society of Superintendents of Training Schools soon realized that there were three ways of establishing university standards for nurses: (1) they had to establish leadership, (2) they had to improve the student body by raising entrance requirements, and (3) they had to improve the quality of the schools by endowments and through recognition by the universities. It was not enough to establish the schools in university hospitals. This had already been done repeatedly without any appreciable effect on the course offered in nursing.

The first step was taken about 1894 when the University of Texas established its school of nursing as a regular division of its medical department. However, its leadership proved insufficient, and the requirements of this school did not meet the general requirements for university students. The plan was frustrated, and the effort has only historical interest now.

TEACHERS COLLEGE, COLUMBIA UNIVERSITY

The first effort of enduring value was the establishment of a course in hospital economics at Teachers College, Columbia University, in 1899. In 1898 Mrs. Robb had read a paper before the American Society of Superintendents of Training Schools recommending that a committee be appointed to study how special instruction could be provided for nurses who wished to prepare themselves for advanced positions. The committee was appointed with Mrs. Robb as its chairman. After having surveyed the field it approached Dr. James S. Russell, Dean of Teachers College, Columbia University, in New York, with its plans. As a result the college was opened to qualified nurses, who could attend all courses that they required. Courses specifically for nurses had to be organized and maintained by the Society.

In retrospect it is hardly possible to realize what a tremendous advance this was. Here was a group, which thirty years before had had little if any professional education or standing, now actually transformed into a group qualified by general and special education to aspire to university degrees. With the opening in 1899 of the course in hospital economics the revolution was practically complete. The work of the following generations consisted merely of extending the advantages thus gained and in building on a firmly established foundation.

Although only two students registered for the new course the superintendents went to work with great enthusiasm; they gave freely and often gratuitously of their time and efforts to make the course successful. Gradually more nurses registered.

In 1907 Mrs. Nutting became the first nurse in the world to become a professor in a university. She established "a new department of household administration which included the division of hospital economics."* Under her guidance the department rapidly developed and achieved international fame, attracting students from abroad who later were to lead nursing developments in their own countries. The first actual head of a training school of nurses in Denmark was a graduate of the New York Presbyterian Hospital and had studied at Teachers College, Columbia University. One of the most important activities of the new department was to establish the Henry Street Settlement in order to develop public health nursing. To accomplish its task, money was necessary. The department was fortunate in receiving an endowment of $200,000 from Mrs. Helen Hartley Jenkins. In 1925 Miss Isabel M. Stewart, who had been Miss Nutting's assistant since 1909, became head of the department.

The purpose of this department was to offer thorough and advanced courses for nurses destined to become heads of nursing schools and who were to seek other advanced positions in teaching and hospital administration. Until the fall of 1964 it offered short and refresher courses for persons who had had some experience in the field. It has succeeded eminently in these tasks and remains the leading institution of its kind in the country and perhaps in the world. In the course of time other colleges and universities have established postgraduate courses of varying scope, many of them excellent, but none of them as completely organized as those of Teachers College, Columbia University.

---

*Roberts, Mary May: American nursing: history and interpretation, New York, 1954, The Macmillan Co.

UNIVERSITY SCHOOLS OF NURSING

Finally some nursing schools became university schools, the superintendents being full professors occupying Chairs of Nursing. Minnesota had the first school of nursing organized as an integral part of a university. This was achieved in 1909 through the efforts of the farseeing Dr. Richard O. Beard of the University of Minnesota. Later the five-year course leading to the degree of Bachelor of Science in Nursing was offered, as well as the three-year course. These five years are a combination of college and nursing education, a system that has been followed by other universities. It changed the status of the fledgling nurse from that of a "pupil nurse" to that of a student.

EDUCATION OF THE PUBLIC HEALTH NURSE

Special training was required for the nurse who was to do visiting nursing, but much more special knowledge was required of the nurse who was to take up preventive medicine. It is one thing to make a bed or to care for the physical needs of a patient, but quite another to examine a class of children and spot the ones who are developing the measles or to visit in a home and evaluate tuberculosis contacts. This was soon realized, but there is, even now, a great deal of argument about what kind of preparation public health nurses should have. Various methods are being tried in various countries. Rather than enumerate in detail how different countries have approached the problem, we shall trace the various lines of thought that have been advanced to solve it.

Many views were advanced, and each has prevailed to some extent. Some have strongly favored complete specialization for all tasks that require but a simple technic. They do not consider basic education in nursing necessary. It has been argued that, to do district midwifery only, it is not necessary to have had a full nurse's course; and many countries have midwives who are not nurses and who are trained not only to see that nature takes her normal course but also to know and recognize complications and to prevent those that can be prevented. Other similar arrangements have been made when a task was big enough to occupy a person's full time and yet special and simple enough to be done without extensive knowledge other than that immediately pertaining to the job. This principle has not gained wide acceptance in the United States.

Most tasks in preventive medicine were not simple. It was generally admitted that the majority of them required some knowledge of anatomy, physiology, hygiene, or pathology, such as was included in the modern nursing course. On the other hand, it was admitted that with the growing importance of public health, almost every nurse would sooner or later come up against some problems of public health. To answer both of these demands it was deemed advisable to include some public health instruction in the undergraduate course. This was done either by affiliation with a visiting nurses' association or through district nursing service maintained by the hospital. Because the emphasis was mainly on hospital training, most of these arrangements were not very satisfactory until the importance of public health was properly appreciated by the teaching staff of the hospital and until the curriculum of the schools had become developed to a point at which such a course could be integrated without being unduly crowded. The first undergraduate courses in this field were given in Boston.

Then as the scope of public health nursing expanded, it was realized that the more or less casual undergraduate contact with the field was not enough. There was enough to learn to justify organized postgraduate courses, and in 1914 Miss Nutting offered a postgraduate course in public health nursing at Teachers College in affiliation with Henry Street Settlement. This was successful, and soon the city of Boston began the special training of public health nursing which, by 1914, had developed into an eight-month course at Simmons College. Later other centers, mostly university schools, developed public health courses. Probably the school offering the course with the widest scope is Western Reserve. This course was established in 1935 and admits college graduates only. Obviously it aims at training nurses for administrative and leadership positions in the rapidly developing field. Thus, as public health nursing has increased in importance, the educational facilities in the field have developed also.

CURRICULUM ORGANIZATION

Another step in advancing nursing education was the gradual improvement of entrance requirements.

While it became known that higher entrance requirements would make for better nurses, it also became clear that a graduated course could best be undertaken if it were preceded by a preliminary course given in the classroom. This was originally a Scotch plan that had been tried in Boston and was reintroduced into this country by Miss Nutting at Johns Hopkins Hospital in 1901. It was found so eminently satisfactory that by 1912 there were 114 schools in the United States giving preliminary courses. These varied in time from a few lecture courses to a regular six-month course. Some included physical and social sciences and practical work, either on mannequins or in the wards themselves, so that when the students entered the wards, they felt more confident and could more quickly adjust to hospital routine. Some times the preliminary course is given at a college that is not an integral part of the school of nursing. In some countries, notably in Finland, this has led to a central school for these preliminary courses, after which the students are distributed to their separate schools. The system of preliminary courses greatly increased the efficiency of the whole course. The principal objection to it has been its cost. It does appear expensive at first sight, although this

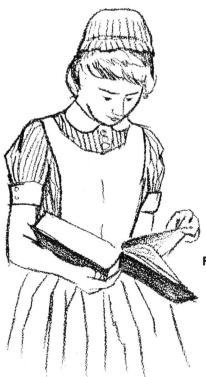

Former Bellevue student nurse

Collegiate student nurse

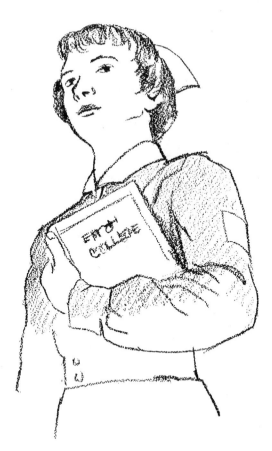

point may be questionable when the gain in efficiency is considered.

THE BROWN STUDY

For many years leaders in the nursing profession believed that schools of nursing should be more closely affiliated with educational institutions. In 1908, mainly through the efforts of Dr. Richard Olding Beard, the school of nursing at the University of Minnesota became part of that University. Particularly since World War I, studies and surveys have been made to find out the place schools of nursing should have in the educational structure of this country as far as both administration and financial support are concerned. The first major study, published in 1923, is called "Report of the Committee for the Study of Nursing Education" made under the direction of Josephine Goldmark. As a result of this study, the Rockefeller Foundation endowed the school of nursing at Yale University.

Continuing interest in the study of nursing education was shown by the Committee on the Grading of Nursing Schools, which worked under the direction of May Ayers Burgess beginning in 1925. One report of this committee, "Nursing Schools Today and Tomorrow," published in 1934, set the blueprint for the organization of the modern school of nursing.

During World War II demands made on nurses increased. As a result of the activities begun by the National Nursing Council, Dr. Esther Lucile Brown directed a study entitled *Nursing for the Future* that has probably had more influence on nursing than anything since the days of Miss Nightingale.

The basic purpose of all nursing education is to prepare qualified graduates to meet the current and future challenge of nursing. Basically, a school of nursing must meet the requirements set up by the State Board of Nursing. Many nursing schools now meet the higher standards required for accreditation by the National League for Nursing. Many nursing programs in colleges are accredited along with the other college curricula by the appropriate regional accrediting board, such as the Middle-States Association of Colleges and Secondary Schools. At the present time students may learn nursing in three general types of schools: diploma, Associate degree, and Baccalaureate. The first two prepare for technical practice, the last for professional practice.

Chapter 17

Nursing publications

As long as nursing remained in the apprenticeship stage and before it began to develop as a profession, there was very little use for publications to express its needs, activities, and progress and to interpret its work to members of its own group, to other professions, and to the community. Florence Nightingale was the first nurse to contribute very much to professional literature.

Today there are many publications in the nursing world. They can be classified as official and nonofficial organs or publications. The official publications of the professional nursing organizations in this country are *The American Journal of Nursing, Nursing Outlook* (with which is combined *Public Health Nursing*), and *Nursing Research.*

A magazine which is controlled, and this usually implies ownership, by the nursing organization which sponsors it, is known as the "official organ" of that association. It is the voice of the association and of the profession, or those branches of it which the association was organized to promote. Like the association itself, the publication is based upon an ideal of service to nurses and through them to the public which they serve. The primary function of a professional publication is to encourage the members to exceed their own best efforts and thus to increase their professional stature.

Professional nursing publications are not pub-

lished primarily for financial profit. However, if there are earnings, they are used to extend the work of the professional group which the publication represents. No individual receives personal financial profit from any earnings of the *American Journal, Public Health Nursing,* or the official bulletins of the state and district nurses associations.*

There are several other nursing organizations that have their own official publications described later in this chapter.

THE AMERICAN JOURNAL OF NURSING

During the history of professional nursing in this country *The American Journal of Nursing* has been its official mouthpiece. As soon as the early leaders began to meet and discuss the need for national organizations, the need for a representative nursing journal was appreciated. In fact, the American Society of Superintendents of Training Schools had considered it, but because they knew the limitations of their scope they thought this project should be delayed until the alumnae association had become a national organization and truly representative of American nurses. One of the first activities

---

*Editorial: What are professional nursing periodicals? American Journal of Nursing **37**:1369, December, 1937.

of the Associated Alumnae was to appoint a committee to investigate how a journal could be started. As the first committee failed, a second was appointed in 1899. Among its members were both Mrs. Hampton Robb and Miss Nutting; only the records of their past courage can explain why these women set out on such a journalistic adventure without experience or outside financial assistance. The *Journal* was started as a joint stock company, the shares were $100 each, to be sold only to nurses—Miss Linda Richards held Share No. 1, Mrs. Robb No. 4, and Miss Nutting No. 6. As the *Journal* grew, it used its savings to buy back the stock, and finally in 1912 it owned all of it so that it is now truly the property of the American nurses, controlled by their association, and its official organ. It states that it has three functions: (1) to be a continuous record of nursing events, (2) to be a means of communication between nurses, and (3) to be a means of "interpreting nursing to the public." It particularly backs legislative efforts to regulate nursing, sponsors the cause of nursing education, and has many other functions of interest to the nursing profession. Miss Sophie Palmer was editor-in-chief of the *Journal* from its first issue in October, 1900, until her death in 1920. Miss Katherine DeWitt came to assist her in 1906 and remained until her retirement in 1932. She held the position of assistant editor, editor pro tem, coeditor, and finally managing editor.

In 1921 Miss Mary Roberts was appointed to succeed Miss Palmer as editor; she retained that position until her resignation in 1949 when she was appointed editor-emeritus. Miss Nell Beeby was editor from 1949 until her death in 1957. Miss Barbara G. Schutt is the present editor. As developments in the profession demanded it, the *Journal* has increased both in content and in variety of subjects discussed. Assistants have been added to the staff as this work increased.

The story of the organizational development of nursing can be traced through the *Journal* from 1900 until the present day. During its early days, nurses were very much concerned about registration and the development of adequate nurse practice acts. In one of the early *Journals* there is an article by Lavinia Dock, "What We May Expect of the Law." Accounts of the development of the Army and Navy Nurse Corps, nursing in the Veterans Administration, and nursing during the wars and in times of disaster appear regularly in this magazine, in addition to the continuous story of what nurses and their organizations are doing.

The *Journal* makes available to nurses all over the country authentic material on new and approved methods of diagnosis, therapy, or prevention, including nursing care. Circulation has now grown to over 250,000 annual subscriptions. In order to help its readers, the *Journal* has a field representative on its staff who meets with nursing groups all over the country, interpreting its activities and program. In addition, an annual index is published during January of each year. A cumulative index in five volumes, the first covering the years 1900 to 1920, the second, 1921 to 1930, the third, 1931 to 1940, the fourth, 1941 to 1950, and the fifth, 1951 to 1960, is another valuable help in using this magazine.

AMERICAN JOURNAL OF NURSING COMPANY

The American Journal of Nursing Company is an incorporated body with its own board of directors elected annually by the board of directors of the American Nurses' Association. It is the publishing corporation for the professional journals.

The American Journal of Nursing Company stock is wholly owned by the American Nurses' Association, and the board of directors of the ANA serve as sole stockholders for the American Journal of Nursing Company. This company also publishes the two other official professional nursing magazines, *Nursing Outlook* and *Nursing Research*.

NURSING OUTLOOK

When the National League for Nursing was formed in 1952, it asked the American Journal of Nursing Company to publish its new official organ, *Nursing Outlook*. Until 1912 articles of interest to public health nurses had been presented in *The American Journal of Nursing*. Since 1909 the Cleveland Visiting Nurses' Association had been editing their own *Visiting Nurse Quarterly*. When the National Organization for Public Health Nursing was formed in 1912, the owners of the *Visiting Nurses' Quarterly* gave this magazine to the new organization and endowed it liberally so that it would not become an economic liability for the new organization. This periodical was a success; in 1918 the name was changed to the *Public Health Nurse,* and it was known by that title until its last issue in December, 1952, when it became the nucleus for *Nursing Outlook,* whose first issue was January, 1953. *Nursing Outlook,* then, like *The American Journal of Nursing,* is owned and published by the American Journal of Nursing Company. The board of directors determines the over-all policy of the magazine. National League for Nursing representatives are on the board of directors. Miss Mildred Hall was the first editor of this new magazine; the editorial staff is made up of professional nurses. Miss Mildred Gaynor was second editor; she retired in 1966. The present editor is Miss Alice Robinson.

Since the National League for Nursing is interested in the development and improvement of nursing service, as well as nursing education, many articles are devoted to the two broad fields of nursing service and nursing education. It will be remembered that the National Organization for Public Health Nursing and the Association of Collegiate Schools of Nursing had non-nurse members as well as agency membership, as does the NLN. The official organ of this new organization, *Nursing Outlook,* therefore includes articles about nursing in relation to the community as well as articles in the field of public health in general and public health nursing in particular.

NURSING RESEARCH

Nursing Research, also published by the American Journal of Nursing Company, appears four times a year. Lucille E. Notter is the present editor. The first issue was published in June, 1952. This magazine actually was started before the National League for Nursing was organized, as an activity of the Association of Collegiate Schools of Nursing. Early in 1952 the ACSN asked the American Journal of Nursing Company to publish a magazine that would be devoted to research in nursing. Its stated purposes were (1) to inform members of the nursing and allied professions of the results of scientific study in nursing and (2) to stimulate research in nursing. It was designed to serve nurses in all fields and branches of the profession and represents the first concerted effort for the establishment of a magazine that had as its primary purpose the reporting of studies. The sponsoring organization was the Association of Collegiate Schools of Nursing; the publisher, the American Journal of Nursing Company. The editorial board consisted of twenty persons representing different branches of nursing and education and coming from different parts of the country.

To finance this project the Association of Collegiate Schools of Nursing gave $900 and the ANA, $500; individual contributions amounted to another $500. When the National League for Nursing, was formed in 1952, into which the Association of Collegiate Schools of Nursing merged, it took over this new magazine. The NLN nominates members for the editorial board, and the American Journal of Nursing Company appoints them. Miss Helen H. Bunge was the first chairman of the editorial board. Members of the editorial board are nurses, educators, or research workers in colleges, universities, or agencies interested in nursing research.

INTERNATIONAL NURSING INDEX

The International Nursing Index is the latest publication to join the official family of the American Journal of Nursing Company. It was first published in 1966 in co-operation with the National Library of Medicine. Over 160 nursing journals received from all over the world are indexed. It is divided by a subject section and a name section.

Before concluding this discussion of official nursing publications, it may be interesting to know that other literature is available from the nursing organizations; for example, *The American Journal of Nursing* publishes an annual index and a cumulative index at the end of every ten-year period. The ANA and the NLN publish bibliographies from time to time. *Facts About Nursing,* a statistical summary, published annually by the ANA, began in 1935 as the *Yearbook on Nursing.* These professional organizations also publish bulletins and books from time to time on subjects of interest to nurses. Various bulletins have been published by the different organizations that came together to form the NLN. These publications are revised quite frequently.

There are many other magazines and journals of interest to nurses. Some of them are directed to people with a major clinical interest, such as: *The Journal of the American Association of Nurse Anesthetists, Bulletin of the American College of Nurse-Midwifery, Journal of Psychiatric Nursing and Perspectives in Psychiatric Care.* Others have an audience that consists of people with a particular functional orientation, as: *American Association of Industrial Nurses' Journal* and the *Journal of Nursing Education.* Still others are directed toward nurses with a particular religious affiliation: *The Catholic Nurse* and *News for Nurses. R.N.* and *Nursing Forum* have a broader appeal to

nurses who are employed in a variety of positions.

BOOKS

When instruction for nurses became organized and particularly when the first schools modeled on the Nightingale plan were started, books became a necessity. Miss Nightingale's *Notes on Nursing, What It Is and What It Is Not,* appeared and became the textbook not only for nurses at the St. Thomas' School for Nursing but also for other schools, both in England and in America, and was translated into foreign languages. Many of the early schools of nursing used medical texts. In this country the first manual for nurses, the *New Haven Manual of Nursing,* was published by the Connecticut Training School in 1879. Other schools, including Bellevue, worked out manuals for nursing. They were what we would now call books in nursing arts. As nursing became organized, as leaders became more sure of nursing needs, and as more leaders appeared, they became articulate in print. One of the early books to obtain wide circulation, believed to be the first nursing text in America, was *Textbook of Nursing* written by a nurse, Clara Weeks Shaw, and published in 1885. It was a standard nursing text for many years. Another early text written by Diane Kimber particularly for nurses concerned the fields of anatomy and physiology. Succeeding editions of that book have continued to be published, and it is now known as Kimber and Gray's *Anatomy and Physiology.* Other well-known texts were Lavinia Dock's *Materia Medica,* Mary Reed's *Bacteriology,* and Harriet Camp's *Ethics.* Mrs. Isabel Hampton Robb wrote two texts, *Nursing Ethics* and *Nursing, Its Principles and Practice for Hospital and Private Use.*

Before World War I, books on clinical subjects written particularly for nurses began to appear. These were usually written by doctors; occasionally by a nurse in collaboration with a doctor. Very few were written by nurses alone. Since World War I, a more dynamic approach to nursing texts and reference books has been noticed. One of the early books giving the new look to texts for nurses was Miss Bertha Harmer's *Principles and Practice of Nursing,* which appeared in 1923. Since then, in nursing as in all other fields the amount of literature available is tremendous, with an increasing amount being written by nurses.

Chapter 18

Nursing during World War I

At the beginning of World War I there were only about 400 nurses in the Army Nurse Corps. During the next year and a half, aided by reserves from the American National Red Cross Nursing Service, the number was increased to over 21,000. A total of 10,000 served overseas. Even during World War I, Army nurses, although members of the Army, had no definite military rank as officers or commissioned personnel. They were, however, subject to military law and had some military privileges. Mainly in recognition for outstanding professional service during the war, relative rank was given to them in 1920.

Although European countries were involved in World War I from 1914 to 1918, American participation in the war was from 1917 to 1918. American doctors and nurses as well as many other professional and technical individuals and services served with European countries, particularly with Great Britain and France. The British medical and nursing services were much better prepared and much larger than the American as far as the military personnel were concerned. Before America entered the war her medical personnel learned much from contact with Great Britain and France.

At the outbreak of World War I in 1914, the American Navy had no hospitals in Europe, but some Navy nurses were temporarily enlisted to serve in France with the American Red Cross. In 1916 the United States Naval Reserve Force was created, including a provision for reserve nurses. The total number was small. By 1917 regular and reserve force nurses totaled only 466. Nurses began to be sent to the Navy's base hospitals in England, Ireland, Scotland, and France. During this same year schools of nursing were established by the Navy nurses at St. Croix and St. Thomas in the Virgin Islands, and one of these nurses was assigned to the Richmond Insane and Leper Asylum as a supervisor.

By 1918 the total number of Navy nurses had increased to 1,386. It was not until 1918 that the base pay was increased to $60 per month.

It was fortunate that Jane Delano was head of nursing in the American Red Cross when the United States entered World War I. She was an experienced nurse administrator and former superintendent of the Army Nurse Corps. The nursing service of the Red Cross immediately became a recognized reserve of the Army Nurse Corps.

In addition to recruiting Army nurses, the Red Cross Nursing Service staffed many American Red Cross installations overseas and recruited nurses for the Navy Nurse Corps and for the United States Public Health Service.

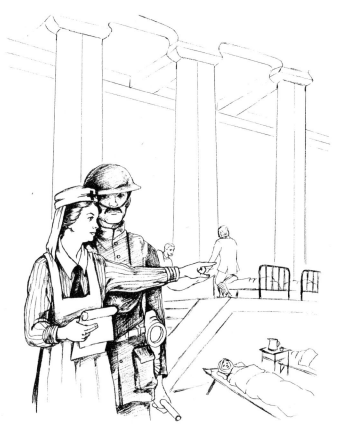

During World War I the wounded were withdrawn from field stations to temporary hospitals set up in large commandeered buildings such as chateaux.

In all, the Red Cross recruited over 20,000 professional nurses during World War I. This was about four-fifths of the total number of professional nurses who served in the World War. During this same period the Red Cross recruited and trained over 2,000 nurses' aides. Of these, about 250 were sent overseas.

The increased importance of home-nursing instruction was evident as the war continued and was emphasized during the influenza epidemic of 1918 and 1919.

ARMY SCHOOL OF NURSING

With the general enthusiasm for the Army created by the war, a move was launched to create an Army School of Nursing. It was organized and opened its doors in 1918

with Miss Annie W. Goodrich as Dean. The course was three years with a special credit of nine months to college graduates. These students were trained in Army hospitals and affiliated with civilian hospitals for such services as pediatrics and public health. In 1921 it graduated its first class of 500 students, probably the largest class of nurses ever graduated. Following this, the classes grew smaller, and the school was closed in 1932 as one of the general economy measures of the time.

VASSAR TRAINING CAMP

In answer to an appeal for college women to assist in the war, Vassar College offered its facilities for the training of college women in the summer of 1918. A twelve-week preclinical course in the basic sciences and elementary nursing was offered as part of a two-year course in nursing for college women. When the summer courses had been satisfactorily completed, students were assigned to selected general hospitals as regular students for the remainder of the nurse program. In all, 430 young women from 115 colleges and universities, representing 41 states, enrolled for the Vassar Training Camp Program. These young women were from many professional fields and created a great interest in nursing in colleges and universities throughout the country.

CONCLUSION

At the end of World War I, Miss Julia Stimson, the first woman major in the United States Army, was Superintendent of the Nurse Corps. She headed the corps from 1920 to 1937 when she was succeeded by Colonel Julia Flikke. Major Stimson felt strongly the anomaly of the nurses' being part of the Army organization and yet being without rank. This was further emphasized by conditions in the British Army in which nurses did have military rank. The defect was remedied in 1920 when the Superintendent of the Corps was created a major, and all nurses below her were given appropriate rank.

Shortly after the Armistice, Miss Delano went to Europe for a tour of inspection of nursing in military hospitals. While there she contracted an ear infection and died of mastoiditis in France in 1919. She was succeeded in her work with the Red Cross by Miss Clara D. Noyes, who had acted as her assistant for several years. In 1919 the League of Red Cross Societies, an international organization, was created to continue the work of the Red Cross in peacetime.

Questions and study projects for unit four

1. Discuss the significance of the World's Fair, 1893, to American Nursing. What leaders are linked with this exposition?
2. Discuss the early professional nursing organizations. How do these organizations differ from labor unions? To what leaders do we owe most in the early days of these organizations?
3. Discuss the origin and early history of professional magazines in nursing.
4. What contributions have been made by Teachers College, Columbia University, to nursing education?
5. Describe the activities of American nurses during World War I. What are some of the major differences between nurse activities during World War I and World War II? (For the complete answer to this, see Unit 7.)
6. Discuss the collegiate movement in nursing and point out some of the difficulties and problems in advancing this, both within and outside the nursing profession.
7. What do we mean by "specialization" in nursing? Discuss how this development is related to (a) nursing service and (b) nursing education.
8. Make an annotated bibliography of recent articles appearing in *The American Journal of Nursing, Nursing Outlook, Nursing Research,* and any other journals available in your library relating to the discussion in this unit.

References for unit four

A new magazine for nursing (editorial), American Journal of Nursing 52:1077, September, 1952.

American Journal of Nursing, 1900-1940, American Journal of Nursing 40:1085-1091, October, 1940.

Anna Caroline Maxwell, R.N., M.A., 1851-1929, American Journal of Nursing 29:187-193, February, 1929.

Ashburn, P. M.: A history of the Medical Department of the United States Army, Boston, 1929, Houghton Mifflin Co.

Bird's-eye view of nursing history (twentieth annual convention of American Nurses' Association), American Journal of Nursing 17:958-966, 1917.

Blair, Mary Stewart: Social trends and nursing organization, American Journal of Nursing 34:141-148, February, 1934.

Chayer, Mary Ella: School nursing, New York, 1937, G. P. Putnam's Sons.

DeWitt, Katharine, and Munson, Helen W.: The Journal's first fifty years, American Journal of Nursing 50:590-597, October, 1950.

Duffus, R. L.: Lillian Wald, New York, 1939, The Macmillan Co.

Dunn, Helen W.: The nursing budget, American Journal of Nursing 63:12, November, 1963.

Esselstyn, Caldwell B.: Trends in financing health care, American Journal of Nursing 63:24, November, 1963.

Forty years of education for nurses at Teachers College, American Journal of Nursing 39:1265-1266, November, 1939.

Gardner, Mary S.: Public health nursing, ed. 3, New York, 1936, The Macmillan Co.

Guild of St. Barnabas, American Journal of Nursing 36:890, September, 1936.

Hampton (Robb), Isabel Adams: Nursing: its principles and practice for hospital and private use, ed. 3, Cleveland, 1909, E. C. Koeckert.

Handbook on Nursing. Compiled by a Committee of the Bellevue School of Nursing, New York, 1878, G. P. Putnam's Sons.

Haupt, Alma C.: Forty years of teamwork in public health nursing, American Journal of Nursing **53**:81-84, January, 1953.

Highlights in the history of the Army Nurse Corps, Washington, D. C., February, 1956, Office of the Surgeon General, Department of the Army.

Lounsberry, Harriet Camp: Making good on private duty, Philadelphia, 1912, J. B. Lippincott Co.

MacDonald, M. G.: Handbook of nursing in industry, Philadelphia, 1944, W. B. Saunders Co.

McGrath, Bethel: Nursing in commerce and industry, New York, 1946, The Commonwealth Fund.

Mary Mahoney Award. Proceedings of the thirty-eighth convention of the American Nurses' Association, vol. 1, House of Delegates, New York, 1952, American Nurses' Association.

Massey, G. Estelle: The National Association of Colored Graduate Nurses, American Journal of Nursing **33**:534, 1933.

Minimum requirements for accredited schools of nursing as approved by the Board of Directors of the A.N.A., May 9, 1918, American Journal of Nursing **18**:1086, 1918.

Munson, Helen W.: The story of the National League of Nursing Education, Philadelphia, 1936, W. B. Saunders Co.

New magazine for nurses: American Journal of Nursing **51**:664, November, 1951.

Nutting, M. Adelaide: A sound economic basis for schools of nursing, New York, 1926, G. P. Putnam's Sons.

Petry, Lucile: One hundred fifty years of service, American Journal of Nursing **48**:434-435, July, 1948.

Poole, Ernest: Nurses on horseback, New York, 1933, The Macmillan Co.

Presenting Nursing Outlook (editorial), Nursing Outlook **1**:21, January, 1953.

Report of the Vassar Nursing Conference, American Journal of Nursing **21**:237, 1921.

Robb, Isabel Hampton: Nursing ethics, Cleveland, 1900, E. C. Koeckert.

Shoemaker, Sister M. Theophane: History of nurse-midwifery in the United States, Washington, D. C., 1946, The Catholic University of America Press.

Standard curriculum for schools of nursing, New York, 1917, National League of Nursing Education.

Staupers, Mabel K.: Story of the National Association of Colored Graduate Nurses, American Journal of Nursing **51**:222, 1951.

Story of the Journal, 1900-1950, ed. 4, New York, 1950, American Journal of Nursing Company.

Story of our magazine, Public Health Nursing **25**:162, March, 1953.

The contribution of the Army School of Nursing. Twenty-fifth annual report of the National League of Nursing Education, New York, 1918, National League of Nursing Education, p. 146.

Thoms, Adah B.: Pathfinders—a history of the progress of colored graduate nurses, New York, 1929, Kay Printing House.

Vassar nursing—preparatory course. A new experiment in nursing education, American Journal of Nursing **18**:1155, 1918.

Vreeland, Ellwynne M.: Fifty years of nursing in the Federal Government nursing services, American Journal of Nursing **50**:626, October, 1950.

Wald, Lillian D.: The house on Henry Street, New York, 1915, Henry Holt & Co., Inc.

Wald, Lillian D.: Windows on Henry Street, Boston, 1934, Little, Brown & Co.

Wales, Marguerite A.: The public health nurse in action, New York, 1941, The Macmillan Co.

Waters, Ysabella: Visiting nursing in the United States, New York, 1909, Charities Publication Committee, p. 42.

Worcester, Alfred: Nurses for our neighbors, Boston, 1914, Houghton Mifflin Co.

Nursing between World War I and World War II

In nursing the time between World War I and World War II was anything but a quiet period. Wars have always accelerated the need for nurses and emphasized the necessity of better nursing service. The old type of nursing education prevalent before World War I was no longer adequate to meet the increasing demands. Increased specialization in nursing service developed rapidly, and the need for a better basic nursing education as well as for the development of postgraduate education was evident. These years are characterized by study and research never before seen in the entire field of nursing. Nursing was truly coming of age.

Chapter 19

Increased specialization in nursing service and nursing education

We now come to a period in the evolution of nursing, which future historians may call the armistice between World War I and World War II. For nursing these were important years, for while in the preceding period nursing had been established as a profession, in this period nurses became aware of the fact that they were a potent social power. Nursing was recognized as something far more comprehensive than taking care of the sick; an equal emphasis was to be placed upon the preservation of health, and out of the feeble beginning of visiting nurses of the past developed the entire field of public health nursing.

In realizing their importance, the nurses also became critical of themselves. It was not enough to have established high aims and standards—the time had now come to formulate and to enforce them. Two great investigations of the nursing field as a whole occurred in this period; Many recommendations resulting from the investigations were put into action.

During World War I nursing was shaken out of any complacency it may have developed. Weaknesses in the form of a poor selection of students and poor training became apparent, in addition to the great scarcity of well-trained personnel. Because of more constructive future planning the public health movement made great advances during and after the war, prevention was emphasized, and more nurses specialized in public health nursing than ever before.

A greater interest in nursing was developed by the community during and after World War I. Professional nurses began to work more closely with educational institutions in solving common problems in education. All of these activities needed financial support, and endowments from private funds and grants from public sources began to be available.

SPECIALIZATION

Traditionally, nursing had offered three main fields of endeavor: hospital nursing (including teaching and administration), public health nursing, and private duty. After World War I nursing in each of the first two areas developed and created a tremendous need for nurses with advanced preparation for special jobs in hospitals, health agencies, schools, and industries. To meet the great need for specialization many courses were worked out, mainly in connection with colleges and universities, to give special preparation.

It is necessary to follow the further development of some of the movements that had started before the war, notably the establishment of schools of nursing within universities. Following the success of Dr. Richard Beard's Minnesota experiment, other schools adopted the idea, and by the year 1920, 180 schools had academic standing, and in 1938, 45 universities were sponsoring complete courses in nursing. They did not all follow the same pattern, nor did they all endeavor to serve the same purpose. So vast had the field of nursing become that many schools could afford to emphasize certain aspects thereof to the neglect of others. Often the schools at the same time achieved the endowment that had been envisioned by Miss Nightingale as a necessity, without which the best work could not be done unless funds were contributed by the university. Some of these endowed schools resulted from the reports we are about to discuss; but they are also the logical consequences of the movement that we have under consideration.

During the years that followed, many schools of nursing were reorganized on a university basis; some courses were four and some were five years in length. At the end of the course students received both a baccalaureate degree and a diploma in nursing.

ENDOWED SCHOOLS

The outstanding attempt at an endowed university school admitting only students with a college degree was the Yale University School of Nursing, which in its organization followed many of the recommendations made by the Committee for the Study of Nursing Education. Its endowment was granted by the Rockefeller Foundation. In this school the balance between the needs of the hospital and the needs of the students was struck entirely in favor of the latter. All theoretical and practical work was planned to fit the requirements of the students. Patients allotted to each student were assigned on this basis and the case method was worked out in nursing. The staff, too,

was chosen for its teaching ability. Miss Annie W. Goodrich was the first Dean of this school.

The experiment proved eminently successful, and in 1929 the school was established on a permanent basis with a large foundation grant. The Rockefeller Foundation was particularly interested because this school was in line with the trend of placing an increasing emphasis on the public health aspects of nursing. However, because of changing needs in nurse education, the corporation of Yale University in 1956 voted to discontinue the basic program and to concentrate on graduate nurse education.

The School of Nursing of Western Reserve University came into prominence in the early twenties; it was made financially independent by the Frances Payne Bolton Foundation. Since then other endowed nursing schools have been established along the same general lines, placing emphasis on education and public health. Some have been established abroad, such as the School of Nursing at Toronto University, Canada.

In addition to endowed schools of nursing many state universities now have well-developed schools of nursing, and some have departments of nursing education. The first of these was, as we have seen, that of the University of Minnesota. It is possible that in the future public support of nursing education through state universities may increase, as provision for meeting the nursing needs of the people is looked upon as one of the functions of the state on the same basis as public education.

The work in these schools has amply proved that superior nursing education is worthwhile. Although the number of endowed schools is still pitifully small, in the future, unquestionably, a number of schools of nursing will be established on a sound financial footing for the purpose of furnishing highly educated nurses for all the positions that are rapidly becoming available for persons capable of filling them. Educational standards are rapidly increasing throughout the country. The doctors, hospital administrators, and business executives with whom modern nurses must deal have increasingly better educational backgrounds and will, more than formerly, expect their nurses to have an adequate educational background.

THE ASSOCIATION OF COLLEGIATE SCHOOLS OF NURSING*

The development of some kind of association between nursing schools and colleges or universities continued. This relationship varied from a very loose, nonacademic tie, in which the school was called a university school merely because the supporting hospital was attached to a medical school, to the establishment of the nursing school as a professional school meeting academic standards set up by the college or university. This situation in university schools of nursing and the variety of standards was studied for several years before the establishment of The Association of Collegiate Schools of Nursing. A first conference held at Teachers College, Columbia, in January, 1933, was formed of twenty-one institutions whose representatives agreed to formulate standards and to set up machinery for the permanent organization, which took place in 1935. The objectives of the Association as stated in the constitution were these:

1. To develop nursing education on a professional and collegiate level.
2. To promote and strengthen relationships between schools of nursing and institutions of higher education.
3. To promote study and experimentation in nursing service and nursing education.

Membership in the Association was restricted to schools or departments on a collegiate and professional level or part of the system of higher education.

*In 1952 this Association merged with two other nursing organizations to form the National League for Nursing.

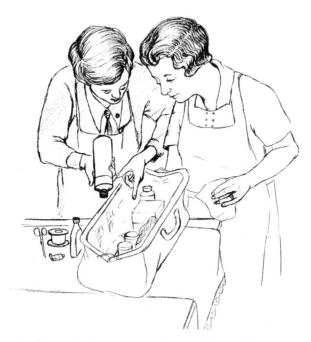

Among the long-standing and still important duties of the visiting nurse is instructing the family and friends in the care of a bedridden patient. The modern nurse still finds this most rewarding, as did the nurse pictured here in the 1930's.

It provided for two classes of membership, as follows:

Active membership shall be open to an accredited school of nursing definitely established as a constituent part of an accredited college or university which offers a combined academic and basic professional program leading to a baccalaureate degree. The organization of the school shall accord with that of other professional schools in the university or college.

Associate membership shall be open to an accredited school of nursing whose professional curriculum meets the standards set by the ACSN, provided that the school (1) is definitely established as a constituent part of an accredited college or university or one of the divisions thereof or (2) maintains a close educational and organizational relationship with an accredited college or university or one of the divisions thereof which makes its resources and facilities available to the school of nursing.

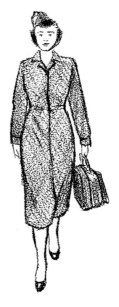

Visiting nurse

SPECIALIZATION IN PUBLIC HEALTH NURSING

We have noted that as the field of public health nursing expanded, many branches became so sharply defined that they appeared almost like small fields in themselves. Nurses who engaged in them found themselves limited in their activities; school nursing, tuberculosis control, and venereal disease control are examples of such fields. For a while it was argued that nurses seeking special preparation in public health should be able to train themselves and to gain recognition in only one of these specialties. Fortunately this view did not prevail. Actually, it was as absurd as to suggest that nurses in their postgraduate training should restrict themselves to dietetics, operating room work, or nursing of contagious disease. Nothing increases the value of a specialized training as much as a broad educational foundation. This is the tendency of modern public health nursing; the undergraduate nurse should receive a taste of it in order to know what it is about. The graduate nurse who decides to make public health nursing a lifework should have a thorough grounding in the entire field be-

fore limiting this work to a special branch. Besides, when working for a big organization like a municipality, the nurse may be shifted from one agency to another. Furthermore, unless a public health agency is established for a very specific purpose, as for instance in compliance with a grant for the elimination of trachoma in a certain region, the broader its scope is, the more useful is it likely to be, for one public health problem rarely exists alone. Most of them are born out of poverty, squalor, and ignorance, which generally will produce more than one plague at a time. Although much specialization may be found abroad in public health nursing, in the United States it is less emphasized except for the purpose of facilitating organization.

Cooperation between the Red Cross and public health nurses did not stop with World War I. When it was over, thousands of nurses, freed from war service, thronged to participate in the rapidly expanding public health activities. Again the task of the cooperating societies was twofold: organization of the field and an endeavor to fill the posts with properly qualified nurses, which in many cases meant that the nurses had to be prepared in this field before they could be appointed. One thing was in their favor; the trend of the times was to give to worthy causes, so that financing was relatively easy. The Red Cross could finance scholarships through which nurses could properly equip themselves. Generally the county was considered the unit suitable for such a project. Child welfare, tuberculosis prevention, and other similar endeavors have prospered under the joint auspices, often in cooperation with special national associations such as the National Tuberculosis Association.

One practical expression of cooperation is the Delano Red Cross Nursing Service established by a bequest from the will of Miss Delano. It provides one or more public health nurses to go into regions in which such work would otherwise not be financially possible. Under its provisions nurses have gone into the mountains of North Carolina, the cold of Alaska, and the islands off the coast of Maine.

The cooperation became international in scope when the Red Cross sponsored public health efforts in war-torn Europe, especially child welfare, and still more so when the above-mentioned courses were established in London under the international auspices of the League of Red Cross Societies. This was an effort that was far more than technical in scope, for it is through such association of young persons from all countries that a foundation can be laid, which perhaps some day may render armed international conflicts not only impossible but unthinkable and relegate them to the dark ages where they rightfully belong. Wars, like squalor and poverty, are largely the children of ignorance. Modern wars may have discouraged such efforts for a time, but there is in them a sterling value that will survive all vicissitudes, and it may be hoped that, when wars are over, friend and foe may again meet to further the common cause of health for all mankind.

INDUSTRIAL NURSING

As children grow up and leave school the majority of them, at least in urban areas, go into industry and business. The logical extension of health service has been to place nurses also in these areas to carry the load, along with the medical service that is now almost universal in large concerns. Here, however, the emphasis is not entirely upon health, for first aid and attention to minor ailments occupy a larger share of the nurse's time. Industrial nursing had its origin at the end of the last century, when some manufacturers employed nurses to visit sick employees. Soon it was discovered that the usefulness of nurses could be greatly expanded within the industrial plant, and by the time of World War I the employment of nurses in industry was quite general. However, in this case the nursing profession found itself closely tied to the economic cycle. When unemployment followed in the postwar period, industrial nursing shared in the retrenchment, and only in the last few years before World War II did industry again make a great demand on nursing. However, with the rising tide of better working conditions and obvious advantage of early health measures, this field may be considered as having been barely explored. It is still in its early stages of organization, some special preparation for it is available at a few universities, and it will undoubtedly prove attractive in the future. In April, 1942, the American Association of Industrial Nursing was organized from a nucleus of several industrial nurses' clubs, which had existed for several years in order to stimulate interest in the special problems of the industrial nurse and to provide a means for the discussion of these problems.

NURSING SERVICE IN THE FEDERAL GOVERNMENT

Nursing in the Federal services has become extremely varied. Nurses are employed in many branches of the Federal Government, all of the positions being classified by the United States Civil Service Commission except those in the Army and Navy Nurse Corps and, since January, 1946, the Veterans Administration. Through the years, positions in these agencies have followed the general lines of specialization existing elsewhere in the wide field of nursing and range from general duty or staff nursing to top administrative jobs.

It was not until 1920 that the first Navy nurses were assigned to serve aboard a hospital ship. This first assignment was on the *U.S.S. Relief.* In 1922 Miss J. Beatrice Bowman was appointed to succeed Mrs. Higbee. During 1920 the Navy Nurse Corps was reduced, in keeping with the total program of disarmament. Educational programs in dietetics, laboratory technic, anesthesia, and tuberculosis nursing were instituted. Salaries gradually increased, gratuity for uniforms was provided, and legislation was passed providing for retirement with pay for members incuring physical disability in the line of duty.

NURSING SERVICE IN THE
VETERANS ADMINISTRATION*

The history of the present Nursing Service of the Veterans Administration has a multiple origin, stemming principally from developments after World War I. Three major changes characterize its development.

The first major change was the creation of the United States Veterans' Bureau on August 9, 1921, to take over the abolished Bureau of War Risk Insurance (created September 2, 1914). Since October 6, 1917, the Bureau of War Risk Insurance had been responsible for providing medical, surgical, and hospital services and supplies to ex-servicemen. Because this Bureau lacked the facilities to carry out this act, the cooperation of the United States Public Health Service had been enlisted. From experience with the Marine hospitals, this Public Health

*From material supplied by Ruth Bayer Scott, Nursing Service, Veterans Administration.

Service was equipped to care also for veterans, being reimbursed from appropriations made to the Bureau of War Risk Insurance.

Miss Lucy Minnigerode, R.N., Superintendent of Nurses of the United States Public Health Service, had the vision and directive skill that enabled her, from modest beginnings, to build a nursing service of 1,880 graduate nurses. Of these, she turned over 1,442 graduate nurses to the United States Veterans' Bureau when it was established by Executive Order of April 29, 1922, and received all hospitals to care for disabled ex-servicemen operated by the United States Public Health Service.

An ex-service nurse, Mrs. Mary A. Hickey, was at the time of the transfer an assistant superintendent in the nursing service of the United States Public Health Service. At the April, 1922, transfer, she became Superintendent of Nurses of the New United States Veterans' Bureau Nursing Service. She was at once responsible for nursing care in forty-seven hospitals, and the follow-up work, which was at that time done by 400 public health nurses who were assigned to fourteen regional districts of the Bureau. This position Mrs. Hickey was to hold for over twenty years—until her retirement on January 1, 1943.

Within these twenty-plus years, the Veterans' nurses grew in number to 4,678, and the hospitals increased to ninety-one.

The second major organizational change was a merger in 1930, with the Veterans Administration arising from the amalgamation of the United States Veterans' Bureau, the Bureau of Pensions, and the National Home for Disabled Volunteer Soldiers. In this consolidation, nurses already on Veterans duty by Executive Order were converted to Civil Service without examination. One nursing service, headed by Mrs. Hickey as Superintendent of Nurses, included all nurses serving the Veterans Administration. The nurses, now in Civil Service, appreciated the opportunity to participate in the Federal retirement plan benefits. By paying into the Civil Service Retirement Fund for earlier years of government service, nurses increased their retirement benefits.

NURSING IN THE UNITED STATES INDIAN SERVICE

The Office of Indian Affairs has had a nursing service for a long time. However, in 1924 with the appointment of Elinor Gregg, Supervisor of Nurses for the Bureau of Indian Affairs, many important and lasting improvements were made; she laid the foundation for the modern program of health work with the American Indian in our states, including Alaska. Nurses are assigned to hospitals on Indian reservations and to other medical stations. Those in the field positions must be public health nurses. In Alaska a physician and from two to six nurses are employed in each of the Government hospitals, and, in addition, public health nurses do rural nursing. Medical care for the Indian has recently been placed under the United States Public Health Section of the Department of Health, Education, and Welfare.

NURSING IN THE CHILDREN'S BUREAU

The nursing division of the Children's Bureau has been greatly expanded in recent years as the Federal Government through grants-in-aid has been reaching into the states to help them plan and put into effect programs for handicapped children as well as maternal and infant welfare services. The Children's Bureau was first proposed by Lillian Wald, a public health nurse. Public health nursing consultants were employed by the Bureau especially after the Sheppard-Towner Act in 1921. In 1935 when the Social Security Act was passed, there was renewed stimulus for improvement of maternal and health services. The Children's Bureau was to administer three types of services as provided for in the Act: (1) maternal and child health services, (2) services for crippled children, and (3) child welfare services.

In 1935 a unit of public health nursing with a director, Naomi Deutsch, was set up.

THE LEAGUE OF RED CROSS SOCIETIES

During and immediately following World War I it became clear that the Red Cross could be an instrument of the greatest social service also in peace. The president of the War Council of the American Red Cross, H. P. Davison, therefore, proposed in 1919 that a "League" of Red Cross societies be formed for the general relief of suffering humanity, the prevention of disease, and the improvement of health—a greatly expanded program. The League is ruled by a board of governors, one from each component society. The secretariat of the League, originally in Geneva, with the International Committee was in 1922 transferred to Paris. By thus enlarging and extending its purpose, the Red Cross now found it easy to extend into South America, which had been less friendly as long as the organization's activities were concerned only with war. The establishment of the League resulted within a few years in the accession of twenty-three new societies and a great increase in its membership.

In order to encourage international cooperation and to exchange experiences, the League has sponsored world international and regional international congresses, and museums have been established for collections of Red Cross material in order that technical improvements in one area can be readily made available to other societies.

For disaster relief the local chapters of the Red Cross are primarily responsible. Each chapter is organized with a group of volunteers ready to respond to any call. Dressings and other relief material are stored in readily accessible places. The various chapters are coordinated to meet an emergency of any magnitude, even on a national scale, such as the great earthquakes in Iran and Japan. Some of the volunteers are lay persons with varying amounts of training in first aid; others are trained nurses and doctors.

Work in public health has been conducted as an educational campaign, more specifically in maternal and child welfare. Close cooperation has been established with other international societies with related purposes, such as The International Union Against Tuberculosis, and societies for better working conditions of seamen. It will be noted that much of this work is in the nature of social service.

Nursing and the League of Red Cross Societies

Of greatest interest for our purpose is the work of the League in the field of nursing. Under its auspices an International Nursing Center was established in London in 1920 under a graduate nurse. The chief purposes in the field of nursing were to encourage the highest standards of nurses' training—especially in backward countries (in some countries this was done by actually sponsoring schools of nursing), by emphasizing the opportunities in public health and preventive medicine for specially trained nurses—and to improve international relationships by offering postgraduate courses to nurses from various countries. This last was done at Bedford College for Women and at the College of Nursing in London. The British Red Cross provided the League with a house in London for the students. By thus acting as a stimulus and by coordinating the field of nursing with all its other activities, the League of Red Cross Societies has tremendously furthered the cause of nursing and has helped to increase the opportunities in the field.

Finally, it must be mentioned that by establishing the Junior Red Cross, the League has strengthened itself by extending its activities to boys and girls who, thus trained in first aid and relief, have become a valuable recruiting ground for the organization.

THE ROCKEFELLER FOUNDATION—THE COMMONWEALTH FUND

The influence of the Rockefeller Foundation has been somewhat different in that it supported largely educational efforts and was even more international in scope than the Red Cross. The Foundation has liberally supported schools of nursing that emphasized the health aspects of nurses' training. We have mentioned what it has done for Yale and Toronto Universities in this field. As this activity was part of an international scheme, it is in line with the work the Foundation has done all over the world. It has been active in furthering education in public health in Brazil, China, Czechoslovakia, and France, to mention but a few countries. Its scope following World War II was broadened in many areas. It also supplied traveling fellowships for the exchange of public health nurses, and it has supported the work of the Nightingale Foundation. Of all the great institutions interested in public health, the Rockefeller Institution takes the widest view of the problem.

The Commonwealth Fund has done similar work. Its activities are, to some extent, international in scope. Most outstanding is the work done in Austria following World War I, especially to further the health of children. In the United States, also, the furtherance of child welfare has been foremost among its activities.

The Commonwealth Fund has been interested in rural health conditions. In 1934 it helped to finance a survey of rural health by the National Association for Public Health.

Many other fields were opening for nurses, but they have developed so naturally and without fanfare and they are still so young that they have no "history." Many nurses now find careers as assistants in doctors' private offices, in department stores, in transportation, especially on ocean liners and airliners, but to some degree on trains—in brief, almost anywhere that people congregate.

Chapter 20

Studies and research between World War I and World War II

In 1920 standards in the best schools of nursing were high, but the greatly increased demands for nursing students during and after World War I had forced many schools to relax their entrance requirements in order to attract more students. Thus, many less desirable applicants were admitted to the schools, resulting in such heterogeneous educational standards that before anything serious could be undertaken, the current state of affairs had to be recorded and analyzed. Then recommendations could be made for standardization and improvements.

The trend was to place even greater emphasis on public health and preventive medicine. This happened to be the exact field in which the Rockefeller Foundation was much interested. It became possible for the Foundation to finance the "Committee for the Study of Nursing Education," which was organized in 1918 as a result of a meeting called by the Foundation and attended by about fifty persons including doctors, nurses, and others interested in public health. The committee was headed by Professor C. E. A. Winslow of Yale University, but most of the work was done by its secretary, Josephine Goldmark, who by her previous training in social research was especially well fitted for the task. Sometimes the committee has been called after her—the "Goldmark Committee." Originally the task of the committee was to study educational requirements for health nursing, but by 1920 it had become clear that this problem was so inextricably tangled with other aspects of nurses' preparation that at a second meeting the inquiry was extended to encompass the entire field of nursing education. Accordingly, the investigation proceeded along wider lines; especially twenty-three hospital schools of nursing, representative of all types and localities, were carefully analyzed, as well as all nursing activities, with emphasis on public health nursing.

FINDINGS OF THE COMMITTEE

The entire investigation resulted in the publication in 1923 of *Nursing and Nursing Education in the United States*. The following three important points were brought out by the investigation:

1. There was widespread neglect of the fields of public health.
2. Many schools were deficient in technical facilities for the teaching of nurses and had instructors inadequately prepared for their tasks. The

course was unstandardized, especially in the relationship of theory to practice.

3. It was general practice for the chief nurse of the hospital also to be the head of the school of nursing. The cause of nursing would be better served by having these two duties vested in separate persons.

The committee then made several recommendations, some pertaining to public health nursing. It was recommended that public health nurses needed a sound basic hospital training of about two and one-third years plus an eight months' course in public health nursing. Although the number of nurses had increased from about 83,000 in 1910 to over 149,000 in 1920, shortages were still apparent in certain areas. This committee pointed out that the old apprenticeship type of training was outmoded in the preparation of the nurse. The committee also recommended that the training of attendants should be developed further. The requirement of a grammar school education and a training program of about eight months' in a good hospital was suggested.

Other recommendations concerned the general education of nurses. The current tendency to lower requirements should be discontinued and efforts made to raise the general standards of nursing education to the level of the best schools. Instructors and other officers of schools of nursing should receive special training to fit them for their tasks. The development of university associations with schools of nursing should be strengthened, and schools should be given adequate financial backing. It was further suggested that "subsidiary nurses" be trained for eight or nine months to carry out non-nursing tasks in institutions and to take charge of patients who do not need skilled nursing care. This meant the introduction of a group of subsidiary workers with a certain elementary training. Within the past few years this group has increased in number and, together with attendants and orderlies, pages, clerks, and secretaries, it has been added to ward personnel to do work formerly done by nurses, while nurses now perform those duties requiring special skill and technic.

The recommendations of this committee have profoundly affected the education of nurses in America. They immediately led to the endowment of the Yale School of Nursing by the Rockefeller Foundation. Their indirect effects extended much farther, and there are few schools of nursing throughout the country that are not better for its efforts.

Chapter **21**

The Committee on the Grading of Nursing Schools

At the beginning of the century the training of medical students in America was very poor. Although some of our doctors were among the best in the world, thousands were so poorly trained that they should not have been entrusted with the simplest medical responsibilities. Yet, they were graduates of "accredited" schools. Because there was no law to force these schools out of business, the American Medical Association, about 1910, investigated all medical schools and graded them A, B, and C. Without legislative efforts the results of this grading were miraculous. A prospective medical student realized that if he graduated from a Grade B or Grade C school, it would lower his professional standing. As a result, poor medical schools either improved to meet acceptable standards or discontinued the course.

The plan was so successful that in 1925 nurses decided to sponsor a Committee on the Grading of Nursing Schools. Its scope was somewhat wider than was suggested by its name, for besides grading schools the committee was also to study in detail the work of nurses and to define the duties belonging within the scope of nursing. It was also to study the supply of nurses and the demands for nursing services, including the

problems of public health nursing. In other words, the committee was to carry further the task that had been started by the Rockefeller Committee. The Grading Committee, however, was only in part financed by outside sources; the nurses raised among themselves $115,000 over a five-year period. The chairman was Dr. William Darrach, but Dr. May Ayres Burgess, a trained educator and statistician was actually in charge of the work.

The committee was naturally comprised of representatives of the three national nursing associations, the National League of Nursing Education, the American Nurses' Association, and the National Organization for Public Health Nursing, and also representatives from the American Medical Association, the American Hospital Association, and the American Public Health Association. Besides these there were representatives of the general public and educators. Miss Mary M. Roberts, editor of *The American Journal of Nursing,* placed the columns of this nursing publication at the disposal of the committee.

The committee worked for about seven years finding facts which were published in three reports. The first, a preliminary report was *Nurses, Patients, and Pocket-*

books, which appeared in 1928. In 1934 *An Activity Analysis of Nursing,* a partial report comprising the studies of Ethel Johns and Blanche Pfefferkorn was published. The final report was *Nursing Schools Today and Tomorrow,* which goes into great detail concerning all the problems involved.

FINDINGS OF THE COMMITTEE

The grading of nursing schools, which was the original purpose of the committee, was not carried out by this committee. In the beginning it was thought that without personal visits to each school by the Grading Committee a just grading would not be feasible, and such a scheme would be too expensive. Later, questionnaires were sent out to the schools and, after a study of these, each school was shown how it stood in relation to other schools. In 1932 a second survey of the schools proceeded along similar lines. The first questionnaire brought to light a great many facts—some of them new even to the trustees of the nursing schools—concerning requirements, equipment, and costs. The result was that many smaller schools decided their effort was not worth the cost and the schools were discontinued. Others realized their defects and had them remedied, with the gratifying results that they were revealed in the second survey.

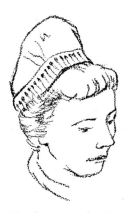

Johns Hopkins graduate nurse

Although the immediate results may not have been as striking as they would have been by grading schools as the medical schools had been graded, this analysis had a profound effect upon the schools during the next ten years, and reforms of various kinds were greatly supported by it. The actual grading of schools was later started by the Accrediting Committee. It was recommended that courses in nursing schools should be on a college level, that entrance requirements for schools of nursing and for colleges should be similar, that close cooperation between the schools should be encouraged, and that they should advance along similar but not identical lines, lest nurses' preparation be frozen; there were still many problems to be solved by experiments. It was also pointed out that improved standards of instruction would lead to improved and greater opportunities for the nurse.

In a practical way the survey inquired minutely into what actual nursing was in the eyes of those who could form an opinion on the question, such as hospital administrators, nurses, doctors, and patients. It also studied the conditions of work, including working hours, remuneration, and opportunities for advancement.

The practical results were the elimination of inferior schools and a temporary decrease in the number of students admitted, with nine-tenths of the schools admitting only high school graduates. The decrease in the number of students led to more graduate nurses being employed in the hospitals. The instruction passed into better qualified hands. Also the entire course is gradually being fitted to the students' needs rather than to the hospitals' requirements.

In this whole reform movement the American Nurses' Association and the National League of Nursing Education have worked closely together. In order to further improve this coordination the NLNE has since 1932 acted as the educational department of the ANA.

ACCREDITING OF SCHOOLS OF NURSING

The Committee on the Grading of Nursing Schools did not, as pointed out, actually grade schools as medical schools had been graded into A, B, and C schools. Too much material had to be studied and evaluated because of the great variety of standards and working conditions found in schools in the United States. However, all this study did lead eventually to the accrediting of nursing schools being undertaken as a project of the National League of Nursing Education.

The aims that were formulated by the Accrediting Committee were stated as follows:

1. To stimulate through accrediting practices the general improvement of nursing education and nursing practice in the United States.
2. To help those responsible for the administration of schools of nursing to improve their schools.
3. To give public recognition to schools that voluntarily seek and are deemed worthy of professional accreditation.
4. To publish a list of accredited schools for the purpose of guidance of prospective students in their choice of schools of nursing and to aid secondary schools and colleges in their guidance programs.
5. To serve as a guide to state accrediting agencies in further defining their standards for recognition of schools and to promote interstate relationships in professional registering of nurses.
6. To make available to institution administrators, students or graduate nurses advanced standing information that will help in evaluating credentials.
7. To provide information which may be made available to lay and professional groups for purpose of developing an understanding of the ideals, objectives, and needs of nursing education.*

The Accrediting Committee worked hard on standards for the evaluation of nursing schools. The school, as a whole, was to be judged, and the list of accredited schools would be those that had satisfactorily met the criteria set up by the committee. The

---

*Editorial: Field work of the Accrediting Committee begins, American Journal of Nursing **38**: 461-462, April, 1958.

Accrediting Committee would visit schools at their request and examine them. The individual school would pay the cost of such evaluation, and the individual school must apply to the committee for accreditation. In 1941 the first list of schools accredited by the National League of Nursing Education was published. Although the war slowed down the work of the committee, it did not entirely stop it; however, because of lack of finances and lack of personnel, the program moved rather slowly during the war years.

CONCLUSION

The period between World Wars I and II is considered by many people as an armistice. However, in the United States the wish of the people to do away with warlike activities as soon after any war as possible was observed in, among other things, the reduction of nurses in the Army and Navy Corps during the 1920's and 1930's.

All surveys that were made during this period pointed to the fact that the nursing profession was aware that it needed to change in order to meet, on the one hand, demands being made by the community for good nursing service and, on the other hand, demands being made by prospective students for a better professional course. A monograph, *Nursing as a Profession,* prepared by Dr. Esther Lucile Brown under the auspices of the Russell Sage Foundation, published in 1936 and revised in 1940, focused attention on some of the problems such as the control of nursing education. In 1936 the National League of Nursing Education published a manual, *Essentials of a Good School of Nursing.* In the same year in cooperation with the Division on Nursing of the Council of the American Hospital Association and a committee of the League, a manual called *Essentials of Good Hospital Nursing Service* was published. These publications pointed out that the major aims of nursing schools and nursing services are different and that these differences must be planned for in the organizations and programs of each.

One of the great handicaps in carrying out some of these programs in nursing education was lack of trained personnel. Again the League tried to help schools and nurses all over the country by publishing, in 1933 a manual, *The Nursing School Faculty: Duties, Qualifications and Preparation of Its Members*. This was revised in 1946. The curriculum in schools of nursing was being readjusted to meet the modern situation. More emphasis was placed on the social sciences. The preventive and social aspects were being integrated in the clinical programs, as well as were mental hygiene and

health teaching. More community experiences were recommended for all students. All of these changes brought up the question of cost. A study made jointly by a committee of the League and the American Nurses' Association resulted in a pamphlet, *Administrative Cost Analysis for Nursing Service and Nursing Education,* published in 1940. The accrediting program of the League was progressing, and collegiate programs were increasing in number. More money, although not nearly enough, was being made available for nursing education, from private endowments and from public sources. This then was the situation at the beginning of World War II.

Questions and study projects for unit five

1. What were some of the outstanding developments in nursing in the period between World Wars I and II?
2. How has the Committee on the Grading of Nursing Schools affected the entire progress of nursing?
3. What has been the development of endowed schools of nursing in this country? What are their greatest contributions to nursing?
4. Describe the accrediting of schools of nursing.
5. In what areas has the Federal Government developed nursing services? Describe them.
6. Show how developments in medicine, public health, and other related social activities in the community affected nursing between World Wars I and II.
7. Make an annotated bibliography of recent articles appearing in *The American Journal of Nursing, Nursing Outlook, Nursing Research,* and any other journals available in your library relating to the discussion in this unit.

References for unit five

Accrediting moves forward, American Journal of Nursing 39:647-648, June, 1939.

Brown, Esther Lucile: Nursing as a profession, ed. 2, New York, 1940, Russell Sage Foundation.

Darrach, William: Implications for nursing in the findings of the Grading Committee, National League of Nursing Education, New York, 1932, pp. 53-60.

Deming, Dorothy: The practical nurse, New York, 1947, The Commonwealth Fund.

Gelinas, Agnes: Nursing and nursing education, New York, 1946, The Commonwealth Fund.

Green, Margaret, Vendegrift, Willie, and Bouwhuis, Clara: Progress and development of the Veterans Administration Nursing Service (mimeographed outline), August, 1948, Washington, D.C., Veterans Administration.

Heinzelman, Ruth, and Deming, Dorothy: How Federal Civil Service works, American Journal of Nursing 46:319, May, 1946; 46:379, June, 1946.

Hodgson, Violet H.: Public health nursing in industry, New York, 1933, The Macmillan Co.

Investigation of problems in nursing education, Nursing Education Bulletin, new series no. 4, New York, 1941, Bureau of Publications, Teachers College, Columbia University.

Koch, Harriett Berger: Militant angel, New York, 1951, The Macmillan Co.

National League of Nursing Education: Annual reports and proceedings, from 1933 on, and other publications including:

A curriculum for schools of nursing, 1927.

Administrative cost analysis for nursing service and nursing education (in cooperation with the American Hospital Association), 1940.

Curriculum guide for schools of nursing, 1937.

Essentials of a good school of nursing, 1942.

Fundamentals of administration in schools of nursing, 1940.

Manual of essentials of a good hospital nursing service (pamphlet, in cooperation with the American Hospital Association), 1942.

Nursing school faculty: duties, qualifications, and preparation of its members, 1933.

Nursing and nursing education in the United States. Report of the Committee for the Study of Nursing Education and Report of a survey by Josephine Goldmark, New York, 1923, The Macmillan Co.

Nursing schools today and tomorrow. Final report of the Committee on the Grading of Nursing

Schools, New York, 1934, Committee on the Grading of Nursing Schools.

Petry, Lucile: One hundred fifty years of service, American Journal of Nursing **48**:434-435, July, 1948.

Stewart, Isabel M.: The Association of Collegiate Schools of Nursing, American Journal of Nursing **36**:45-47, January, 1936.

Stewart, Isabel M.: The philosophy of the collegiate school of nursing, American Journal of Nursing **40**:1033-1036, September, 1940.

Stewart, Isabel M.: The Indian Service in Alaska, American Journal of Nursing **42**:1114, October, 1942.

Stewart, Isabel M.: The education of nurses, New York, 1943, The Macmillan Co.

Twenty-five years of nursing education in Teachers College, 1899-1925, Teachers College Bulletin, seventeenth series no. 3, New York, 1926, Bureau of Publications, Columbia University.

Vreeland, Ellwynne M.: Fifty years of nursing in the Federal Government nursing services, American Journal of Nursing **50**:626, 1950.

Wiedenbach, Ernestine: Toward educating 130 million people, American Journal of Nursing **40**:13-18, January, 1940.

Witte, Frances W.: Opportunities in graduate education for men nurses, American Journal of Nursing **34**:133, 1934.

Nursing during World War II

"In the continuing world struggle between dictatorship and democracy, it is important to study and to reevaluate the lessons that have been learned in periods of national emergency. One of these is that democracies are able to mobilize their resources to achieve a mission in which all citizens are united.

"The nurses of this country—and those who worked with them in planning, organizing, and directing their voluntary mobilization in World War II—may well be proud that the unprecedented needs for nursing services both in the war theaters and at home were met. Contributing in a major way to this achievement was the United States Cadet Nurse Corps."*

*United States Cadet Nurse Corps, 1943-1948, Federal Security Agency, United States Public Health Service, Washington, D. C., 1950, Government Printing Office, p. v.

Chapter 22

The National Nursing Council

The United States was not actively engaged in World War II until the end of 1941. However, by the middle of 1940, the Nursing Council of National Defense (forerunner of the National Nursing Council for War Service, Inc.) was organized by the six national nursing organizations. Julia C. Stimson was president, and Alma Scott was secretary. These six national nursing organizations were the American Nurses' Association, the National League of Nursing Education, the Association of Collegiate Schools of Nursing, the National Organization for Public Health Nursing, the American Red Cross Nursing Service, and the National Association of Colored Graduate Nurses. One of the main purposes of this Council was to serve as a coordinating agency made up of representatives from professional nursing organizations and later representatives from hospital and medical groups and the general public. The major activities that began at once included recruitment of student nurses and the classification of all graduate nurses in the country as to their availability for military service. Under the direction of the Nursing Division, Procurement and Assignment Service, War Manpower Commission, considerations of whether the nurses were essential on the home front were made. The Council cooperated with the Red Cross in recruiting nurses for the Army and Navy Nurse Corps.

INVENTORY OF NURSES

The national inventory of nursing personnel showed that there were about 100,000 nurses under 40 years of age and unmarried, who were potential recruits for the Red Cross Nursing Service, first reserve. This national survey also revealed an acute shortage of nurses. In July, 1941, through the efforts of the National Nursing Council and the Committee on Educational Policies and Resources and with the cooperation of the United States Public Health Service, under the sponsorship of Representative Frances Payne Bolton of Ohio, Public Law 146 was passed by Congress. This provided for the first Government funds for the education of nurses for national defense, and under the terms of the Act, 1,000 graduate nurses were given postgraduate preparation and 2,500 inactive nurses were given refresher courses. Over 200 basic schools of nursing were given financial assistance, which enabled them to increase their facilities and their enrollment. During 1942 the Council worked in cooperation with the Armed Forces trying to meet the demand. Recruitment was stimulated by advertising, and schools were helped in adopting an accelerated program. State

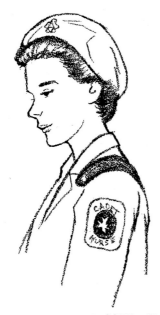

Cadet nurse—World War II

and local councils were given assistance in recruiting graduate and student nurses. During this period the Council's main financial support came from the Kellogg Foundation. The Milbank Memorial Foundation also helped as did the professional nursing organizations.

Early in 1942 the plan that eventually produced the United States Cadet Nurse Corps was discussed, and in July the bill that has become known as the Bolton Act became a law. The main purpose of this Act was to prepare nurses in adequate numbers for the Armed Forces, Government and civilian hospitals, health services, and war industries, through appropriations to institutions qualified to give such preparation. The program was carried out by a newly created Department of Nursing Education in the United States Public Health Service, with Miss Lucile Petry as Chief Director, responsible to Surgeon General Parran.

LOCAL NURSING COUNCILS

The National Nursing Council for War Service, Inc., stimulated the organization of local nursing councils for war service. Dis-

trict and state nursing associations assumed leadership of these councils and provided a channel for better distribution of professional nurses and auxiliary help for military and civilian nursing needs. Through these councils the needs and resources of communities all over the country were studied, in many instances for the first time. A great deal of help was given to the local groups by the National League of Nursing Education and by the Nursing Division of the United States Public Health Service. The National Council had given a great deal of attention to the training and use of practical nurses and to the training of nurses' aides. Working with the Red Cross Nursing Service, more than 100,000 nurses were actually certified during the war, and more than 200,000 nurses' aides were recruited and trained all over the country. As the war went on, the National Nursing Council for War Service, Inc., had representatives from the six national nursing organizations already mentioned and in addition included representatives from the Council of Federal Nurse Services; the Division of Nursing Education, United States Public Health Service; Nursing Division, Procurement and Assignment Service, War Manpower Commission; Subcommittee on Nursing, Health, and Medical Committee; International Council of Nurses; the American Hospital Association; and members-at-large. All during the war the National Council provided a splendid way of integrating and coordinating the programs of organized nursing and of fulfilling the war needs, both civilian and military.

CONCLUSION

In 1943 when the Federal nursing programs were established, the National Council members voted to keep the Council incorporated and active for the duration of the war and six months thereafter. Soon after V-J Day the Kellogg Foundation guaranteed to finance the National Council programs through the middle of 1946. The name was changed to the National Nursing Council.

Chapter 23

The Federal Government and the
financing of nursing education

The participation of the Federal Government and the financing of nursing education culminated in the Cadet Nurse Corps. This participation was made possible by the Bolton Act (sponsored by Mrs. Frances Payne Bolton, Congresswomen from Ohio who had been interested for years in nursing education) which was passed in July, 1942. However, a great deal of planning and work had been done before July, 1943. The need for more nurses had been apparent long before Pearl Harbor. In early 1940 nursing organizations, Government agencies, hospital administrators, and interested people in the community were beginning to think and to plan toward alleviating the nurse shortage. The needs of the country had been defined as follows:

1. To step up recruitment of student nurses.
2. To educate further and better prepare graduate nurses.
3. To induce professionally inactive nurses to return to service and if necessary to take refresher courses.
4. To train and use voluntary nurses' aides under professional supervision.*

---

*Federal Security Agency, United States Public Health Service: United States Cadet Nurse Corps, 1943-1948, Washington, D. C., 1950, Government Printing Office, p. 4.

The first national inventory of nurses was taken in 1941, directed by Pearl McIver of the United States Public Health Service and largely financed by that agency. The cost of the survey was $100,000, of which the American Red Cross contributed $5,000 and the Health and Medical Committee $10,000. This inventory showed that in 1941 there were 289,286 registered nurses in the United States. Of these, 171,055 were actively practicing nursing.

FEDERAL AID BEGINS

During World War I the Army had its own school of nursing, and the Vassar Training Camp helped to increase the number of nurses. It was felt, however, that similar efforts would not be adequate during World War II. As a result the Federal Government appropriated more than $175,000,-000 for nursing education during World War II. Most of this was used for student nurses in the Cadet Corps. The first proposal for Federal aid resulted in $1,200,000 being appropriated in the Labor-Federal Security Agency Appropriation Act of 1942, seventy-seventh Congress. This Act provided for three types of education: (1) refresher courses for inactive registered nurses, (2) postgraduate education in special fields for graduate nurses, and (3) increased student enrollment in basic nursing schools. The Surgeon General of the United States Public Health Service had authority to establish regulations for the administration and allotment of funds. This was two years before the creation of the Cadet Nurse Corps. Institutions offering postgraduate training had to meet standards equal to those recommended by the National League of Nursing Education and the Association of Collegiate Schools of Nursing. Criteria for standards were those published by the National League of Nursing Education in *Essentials of a Good School of Nursing* and *Essentials of a Good Hospital Nursing Service*. Schools of nursing associated with hospitals having a daily average of 100 or more patients in the four basic services were eligible to apply for aid. These funds were used for tuition scholarships for the maintenance of students added to the normal enrollment for the school, for necessary additional instructors and instructional facilities, and also for affiliation in special services. Funds could not be used for the construction of buildings but could be used for securing additional living quarters. Cash allowances to students were not provided at this time although they were later under the Cadet Corps.

CADET NURSE CORPS

The Bolton Act became law on July 1, 1943. It provided for a uniformed Cadet Nurse Corps and for grants for postgraduate education. Any state-accredited school was eligible to apply for funds, provided a three-year course was accelerated to thirty months. Under the Act the school arranged for senior Cadets to serve in either a Federal hospital or other health agency. The Federal Government paid for tuition, fees, and maintenance of students for the first nine months of training. An initial appropriation of $65,-000,000 was begun July, 1943.

This program was administered in the United States Public Health Service under the Surgeon General. In order to handle the administration, a Division of Nursing Education was established in July, 1943, with Lucile Petry Director of this new division. Some of the outstanding nurses who worked with her in this program were Eugenia K. Spalding, Mary J. Dunn, and Pearl McIver. With this accelerated program the following regulations were established to maintain standards. The school must:

1. Be state accredited.
2. Be connected with a hospital approved by the American College of Surgeons or with a hospital of equivalent standards.
3. Maintain adequate institutional facilities and personnel.
4. Provide adequate clinical experiences in the four basic services—medicine, surgery, pediatrics, obstetrics.
5. Provide maintenance and a stipend of $30 for all senior Cadet nurses or arrange for their requested transfer to federal or other hospitals.
6. Provide satisfactory living facilities and an adequate health service for students.
7. Provide for an accelerated program.
8. Restrict its hours of practice.*

Standards devised by the National League of Nursing Education were used. The goal of 65,000 new students for the year was set, and a total of almost 170,000 cadets joined the Corps during its short existence. Of these, 65,986 withdrew before finishing the course. This was a mortality of about 33%, which was slightly lower than that reported for all students enrolled in schools during the same period and only 4% higher than the prewar rate. The reasons for withdrawal were the usual ones—some slightly accentuated by the war—homesickness, marriage, failure in studies, health reasons, and, of course, when hostilities ceased many left the program.

One of the main objects of the Cadet Nurse Corps was to accelerate the length of the course. Acceleration of such programs

---

*Federal Security Agency, United States Public Health Service: United States Cadet Corps, 1943-1948, Washington, D. C., 1950, Government Printing Office, p. 23.

had become common during the war—for example, medicine and engineering. Because many states required thirty-six months for graduation, planners for the accelerated program were faced with a dilemma. The compromise made was that a senior Cadet period of six months be spent in a military or essential hospital or health agency. The acceleration of the program resulted in a great deal of discussion both during and after the war. Many leaders believed that two years was adequate time for the nurse course, if so-called noneducational duties were kept to a minimum. Others believed that the shortened period was justified only during the emergency.

The Bolton Act provided that the program should be open to all regardless of race, color, or creed. It is interesting to note that twenty-one Negro schools of nursing participated in the program and that thirty-eight other schools admitted Negro girls as regular students. This precedent has continued in most schools that participated during the war.

With the great increase in the number of nursing students, dormitory facilities were vitally needed. Under the Lanham Act (National Defense Office) funds were made available for living quarters, libraries, and class and demonstration rooms in nursing schools. It is interesting to note that $29,-657,785 was appropriated for this purpose. At the end of the war, many schools of nursing had better physical facilities than they had ever had before.

The Nurse Training Act of 1943 created the Cadet Nurse Corps and also provided for the continuation of refresher and postgraduate training of graduate nurses, which had been begun as part of the war effort. These programs for graduate nurses had to meet the standards of or be approved by the National League of Nursing Education, the National Organization for Public Health Nursing, and the Association of Collegiate Schools of Nursing.

CONCLUSION

When Japan surrendered in August, 1945, recruitment to the Cadet Corps was terminated at once, and no more students were admitted after October 15, 1945. Provision was made for students already in training to complete their course, and the last Cadets were graduated in June, 1948. In the Cadet Nurse Corps, 169,443 student nurses had been enrolled in 1,125 nursing schools; of these, 124,065 had graduated.

Chapter 24

Military nursing

Nursing in World War II differed from nursing in any other war, as do all activities of war. Tremendous advances in medical science and the widespread activities of a great variety of fighting men presented a challenge and a great responsibility to the Army and Navy Nurse Corps. In World War II the Army and Navy nurses served in every part of the world. World War II has often been described as a total war, and for that reason the nurse had to be trained under combat conditions and had to know how to adapt her technics to meet changing situations. The medical department worked as a team so successfully that 97% of all casualties were saved, and the death rate from diseases was reduced to one-twentieth of what it had been in World War I. Full military recognition was given to the nurses during World War II in 1944, and they became a permanent part of the regular military force. Colonel Julia O. Flikke, Superintendent of the Army Nurse Corps from 1937 to 1942, was the first woman to be a colonel in the United States Army. In 1942 she was succeeded by Colonel Florence A. Blanchfield. Training for all military nursing personnel was the responsibility of the Office of the Surgeon General. Direction of the Navy Nurse Corps was under Chief of the Bureau of Medicine and Surgery.

With the outbreak of World War II, members of the Navy Nurse Corps found themselves in the center of initial activity. When the Japanese attacked and took Guam in December, 1941, five nurses were taken prisoner. Just about one year later they were returned to the United States aboard the exchange ship *Gripsholm*. At Manila eleven nurses were captured in 1942 and were held as prisoners of war for thirty-seven months.

By July, 1942, a total of 1,778 nurses were on duty with the Navy; 827 were United States Navy, and 951 were United States Naval Reserve. In that year legislation was passed giving Navy nurses relative rank, from ensign through lieutenant commander. The base pay for an ensign was increased from $90 to $150 a month. Sue Dauser was Superintendent of the Navy Nurse Corps at that time and took oath as its first captain. She was the first woman captain of the American Navy.

Early in 1944 student nurses under the Cadet program reported to Naval hospitals to begin a six months' practice period during their senior year. By 1945 the Navy Nurse Corps had increased to over 11,000, including both regular and reserve Corps members on active duty. In the United States they served in forty Naval hospitals, 176 dispensaries, and six hospital Corps schools. They served aboard twelve hospital ships and at land base establishments in many foreign countries.

In 1944 the destroyer *U.S.S. Higbee* was launched. This was the first combat ship to be named for a woman of the service.

When the surrender was signed aboard the *U.S.S. Missouri,* Navy nurses were stationed aboard three hospital ships of the Third Fleet, waiting to go ashore to Allied prisoners and to help evacuate them from Japan.

In line with other military developments, training for the air evacuation of casualties became increasingly important, and the first Naval school for the instruction of nurses in the air evacuation of casualties was opened. Instruction and developments during World War II were rapid and followed developments in general Naval science as indicated by the over-all military plans and programs.

All during the war basic training or indoctrination courses were given to nurses in the Army and Navy. Education in various nursing specialties, particularly in such areas as psychiatric nursing, was provided as needed. It was not until April, 1947, through Public Law 36, that a permanent Nurse Corps for the Army and Navy was established by the Government.

This Act has removed the need for the Red Cross to maintain a roster of reserve nurses for the Army and Navy. The Red Cross nursing program has been organized since the end of the war. At present the Red Cross program has the following objectives: continuing development of nursing service for times of epidemic disease or other national emergency, voluntary community service such as teaching home nursing courses, and the development of the National Blood Bank Program of the American Red Cross.

RECRUITMENT PROBLEMS

In the period immediately before the outbreak of war there had been discussion among nursing leaders and the Surgeon General of the advisability of having either an Army school of nursing or some kind of summer training camp for nurses similar to the Vassar Training Camp of World War I. Neither of these ideas seemed to be completely satisfactory, although in the summer of 1941, Bryn Mawr College contributed its campus and plant to this project, in cooperation with the Red Cross. However, only thirty students instead of an anticipated two hundred registered for the course. This country was not yet at war, and enthusiasm for such activities had not developed.

In the summer of 1941 some American nurses went overseas with the American Red Cross–Harvard Field Hospital Unit. This unit was intended primarily to function in England as a research center in communicable diseases; when fully staffed it included sixty-three nurses. In crossing to England five nurses and a house mother were lost because of German submarine activity. The bombing of England had increased during 1941, and many of these American nurses worked in British hospitals and air-raid shelters.

The Red Cross, in cooperation with the Office of Civilian Defense, developed a program for training nurses' aides. This program was actually carried out by Red Cross chapters all over the country and greatly relieved the pressure in civilian hospitals. During World War II the Red Cross certified almost all of the over 77,000 nurses who served with the Armed Forces. The need for extending the nurses' aide program during World War II was evident. The Red Cross Volunteer Special Service, in cooperation with the Office of Civilian Defense, recruited and trained more than 200,000 nurses' aides. This training course supplied the country with a large group of volunteer nurses' aides who gave invaluable service in relieving the shortages in hospitals and health programs that resulted from the large numbers of nurses serving in the Armed Forces.

Instruction was given in two home nursing programs: the Home Care of the Sick, and Mother and Baby Care. Many of the teaching technics that were being used successfully in industry to teach skills safely and quickly were used in this instruction.

The Nursing Service of the Red Cross during World War II also recruited nurses to serve in the blood collection centers, which had been established to procure blood to meet both military and civilian needs.

After Pearl Harbor the number of professional nurses enrolling with the Red Cross for work with the Armed Forces increased rapidly. At times there was some resentment on the part of nurses who did not understand the background about why they had to enter the Armed Forces through the Red Cross. The Surgeon General's Office had stated repeatedly that it did not want to assume the responsibility of recruiting nurses; the situation was clarified a great deal in 1942 when the Surgeon General's Office made an announcement that the Red Cross

was the official recruiting agency of the Army Nurse Corps. The Navy Nurse Corps did not work as closely with the Red Cross as the Army Nurse Corps did, and by the end of 1946 the Navy Nurse Corps had taken over the processing of its own applicants. In spite of all these activities the number of nurses actually in service lagged behind the number needed. Although in the spring of 1944 the goal of 40,000 nurses for the Army had been reached, the Surgeon General was already requesting 10,000 more. The critical situation on the battlefields was acknowledged by the leaders of this country as never before, and in January, 1945, when he gave his annual message to Congress, the President requested a draft of nurses. Three days later a draft bill was introduced into the House of Representatives. The nursing organizations at once took a stand in favor of a National Service Act for

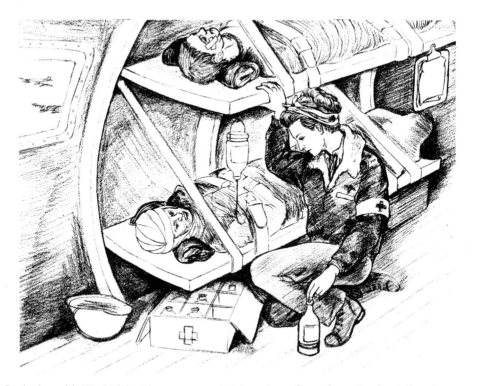

Beginning with World War II, many wounded have been flown from the front lines to permanent hospitals well away from the battle zone.

all men and women, not only for nurses. The bill was discussed for three months, during which time the Red Cross Nursing organizations and others made a supreme effort to recruit an adequate number of nurses. Fortunately, the war in Europe came to an end, and in May, two weeks after V-E Day, action on the bill was dropped.

CONCLUSION

During World War II nursing in every branch of the Armed Forces matured, and the Army, the Navy, and the Air Force found that more and more nurses were proving themselves in the medical and health areas of their respective military programs.

It was not until April, 1947, through Public Law 36, that a permanent Nurse Corps for the Army, Navy, and Air Force was established by the Government. This removed the need for the Red Cross maintaining a roster of reserve nurses for the Armed Forces. Therefore, since May, 1947, the Red Cross Nursing program has been different from the one that existed prior to this time.

After World War II the G. I. Bill of Rights made it possible for many nurses who had served during the war to attend college and to become better qualified as leaders in the field. More recently the Federal Government, through Public Law 911, has provided grants to graduate nurses and to schools so that an increasing number of graduate nurses can become better prepared for the demands made of them.

Questions and study projects for unit six

1. Discuss the National Nursing Council for War Service, Inc. Why was it organized, what were its achievements, and what did it lead on to?
2. Discuss the association of the Red Cross with the Army and Navy Nurse Corps during World War II.
3. How did the National Nursing Council for War Services, Inc., function?
4. Discuss the activities of the nurse in World War II and compare these activities, both civilian and military, with nursing during other wars. Why was World War II different?
5. Make an annotated bibliography of recent articles appearing in *The American Journal of Nursing, Nursing Outlook, Nursing Research,* and any other journals available in your library relating to the discussion in this unit.

References for unit six

Archard, Theresa: G. I. Nightingale, New York, 1945, W. W. Norton & Co., Inc.

Army Nurse, United States Army Nurse Corps, Washington, D. C., 1944.

Baehr, George: Mobilization of the nursing profession for war. Proceedings of the thirty-third convention of the American Nurses' Association, New York, 1942, American Nurses' Association, p. 153.

Bolton Bill, American Journal of Nursing 43:617, July, 1943.

Bradley, LaVerne: Women in uniform. Insignia and decorations of the United States Armed Forces, revised edition, Washington, D. C., 1944, National Geographic Society, pp. 159-98.

Connelly, Ellen H.: Shipmates in white, American Journal of Nursing 49:204, April, 1949.

Cooper, Page: Navy nurse, New York, 1946, McGraw-Hill Book Co., Inc.

Flikke, Julia O.: Nurses in action, Philadelphia, 1943, J. B. Lippincott Co.

Marsh, Penny, and Lee, Ginger: Wartime nurses, New York, 1943, Dodd, Mead & Co., Inc.

Miller, Jean Dupont: Shipmates in white, New York, 1944, Dodd, Mead & Co., Inc.

National Nursing Planning Committee, American Journal of Nursing 45:513, 1945.

Newell, Hope: The History of the National Nursing Council, New York, 1951, National Organization for Public Health Nursing.

Nurse Draft Bill passed by the House, American Journal of Nursing 45:255, 1945.

Nurses United for War Services, Public Health Nursing 36:340, 1944.

Nursing needs and nursing resources, American Journal of Nursing 44:1044, 1944.

Nursing in War Manpower Commission (with organization chart), American Journal of Nursing 43:741, 1943.

Redmond, Juanita: I served on Bataan, Philadelphia, 1943, J. B. Lippincott Co.

Schaffter, Dorothy: What comes of training women for war, Washington, D. C., 1948, American Council on Education.

United States Cadet Nurse Corps, and other Federal nurse training programs, United States Public Health Service pub. no. 38, Washington, D. C., 1950, United States Government Printing Office.

War Manpower Commission; Classification, clearance and appeals procedure, American Journal of Nursing 43:885, 1943.

Unit **seven**

Contemporary developments and trends

"The leaders of the nursing profession were faced with a serious dilemma. Since the days of Florence Nightingale, they had insisted that nurses, and nurses alone, must determine how to discharge their responsibilities to society. Although every profession has the ultimate responsibility and autonomy for determining its own role, the leadership in nursing was becoming increasingly aware that many problems with which they had to grapple were only in part professional and not subject to assessment and solution by nurses alone. Because many crucial issues had major ramifications in medicine, government, education, administration, and economics, it seemed wise to elicit the assistance of experts in these other fields.*

---

*The Committee on the Function of Nursing. Eli Ginzberg, and others. A program for the nursing profession, New York, 1941, The Macmillan Co., pp. vii, viii.

Chapter 25

Major trends affecting
health care

The community's interest in matters of health has always been accelerated by war; even when the acute war need is past, that interest is found to be at a higher level in all matters of health at the end of a war than at the beginning. Since World War II, the field of public health has expanded in many directions. Many communities have increased the size and scope of existing health facilities or have built additional ones with the aid of funds from both voluntary and governmental sources. The bulk of the middle class American population is covered by some form of health insurance either to pay possible hospitalization expenses or to provide for payment of other medical expenses. Mass media bombard us with information and misinformation about health and illness. All of these factors contribute to an increase in the utilization of existing health facilities and a public demand for quality.

MAJOR TRENDS

Major factors influencing health care and the provisions of health services are among the following.

1. There has been a surge of knowledge within the health sciences concerning people and diseases. This increased knowledge has led to technological development which refines the quality of care that can be provided for people but makes the administration of that care far more complex than it was ten or fifteen years ago.

2. A true revolutionary change has taken place in diagnosis and treatment, resulting from the numbers of people outside the medical field who have contributed to scientific discoveries of biochemistry, technological equipment, and the psychosocial aspects of medicine. This is particularly true of many of the newer drugs, beginning with the discovery of penicillin by Sir Alexander Fleming, a biologist. Renal dialysis, the heart-lung machine, various monitoring devices, closed circuit television, computers, and radioactive isotopes are only a sampling of the complex treatments and equipment invented or perfected by nonmedical workers and used in present-day hospitals.

3. The provision of health services has changed radically as a result of increased knowledge and the use of

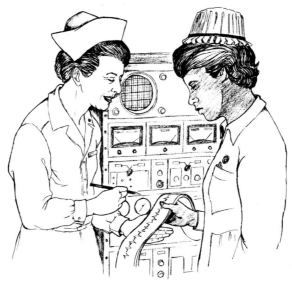

The nurse plays a vital role in those aspects dealing with patient care as the use of technological equipment increases.

newer technological devices. Utilization of the knowledge and management of the machines require rigorous scientific training of responsible health personnel.

4. A recent basic change in the way in which Americans view health has exerted a profound change on the provision of health services. When health is seen as a right, rather than a privilege, then society assumes an obligation to provide this service to its members, regardless of their ability to pay for it. The British Health Service exemplifies one form of this. In the United States, Medicare on the Federal level provides financial access to this right for all of our citizens over age 65. There has been discussion of proposing legislation which would provide similar facilities for dependent children as well. These forms of health insurance not only make care available to the particular citizens for whom it is designed, but also serve to upgrade the quality of the facilities of care in

many regions. Indirectly, therefore, all people are benefited through these official governmental actions.

5. Because of the nurse shortage, more and more schools of practical nursing have been established and continue to grow at an accelerated rate. These have been encouraged and supported by Federal funds. A whole corps of auxiliary personnel, such as aides and volunteers, has been added to the staff of hospital wards.

6. The pattern of incidence of patient illness has undergone vast change in the last generation. The emphasis in hospitals is upon early discharge. The patient's condition is followed by health workers including the public health nurse. The treatment of long-term illness is the utilization of outpatient and extended care facilities.

7. The patients' expectations have also changed. Because of effective means of communication, patients know more about particular diseases. The World Health Organization's concept

of health has become operational; we no longer think of health in terms of the absence of disease but as a state of physical, mental, and social well-being.

8. More people now receive direct medical supervision. In other words, more people are being cared for constantly. Almost all industrial plants have nurses educated to follow the entire work force. Colleges, for the most part, now have a medical officer. Grade school children are placed under supervision at the time they enter school, and their health records are kept for them through elementary school, high school, college, and at work. In the larger cities, these children have already been registered at well-baby clinics shortly after birth. Medicare now assures retired workers of the financial ability to continue to receive competent health supervision.

9. The continued emancipation of women has had its effect upon health care. Although more and more women enter the labor market, the opportunities for employment in service occupations are increasing. Unfortunately, the predominantly female occupation of nursing no longer has the first claim on young women it previously enjoyed. The percentage of eligible young women electing nursing as a career has steadily declined over the past decades from 7% in the 1950's to 5% in the 1960's. The Bureau of Labor Statistics of the Department of Labor projects an increase in the demand for workers in the health service industries of about 45% between 1966 and 1975 (from 3.7 to 5.35 million).

10. The phenomenon of the "college-bound" youth in America probably accounts for the tremendous growth of the junior/community colleges.

Growth of nursing programs within these institutions has been projected to increase 445% by 1970. Besides nursing, many other health careers have established educational programs under the aegis of the junior/-community college. The Department of Health, Education and Welfare lists twenty-seven categories of health workers, both professional and technical.

11. The population explosion which occurred following World War II gave great impetus to development of the family planning movement. Contraceptive technics had been available for a selected segment of the population prior to this time. As the number of babies being born increased, the desire on the part of society to limit the population explosion as well as the choice on the part of parents to space their children spurred the development of more effective technics as well as more universal dispersal of information about these technics.

These trends all demonstrate the dynamism of health care and the internal and external pressures upon nursing and other health services to change. What is true today most certainly will not be valid ten years from now. This compounds the existing internal struggle in nursing to identify its unique role within the health team and to differentiate the preparation and function of its various practitioners.

CONTEMPORARY SOCIAL AND HEALTH PROBLEMS

Between 1900 and 1952, the nation's population doubled; in the past fifteen years the birth rate has continued to increase; people are living longer. Statistics show that the number of individuals 65 years of age or over had grown from 3 to 11½ million and by 1960 had reached 15½ million. Hospital admissions in 1966 totalled over

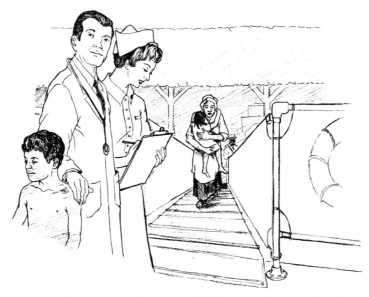

Health teams, such as those provided by project HOPE, expand good will and provide much needed medical care in less fortunate areas of the world.

29 million. In addition there were more than 100 million visits to outpatient and emergency departments.

This utilization of health agencies has been the result of health education, the growing confidence in hospitals by all people, the complicated medical and health treatments that necessitate a hospital environment in which to operate, and insurance and hospital plans that enable individuals to pay for hospital care. New medical technics and drugs have helped to shorten the average patient's stay in the hospital from eighteen to eight days. While in the hospital most patients need skilled nursing care.

Public health services have been extended in all communities; industrial nursing, school nursing, and bedside nursing in the home have increased as rapidly as trained personnel and institutions are available. The requirements of the military and the Veterans Administration continue to increase and make demands upon professional and nonprofessional nursing personnel.

Life expectancy in the United States has increased. With more individuals living to be over 60 years of age, the incidence of degenerative diseases is on the increase. The development of communicable disease control and better child welfare programs have resulted in a great decrease in contagious diseases. Such conditions as smallpox, diphtheria, and typhoid fever have been almost eliminated in many communities. Heart disease, cancer, and kidney disease rank high as the causes of death. Chronic illnesses associated with degenerative diseases are more frequent.

Changes in morbidity and mortality patterns mean that the nurse needs a different type of preparation now than twenty-five or fifty years ago. Prevention and better treatment are slowly taking the place of custodial care of the mentally ill. However, many states are still so hampered by the lack of finances, trained personnel, and adequate institutions that custodial care for the mentally ill and for patients with chronic illnesses still prevails. There has been a real reduction in maternal and infant mortality as well as improvement in the diagnosis and treatment of many heretofore incurable conditions. Chemotherapy has revolutionized the treatment of many severe illnesses.

The effects of President Truman's Commission to Study the Health Needs of the Nation are still being felt. A great deal of this report dealt with health personnel, that is, physicians, dentists, nurses, and paramedical technicians. This report emphasized the concept of the medical team with doctors and nurses serving as leaders of teams with other auxiliary medical workers and technicians. As medicine has become more specialized, a need has been created for workers with special education in many fields closely allied to medicine. With the expansion of preventive, psychiatric, and rehabilitative services has come a demand for auxiliary workers in these fields. As a result, there are more than thirty paramedical specialists, such as medical laboratory technicians, x-ray technicians, dietitians, physical therapists, speech therapists, medical record librarians, social workers, clinical psychologists, hospital administrators, and many others whose education ranges from one year after high school to several years after college. Such education is invariably expensive and often beyond the financial ability of an average student. The Federal government has assumed an increasing share of the costs of both professional and technical education in the health fields through direct scholarship aid as well as through indirect subsidization of both students and schools via project and construction grants and loans. Much of this Federal assistance has been provided through the Bureau of Health Manpower under the Health Professions Educational Assistance Act of 1963, the Nurse Training Act of 1964, and the Allied Health Professions Personnel Training Act of 1966. In the fiscal year 1967, Federal aid for health service personnel totaled $400 million.

One problem in all communities is that of providing adequate facilities and educating adequate personnel to use the facilities and to provide the type of medical health care we now know individuals and communities need.

Changes in the patterns of illness have created the need for not only a different kind of education but also a different type of hospital construction; for example, instead of hospitals for communicable diseases, more facilities are needed for extended care of the mentally and physically disabled and chronic custodial care.

One of the great difficulties in providing adequate care for everyone in the United States is that health workers and health facilities are located in the urban centers. A better distribution of health institutions and health personnel is a problem that is being studied by medical, health, and nursing organizations—state, regional, and Federal. To study this problem, the Hill-Burton Act, 1946, provided assistance to the states to plan and provide modern hospitals and public health facilities. States, with the help of the Federal Government, made studies, and Congress authorized an appropriation for the construction of hospital and allied facilities.

Not too long ago nurses, graduate and student, did all the nursing necessary in both hospital and community. Nursing was relatively simple and usually included personal hygiene measures and technics to make the patient comfortable, such as bathing, changing his position, and giving a few medications, usually by mouth. Nursing has increased in complexity as nurses have assumed such functions as the administration of parenteral medication, collection of specimens, and participation in the performance of complicated diagnostic tests as well as therapeutic procedures, all of which require increased vigilance and careful observation of the patient.

In order to carry out the increased number and variety of activities, more personnel are needed to help at the less technical level. Therefore, the practical nurse and the nurses' aide, the ward clerk, the unit manager, and the messenger have been added to the team. Until quite recently there was some resistance to the practical nurse. At first the practical nurse was an untrained

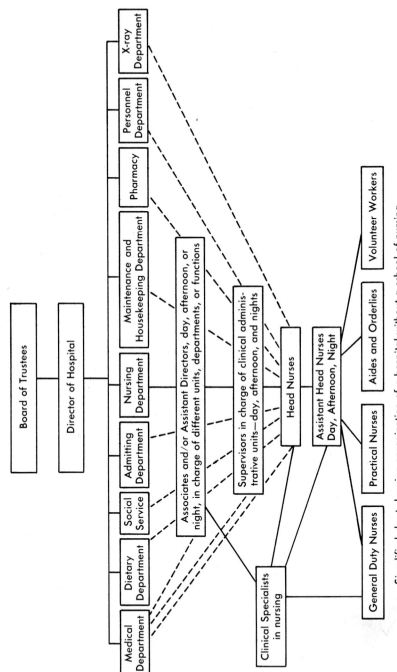

Simplified chart showing organization of a hospital without a school of nursing

person who, because of her aptitude for nursing and her interest in it, became a useful person in the hospital and community. As the duties given to the practical nurse increased, it became apparent that a formal course of education must be worked out and that this group should be licensed.

Since World War II the number of approved schools of practical nursing has increased nationally. Most of these have developed in the vocational department of the board of education. Many obtain funds from the Federal Government, as well as from the state, in order to develop a program. All of this instruction in approved schools for practical nursing is under the direction of professional nurses. Today all states have some type of licensure for nurses.

INFLUENCE OF HOSPITALS AS MAJOR HEALTH FACILITIES

In most public health work the hospital looms in the background either for diagnosis and treatment or for the care of specialized conditions. Even now the large majority of active nurses spent their lives in close contact with the hospital.

In the evolution of the hospital several influences operate with varying force at different periods.

1. The community has always found it expedient to isolate its members if they suffer from loathsome or contagious diseases; thus, pesthouses, leper houses, and lunatic asylums developed. To this day the motive of the isolation hospital is quite as much protection of society as it is care of the patient.
2. The second important motive is charity toward the sick, particularly the sick poor. This was an important motive as early as in the ancient Indian hospitals. It was all-important in the hospitals of the Middle Ages under the auspices of the Church and was strongly emphasized when nursing was "born" again a hundred years ago. It

was important to Miss Nightingale and those she inspired. In the modern hospital, personal charity is most apparent in the strictly denominational hospital; in the others, nondenominational, university, or government (city, state, or Federal) hospitals, the directly charitable relation has yielded to an impersonal acknowledgment that the community must look after its citizens when they are sick and cannot take care of themselves. It is a kind of twentieth century version of altruism, which, although less personal, may be more acceptable to the patient who receives it.

3. The third motive is the facilities for instruction that the hospital offers. Although doctors were not necessarily a part of the primitive hospital, they became increasingly important in it. The modern hospital is unthinkable without a medical staff. The establishment of medical schools within, or closely allied to, hospitals greatly stimulated the growth of hospitals. As medical training became more complicated, the demands on the hospital grew; today almost every outstanding hospital is committed to the training of doctors. A similar relationship of nursing schools to hospitals developed much later. Until recently, organized nursing education had been financed by hospitals.
4. The hospital is essential for expansion of medical knowledge. Originally a doctor grew wiser from personal experience supplemented by books. Thus, wisdom is acquired; however, the validity of clinical impressions must be tested before they can be accepted. It became necessary to rely not on individual scattered clinical impressions but on large numbers of cases observed under more or less similar conditions. The modern hospital has facilities for carrying out in-

vestigative procedures that would be impractical or impossible at home.

5. Finally, in recent years the best practice of medicine has required a large number of technical procedures that necessitate a specially constructed plant. It is difficult to arrange, outside the hospital a substitute for the modern operating room, x-ray department, clinical laboratory with all its branches, and the nutrition department. Although these departments have reached their present high state of development within the memory of living man, they have, nevertheless, grown to become one of the most important reasons for the existence of the modern hospital.

With all this, the hospital is an expensive business. Three billion dollars are invested in American hospitals, and the cost per patient is more than four times what it was fifty years ago. This increased cost of medical care has created a new problem, which has been subjected to repeated analysis. The old voluntary hospital, run entirely on gifts, is almost obsolete. Increasing costs threaten to exceed voluntary contributions, and increasing taxes prevent the accumulation of wealth, out of which gifts can be made. The hospital financed by local or Federal government has generally been restricted to providing care for the indigent; yet most people who become sick cannot pay the entire cost of the medical aid that they receive. The financial structure of hospitals is constantly changing to meet these difficulties; public funds are available to an increasing extent to fill the gap between the amount patients can pay and the cost of their care. The hospital is becoming a public service. On the other hand, attempts are being made to spread the cost over large groups of persons by group hospital insurance schemes. When each person pays a little each month, funds can be accumulated to carry the load for the individual when he is least able to shoulder it. During World War II and in the postwar period a great increase in community interest called attention to the need for volunteer workers. Individuals for the first time in history began to learn about their hospitals by working in them. Individuals who are asked to support hospitals naturally have become interested. They want to know how the hospital is being administered and believe they should have a share in knowing how their money, whether tax or voluntary contributions, is being spent.

Hospitals may be classified in two general ways—first by type of service offered and second by ownership or control. In 1951 the American Medical Association found that nongovernment, or private hospitals comprise almost 70% of the hospitals in this country and government hospitals, 30%. Church and religious groups have from pioneer days controlled and administered many of our hospitals. This is reflected by the national hospital organizations; the American Hospital Association, the Catholic Hospital Association, and the American Protestant Hospital Association. The modern hospital is a diagnostic, therapeutic, preventive, rehabilitative, and educational institution, as well as one carrying on the traditional functions of providing health facilities and services. With medical progress, specialization within the hospital has revolutionized hospital administration and construction. The chart on p. 176 shows the many different departments necessary in the modern hospital. All this has added tremendously to the cost of hospital care. So much money has been invested in the modern hospital that, unless very careful and skillful administration exists, the cost of medical care could be exorbitant.

The patient today knows about many new diagnostic and therapeutic aids and demands them; therefore, the modern hospital has to be equipped to give such service. The hospital has to meet standards set by the state, by the American Hospital Association, and by the American College of Surgeons. One of the most outstanding achievements of the American College of Surgeons has been hospital standardization. This movement, begun in 1918, was aimed at giving the patient the best professional, scientific, and humanitarian care possible. A survey made by the American College of Surgeons in 1944 showed that 80.6% surveyed met the high standards. The Catholic Hospital Association and the American Protestant Hospital Association cooperate in maintaining these standards. Because of advances in transportation, modern medical centers are usually located in large cities where not only professional personnel but also scientific and technical equipment are concentrated. Today, the large modern hospitals are usually situated in urban centers, with smaller hospitals in outlying towns, from which patients are brought for the more complicated treatments and surgical operations.

The educational and community functions of the modern hospital have been well expressed by a leading hospital administrator as:

1. Develop public understanding and appreciation of hospital service.
2. Foster an attitude of genuine good will on the part of the public toward the hospital.
3. Stimulate a more accurate analysis of community needs and institutional resources so that the hospital may assume its rightful place in the life of the community.
4. Promote a greater desire on the part of the personnel to understand the work of the hospital and to effect closer contact between the personnel and the public.
5. Cooperate with other health agencies in the community so as to meet more adequately the health and welfare needs of the community.
6. Clarify to the public and to governmental bodies the status of voluntary hospitals so that the many economic problems now being controversially discussed may be solved in the most desirable manner.
7. Effect a thorough understanding as to the legitimate reasons for hospital construction, make known the disadvantages of overhospitalization, and stimulate the greater use of existing hospital facilities.

8. Remove the influence of politics from governmentally owned and controlled institutions.
9. Explain the reasons for hospital standards —what they are, how they protect human life and promote safer and more adequate care of the sick and injured.
10. Encourage the public to look to national organizations cooperating with hospitals for information and guidance in problems of health and welfare.
11. Clarify to the public the position of the hospital as the principal source of skilled and continuous nursing so that it may be generally understood that this service is available to the community.
12. Improve the health and welfare conditions of the community by encouraging the use of hospital facilities in the periodic health examination.
13. Promote closer cooperation and integration of all hospitals in each community and entirely eliminate any spirit of competition.
14. Encourage the use of the hospital by people previously fearful of institutional care.
15. Stimulate voluntary contributions and public and private endowments.*

CONCLUSION

A dynamic society and a period when rapid change is taking place result in strain on existing institutions and professions. This is noted particularly in such traditional institutions as the hospital and such traditional professions as medicine and nursing. No longer is the old method of treating disease adequate and no longer is the old method of educating doctors and nurses satisfactory to meet the demands placed on these workers by society. Hospitals, health agencies, and professional organizations are striving hard to change in constructive ways in order to meet these needs. National and state medical, nursing, and health professions are constantly studying the activities of their workers and striving to adjust the educational qualifications so that they will be able to function more effectively in contemporary society.

*MacEachern, Malcolm T.: Hospital organization and management, Chicago, 1940, Physicians' Record Co., pp. 796-797.

Chapter 26

Contemporary nursing

The demand for nurses continues to outrun the supply. Increasing demands from hospitals and expanding community health services, industry, military services, and international programs have all contributed to this shortage. It is important for young people to know that opportunities in nursing are likely to continue and to expand in the coming years.

In 1963 the consultant group to the Surgeon General of the United States in forecasting the health needs of the nation in 1970 predicted that 850,000 nurses would be needed, including 300,000 with academic degrees. A little over 300,000 nurses were actively engaged in giving service to civilians in 1950. In 1962 the number was 550,000, but this number is probably inaccurate because it includes 70,000 part-time workers.

Since World War II, new hospitals have been built in many communities, and old hospitals have increased their facilities. It has not been uncommon to find that many institutions have not been able to expand as rapidly as needed because of the scarcity of nurses and other health personnel. Many agencies, both civilian and military, yearly report shortages. It must be remembered that the problem of nursing shortage is one of quality as well as quantity.

There are demands for nurses with the broad training that can be obtained in collegiate programs. Graduate programs equip individuals for leadership, particularly in administrative, supervisory, teaching, and clinical specializations. Because of the development of specialization in functional areas as well as in the clinical areas, great demands are placed upon nurses for additional education and experience. Thus, the young person wishing to function effectively today in any clinical area finds that he or she must take postgraduate work. It is an era of specialization, and the great wealth of information that must be mastered by anyone practicing in a special field necessitates education beyond what it is possible to give to any undergraduate nursing student. The effective nurse today must know a great deal more than the nurse of twenty-five years ago.

Newly discovered drugs and treatments, the implementation of the concept of the relationship between emotions and physical illness, and new knowledge about people and disease have necessitated programs of continuing education for all workers in the health fields.

In order to utilize to a better extent all professional workers, studies are being made to find out more effective ways of using all personnel to meet health needs. Practical

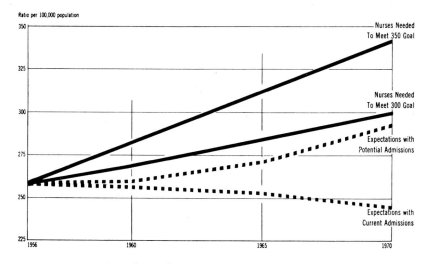

Matching the goals with expectations

(From Nurses for a Growing Nation, National League for Nursing, New York, N. Y.)

nurses, hospital aides, clerical workers, and other professional workers, such as dietitians, social workers, and occupational therapists, can often work on a team basis with the nurse and the doctor to provide better care than we have been accustomed to in the past.

The nurse shortage in 1953 was attributed to five major factors.

1. The shortage of young women in the population.
2. The increase among young women with home responsibilities.
3. Nurses' salaries and the cost of education.
4. Higher professional requirements.
5. The present utilization of professional nursing personnel.*

These factors were valid because of the maturation of the decreased number of "depression babies" from the early 1930's. However, at this time, although there is no shortage of young women in the popula-

tion, nursing is not attracting a proportionate number of young people.

In February, 1963, The Surgeon General's report identified the following as problems and reasons for the continuing shortage:

Too few schools are providing adequate education for nursing.

Not enough capable young people are being recruited to meet the demand.

Too few college-bound students are entering the nursing field.

More nursing schools are needed within colleges and universities.

The continuing lag in the social and economic status of nurses discourages people from entering the field and remaining active in it.

Available nursing personnel are not being fully utilized for effective patient care, including supervision and teaching as well as clinical care.

Too little research is being conducted on the advancement of nursing practice.*

The increase in the number of nurses has been almost double that of the population

---

*Professional nursing occupations, Medical Services Series, Bulletin No. 203-3, revised, United States Department of Labor, Women's Bureau, Washington, D. C., 1953, Government Printing Office, pp. 20 ff.

*Report of the Surgeon General's Consultant Group on Nursing, United States Department of Health, Education, and Welfare, Public Health Service, Public Health Publication No. 992, Feb. 1963.

increase in the past decade, and there is still a decided shortage. To add further complications, every prediction indicates a continuing population explosion that will demand more needs for nursing care. Even the very modest proposed goal of 300 nurses per 100,000 population in 1960 reached only 282 per 100,000.

CHANGING PATTERNS IN EDUCATION

Modern nursing has evolved out of the religious, militaristic and social backgrounds described earlier. Because of the Nightingale type of preparation in the United States, nursing education developed within the hospital. Much of this education, until the last quarter of the century, was based on the apprenticeship system; the student worked in the hospital and by doing more work than was necessary for her nursing education, paid for her room and board and part of her instruction. A similar system exists in some schools of nursing today. Other nursing schools have worked out a type of affiliation with an educational institution in which the student's program is based on her educational needs. Hospital schools, in order to meet the requirements set by the state and the accreditation standards established by the National League for Nursing, have carefully worked out educational programs.

The first schools of nursing in the United States were organized on "The Nightingale System." When the schools first tried to become independent under the support of committees of women, the economic problem of supporting them became too great. Therefore, the pattern in America was for hospitals to support and control schools of nursing. When a hospital sponsors a good school of nursing, however, it finds that funds must be set aside for this purpose. Although nursing schools originally developed as educational institutions, they were not supported or administered by educational institutions, but by hospitals, whose main focus of interest and concern must always be the care of the patients. It was within this

setting that the diploma programs, the oldest form of nursing education in the United States, developed. In 1967 there were 797 such programs in the United States. Baccalaureate programs, in which a student enrolls as a regular college student and earns a college degree as well as being eligible to sit for licensure examinations, were the second form of educational program in nursing to develop. Originally most of these were five years in length, and consisted of two years of college and three in a hospital. There has been extensive change in the curricula of these schools, particularly since the end of World War II. Most students study nursing as well as other subjects in a program which may vary from four academic to five calendar years. In October, 1967 there were 36,599 students enrolled in baccalaureate programs.

The Junior College

The junior or community college has evolved over the last half century into the most dynamic force in higher education today. Some of the early colleges limited their role to providing the first two years of a baccalaureate program. The original plan has been altered by the social forces of population and the postwar demand for college opportunity for all youth. Thus, while the original concept of liberal arts and general education courses for transfer purposes is still a part of the junior college, most of the institutions now emphasize studies that prepare men and women to take jobs immediately in industry, government service, and service occupations—such as hotel managements. This basic change in philosophy is dramatized by the growth of junior colleges within the last decade. Over 200 junior colleges have been established since 1952, when there were 597, bringing the number to over 800 in 1967. This basic change in philosophy made it possible for nursing education to establish itself within this arm of higher education.

In 1951 Dr. Mildred Montag published

Table 26-1. Graduations from basic nursing programs that prepare for beginning practice as registered nurses

Academic year	Associate degree		Diploma		Baccalaureate		Total	
	No. of programs	No. of graduations	No. of programs	No. of graduations	No. of programs	No. of graduations	No. of programs	No. of graduations
1956–57	28	276	944	26,141	167	3,478	1,139	29,855
1957–58	38	425	935	26,314	172	3,650	1,145	30,389
1958–59	48	462	916	25,907	171	3,943	1,135	30,312
1959–60	57	789	908	25,288	172	4,136	1,137	30,213
1960–61	69	917	883	25,311	174	4,039	1,126	30,267
1961–62	84	1,159	874	25,727	178	4,300	1,136	31,186
1962–63	105	1,479	860	26,438	183	4,481	1,148	32,398
1963–64	130	1,962	840	28,238	188	5,059	1,158	35,259
1964–65	174	2,510	821	26,795	198	5,381	1,193	34,686
1965–66	218	3,349	797	26,278	210	5,498	1,225	35,125
1966–67	281	4,654	767	27,452	221	6,131	1,269	38,237

her doctoral thesis "The Education of Nursing Technicians." This thesis introduced a new member of the nursing team—the nursing technician whose duties would be more limited than those of the professional nurse, but would require broader knowledge and skill than the practical nurse.

Dr. Montag proposed that the program for educating the nurse technician be two academic years in length in a collegiate framework, hopefully within a junior college.

Late in 1951, philantropic funds were made available for the Cooperative Research Project in Junior and Community College Education of Nursing. Dr. Montag was the project director. Seven junior colleges and one hospital school were selected for two year pilot programs. From this original group of seven programs in 1952, the number has grown to over 355 in January of 1969.

FINANCING OF NURSING EDUCATION

One great stumbling block in the development of collegiate programs in nursing has been finances. The traditional pattern was that the student through an apprenticeship or intership gave service to the hospital and thus paid for her education. In many di-

ploma schools, tuition is very low or, in some cases, nonexistent.

As nursing education moves from the hospital-controlled schools into colleges or universities, students must assume financial responsibility for their education. In the United States, state and city colleges provide less expensive education than private institutions. Many scholarships, loan funds, and fellowships exist for students of nursing as well as for other students.

Most leaders in all of the health related occupations and professions believe, that education should be the responsibility of the educational institutions of the country, both public and private, and that preparation for nursing should be considered as education rather than as work experience. They believe that these programs should be administered and controlled by educational institutions, that money from public and private sources should be available for all nursing education, and that funds should be available for the development of instructional facilities and for research. The question may be asked, "Who should pay for nursing education? The student? The patient? Educational institutions? The public?" The public pays a large share of the bill for educating teachers and preparing workers for other professions;

it must also be prepared to pay for the education of nurses. Nursing service is one of the greatest needs in all communities today. Communities should be prepared to bear the expense of preparing workers in this field. Many experiments are currently being conducted in this field. Reevaluation of old types of programs and experimentation with new forms are evident in many places. For example, tuition cost for students enrolled in nursing curricula located within most community colleges is borne one third by the student, one third by the local community, and one third by the state.

Many schools of nursing have reported in the last few years that they cannot enroll as many nursing students as they would like, because of the lack of qualified faculty. In 1956, the *Professional Nurse Traineeship Program* under Title Two of the Health Amendment Act (Public Law 911) provided funds for graduate nurses for advanced preparation in teaching, administration, and supervision. This program is administered by the division of nursing resources of the United States Public Health Service. It was designed to help relieve the shortage of well-prepared nurses in these three important positions.

In a statement released in June, 1964, Surgeon General Luther Terry reported that over 24,000 registered nurses had studied under this program. Ten thousand nurses pursued full-time academic study at colleges and universities to prepare for teaching and/or administration, and 14,000 nurses took intensive short-term courses to improve and update their skills. Dr. Terry said, "The training of nurses is a national concern because nurses now require more knowledge than ever before, to be able to use the advanced techniques which modern medical science makes possible."

Trainees under this program operate in 56 schools of nursing and schools of public health in this country and in Puerto Rico. Each trainee receives tuition and fees, transportation to the institution and to and from field practice centers, and an allowance for living expenses and for legal dependents. In 1969, the stipend allowances were radically revised. Baccalaureate and higher degree programs have protested this action.

In order to be eligible for this program a graduate nurse must be a citizen of the United States or have declared the intention of becoming a citizen, must be a graduate of a state-approved school of nursing, and must be enrolled in a program preparing the nurse to become a clinical specialist, teacher, supervisor, or administrator. Another program, under Title One of Public Law 911, provides funds for graduate nurses to prepare for staff level positions in public health nursing.

In 1964 Public Law 88-591 was passed by Congress and signed into law. It became known as the Nurse Training Act of 1964. Its purpose was to increase the supply of well-prepared nurses in the United States through a program of Federal assistance to schools of nursing and students of nursing. The major points of the law consisted of the traineeship program, projects grants for improvement in nurse training, nursing student land program, payments to diploma schools of nursing, and construction grants program for schools of nursing. It was a giant step in giving nursing education a broader financial basis from which to move in providing better and more knowledgeable patient care.

The act was originally intended to last for five years but from the evaluation report submitted in the Spring of 1968, there is every indication that it will be renewed and expanded.

This period of rapid changes in nursing coincides with rapid changes in social and economic conditions in the United States. Nursing education today must prepare the nurse to meet the challenge that is made by society. It may be said that the future of nursing education in America is likely to be characterized by changes in line with the general system of education but still retain fundamental principles from the heritage of the past. Brown's *Nursing for the Future* proposed that all nursing programs be developed as rapidly as possible within and as a part of the educational system in this country and be organized, administered, and controlled by educational institutions as are educational programs for other occupations.

PROFESSIONALIZATION OF NURSING AND THE NURSING TECHNICIAN

Many articles in nursing literature, particularly in *The American Journal of Nursing* and *Nursing Outlook,* discuss nursing as a profession. Many people have tried to answer the question, "What makes an occupation a profession?" Sociologists point out that professionalization of an occupation arises to protect both the worker and the public. When great responsibility and trust as well as technical knowledge are involved, practice must be limited. The professions well established for centuries were medicine, law, and the ministry. Only individuals properly qualified by training and by character were allowed to enter these professions. During the twentieth century many other occupations have become professionalized. Nursing is one of these. The selection of candidates to practice nursing is complicated. Professional nursing organizations are constantly alert to standards of education and standards for practice.

It is emphasized by scholars of history and other social sciences, that professional organizations have a responsibility to their members and the public to set standards for admission, to control education, to impose a code of ethics, and to safeguard the conditions under which its members practice. The standards set by the profession benefit the public served.

Brown describes the professional nurse as follows:

In the latter half of the twentieth century the professional nurse will be one who recognizes and understands the fundamental health needs of a person, sick or well, and who knows how these needs can best be met. She will possess a body of scientific nursing knowledge which is based on and keeps pace with general scientific advancement and she will be able to apply this knowledge in meeting the nursing needs of a person and a community. . . .

She must be able to exert leadership in at least four different ways:

1. In making her unique contribution to the prevention and remedial aspects of illness
2. In improving those nursing skills already in existence and developing new nursing skills
3. In teaching and supervising other nurses and auxiliary workers
4. In cooperating with other professions and planning for positive health of community, state, national and international levels. . . .

The professional nurse must be able to evaluate behavior and situations readily and to function intelligently and quickly in response to their variations. She must recognize physical symptoms of illness that are commonly identified with organic changes. She must also recognize the heretofore less considered manifestations of illness such as anxieties, conflict, and frustrations which have a direct influence on organic changes and are now thought to be the result of an incompatible interaction between a person and his environment. . . .

The nurse must be able to direct her actions and her verbal expressions on the basis of a sound understanding of human behavior and human relationship.*

The struggle to differentiate the functions and practice of the technical and professional nurse is reflected in the number of meetings, seminars, and studies devoted to this subject.

Dr. Ruth Matheney, in a historic paper presented at a meeting of the Councils of Associated Degree Program and Baccalaureate and Higher Degree Programs at the National League for Nursing Convention in 1967, lists several functions of the technical nurse. These include:

1. Identifying nursing problems; for the technical nurse this includes the common, recurring problems (e.g. maintenance of

*Brown, Esther Lucile: Nursing for the future, a report prepared for the National Nursing Council, New York, 1948, Russell Sage Foundation, pp. 73-74.

oxygen, nutrition, elimination; prevention of cross infection).

2. Selecting appropriate nursing action; for the technical nurse this includes listening, observing, environmental manipulation, feeding, and other nursing measures.

3. Providing continuous care for the individual's total health needs; for the technical nurse this includes referral to other members of the health team and to other health agencies.

4. Providing care to relieve pain and discomfort and promote security; for the technical nurse this means measures of physical hygiene, maintenance of body alignment, keeping channels of communication open, and avoiding adding to patient stress.

5. Adjusting nursing plans to the patient as an individual; for the technical nurse this includes recognizing and utilizing the significance of the patient as a person and a social being.

6. Helping the patient toward independence; for the technical nurse this means helping the patient to help himself when he is ready.

7. Supporting nursing personnel and family in helping the patient to do for himself that which he can; for the technical nurse this means listening, suggesting, and informal teaching with nursing personnel and patient families and referral to other members of the health team (such as the professional nurse or physician) where indicated.

8. Helping the patient to adjust to his limitations and emotional problems; for the technical nurse this means creating an environment where the patient is free to focus on feelings and reactions, and referrals to appropriate members of the health team where indicated.

The ANA position paper

In December of 1965 the American Nurses' Association, through its Committee on Education, set forth its position concerning education for the practice of nursing. The Association believes that:

The education for all those who are licensed to practice nursing should take place in institutions of higher education.

The minimum preparation for beginning professional nursing practice at the present time

should be baccalaureate degree education in nursing.

The minimum preparation for beginning technical nursing practice at the present time should be associate degree education in nursing.

The education for assistants in the health service occupations should be short, intensive, preservice programs in vocational education institutions rather than on-the-job training programs.*

Following months of discussion by units across the country the House of Delegates of American Nurses Association unanimously approved the work of the Education Committee at the San Francisco Convention in May, 1966.

The NLN position

In May, 1965, at the biennial convention, the following resolution was adopted by the NLN membership:

The NLN in convention assembled recognizes and strongly supports the trend toward college-based programs in nursing. The NLN recommends community planning which will recognize the need for immediate expedition of recruitment efforts which will increase the numbers of applicants to these programs and implement the orderly movement of nursing education into institutions of higher education in such a way that the flow of nurses into the community will not be interrupted.

To forward the continuing professionalization of nursing reflected in this statement, the National League for Nursing shall sponsor a vigorous campaign of interpreting the different kinds of programs for personnel prepared to perform complementary but different functions.

The NLN strongly endorses educational planning for nursing at local, state, regional, and national levels to the end that through an orderly development a desirable balance of nursing personnel with various kinds of preparation become available to meet the nursing needs of the nation and to insure the uninterrupted flow of nurses into the community.

Is nursing a profession?

In 1915 Dr. Abraham Flexner read a paper before the National Conference of

---

*American Nurses Association First poisition for nursing education, American Journal of Nursing, December, 1965, pp. 107-108.

Charities and Correction in which he set down certain criteria that have ever since formed a basis for judging whether an occupation has attained professional status or not. According to his interpretation of the professions:

> . . . (1) they involve essentially intellectual operations accompanied by large individual responsibility; (2) they are learned in nature, and their members are constantly resorting to the laboratory and seminar for a fresh supply of facts; (3) they are not merely academic and theoretical, however, but are definitely practical in their aims; (4) they possess a technique capable of communication through a highly specialized educational discipline; (5) they are self-organized, with activities, duties, and responsibilities which completely engage their participants and develop group consciousness; and finally (6) they are likely to be more responsive to public interest than are unorganized and isolated individuals, and they tend to become increasingly concerned with the achievement of social ends.*

STATE BOARDS

In most states today licensure is required to practice nursing. Licensing is necessary for the protection of the nurses as well as

*"Is Social Work a Profession?" in Proceedings of the National Conference of Charities and Correction, 1915, pp. 578-581.

the patients, the community, and employment agencies. Until 1944, each state made up its own examinations; as a result they were quite varied. A very important educational advance was made when the National League of Nursing Education (one of the organizations that became the National League for Nursing in 1952) developed, through its evaluation and guidance service, examinations that could be used by all the states. These examinations are composed by experts and distributed to the states where they are administered in local centers. The papers are returned to headquarters for grading and evaluation. This is known as the State Board Test Pool, and is controlled by the Council of State Boards, which is under the jurisdiction of the American Nurses' Association. At the present time, some states are developing very strong departments or divisions of education. The state boards automatically come within this central control with some of the lines of authority not clearly defined.

The rapidly expanding junior college programs have, in many instances, encouraged the state boards and nurse educators to reexamine minimum requirements and the methods in which to achieve the educational goals.

Chapter 27

A survey of nursing practice

Demands for nursing services are constantly increasing, and specialization has entered the wide field of nursing. Opportunities in nursing are greater today than ever before and seem to be increasing constantly. Not only is there a need for many more nurses than are now available, but many nurses are needed in such clinical specialties as, medical-surgical nursing, maternal and child nursing, psychiatric nursing, rehabilitative nursing, and community or public health nursing. In addition, there are such specialized fields as the military, government health field research, the Peace Corps, and international organizations like the World Health Organization, which require nurses who can function as supervisors or educators.

Traditionally, nurses have worked in hospitals or other institutions, in private homes, or with the military in giving care to patients. As the field of health services developed, expanded, and became specialized, variations and job combinations extended far beyond the relatively simple nursing situations of fifty years ago.

CLINICAL SPECIALISTS

One of the newest and most exciting developments within nursing today is the development of the nurse clinician, or clinical nursing specialist. This evolving functional role, which is being established on an equal basis with the teacher and supervisor, requires postgraduate educational preparation, usually on the master's level or beyond. Education at this level is financially available to almost any qualified applicant because of the large numbers of scholarships, fellowships and educational grants and loans. An extensive list of these is available from the Committee on Careers, a joint ANA-NLN committee.

SPECIAL FIELDS OF NURSING PRACTICE
Anesthesia

Since the 1880's nurses have been administering anesthetics in America and postgraduate instruction of nurses in anesthesiology was instituted about the same time. The first schools for teaching this specialty for nurses, however, were not organized until about 1910. Membership in the American Association of Nurse Anesthetists is open to all qualified nurse anesthetists.

Many states by law allow the administration of anesthetic by nurses. A case in the Supreme Court of California in 1946 decided that administration of anesthetic by a nurse was not contrary to the Medical Practice Act of that state. In no other state has the legality of nurse anesthetists been tested. As in other specialties in nursing, there is great need for nurse anesthetists, not

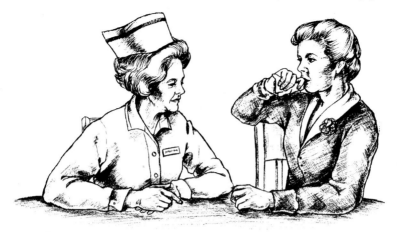

The personalized attention of nurses facilitates the recovery of many psychiatric patients.

only in civilian but also in military hospitals. The professional organization of this group is the American Association of Nurse Anesthetists, which publishes a quarterly journal, *Journal of the American Association of Nurse Anesthetists.*

Industrial nursing

Industrial nursing has expanded, as has industrial medicine, from first-aid stations to a complicated practice of industrial health. This field has been given great impetus since World War II. It is estimated that there are over 12,000 industrial nurses in this country. The industrial nurse needs technical skill to deal with diagnostic and treatment situations. She must come in close contact with all workers and their health problems. Knowledge of the health problems of the worker and his family combined with a knowledge of community resources helps industry to maintain health and individual productivity on as high a level as possible.

Requirements in this field are that the person be a registered nurse with a foundation of nursing skill in modern health work. Current state registration is necessary. In industrial work, the nurse must like people, be able to work effectively on the health team, and be able to work well with patients' families. Industrial nursing is ex-tremely varied; for example, the industrial nurse may work in an industrial hospital or in an industry in which the services are comparable to those in outpatient departments.

Nurse-midwifery

The first school for nurse-midwifery in the United States was opened in 1932 by the Association for the Promotion and Standardization of Midwifery, Inc., in cooperation with the Maternity Center of New York. In 1935 the Lobenstein Midwifery Clinic was consolidated with the Maternity Center Association. During the first twenty years this school graduated 231 nurse-midwives, but with the growing recognition of the place of this professional worker, the demand for graduates has always far exceeded the supply.

At present three universities offer courses in nurse-midwifery. The one at the Johns Hopkins University School of Medicine and the one under the Faculty of Medicine of Columbia University have been developed in cooperation with the Maternity Center Association of New York. A third program is part of the facilities of the Yale Medical Center.

Schools preparing for the practice of nurse-midwifery are also operated by the

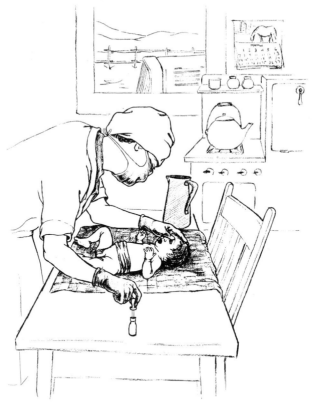

In certain rural areas of the United States where medical care is scarce, the nurse midwife often performs home deliveries.

Frontier Nursing Service in Lexington, Kentucky and in Santa Fe, New Mexico. Historically, practice of this specialty has been in rural areas where there was inadequate prenatal care. A fascinating account of the development of the Frontier Nursing Service is found in *Nurse on Horse Back,* by Florence Breckinridge, founder of·the Service.

Nursing in the Department of Health, Education, and Welfare

Under the Department of Health, Education, and Welfare, a nurse may work in one of the public health service hospitals serving seamen, personnel of the United States Coast Guard, officers of the Coast and Geodetic Survey, Federal employees injured at work, and public health officers. The nurse may also work with the American Indian in one of the fifty-six Indian hospitals and clinics scattered through our states. Since 1956 the responsibility of the health of the Indian has been placed in the Department of Health, Education, and Welfare.

In 1953 the Clinic Center opened in Bethesda, Maryland, as part of the National Institutes of Health of the United States Public Health Service. The National Institutes of Health include several institutes: heart, cancer, mental health, arthritis and metabolic diseases, neurology and blindness, and allergies and infectious diseases. In the large 500-bed hospital, research and clinical care of patients are closely integrated. The nurse is a member not only of the patient care team but also of the research team.

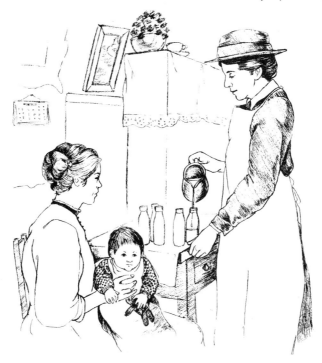

In the early 1900's the baby welfare nurse played an important role in starting a baby off on a long and healthy life.

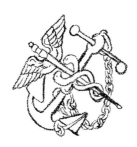

**United States
Public Health Service insignia**

Members of the United States Public Health Service do valuable work in the field of public health nursing by participating in studies, working on health teams in various control programs, and, when qualified, by serving as nurse consultants.

The United States Public Health Service has expanded its overseas program since World War II. These nurses serve in many areas of Latin America, Africa, the Near East, and the Far East. In the United States Public Health Service a graduate nurse, male or female, may enter either by appointment to its commissioned corps as a regular or reserve officer or through Federal Civil Service employment.

The army nurse corps

The Army Nurse Corps is the oldest of all the women's military services and is made up entirely of registered nurses representing all fields of nursing.

The Army-Navy Nurses Act of 1947 granted to nurses permanent commission status in the United States Army. An Army Nurse Corps section was established in the Officer Reserve Corps. Colonel Florence A. Blanchfield worked hard to achieve this and was the first woman to receive permanent

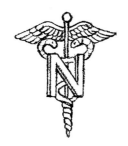

Army Nurse Corps insignia

commissioned rank of colonel. Not only the variety of service but also the security found in the military nursing fields may be attractive; for example, personnel policies, complete hospital, medical, surgical, and dental care when needed, limited health services for dependents, generous retirement benefits after twenty years of service, substantial allowance for initial purchase of officer's uniform, and, of course, pay increases for all grades, depending upon length of service.

In addition to such positions as head nurse, chief of nursing service, instructor, general duty nurse, and supervisor, many specialized positions such as an Army health nurse, chief of nursing personnel, and nurse education coordinator exist. Specialists are needed in various fields and are given instruction by the Army; for example, in operating room technic and management, in anesthesiology, in neuropsychiatric nursing, and in nursing and hospital administration. Through the Army's information and education program, Army nurses may enroll in extension and other collegiate courses at reduced rates.

Army nurses may serve in America or in any of the foreign stations in which the United States Army functions. Applicants must be registered professional nurses, citizens between the ages of 21 and 45, physically and professionally qualified, and graduates of schools acceptable to the Surgeon General. Married nurses are accepted for reserve appointments or extended active duty if they do not have dependent children

under 18 years. Applicants must pass a physical examination conducted at an Army or Air Force medical center or by a civilian physician at no expense to the government. For appointment as a second lieutenant, the nurse must be a high school graduate, have graduated from a basic nursing program, and meet citizenship and physical qualifications and moral requirements specified. As a first lieutenant, the young nurse must meet the above requirement, be registered in the United States or United States territory, and have fifteen semester hours in an accredited college or university, and three years' professional experience. A nurse currently certified by the American Association of Nurse Anesthetists with three years' professional experience in anesthesiology or experience within twenty-four months prior to the appointment may also be appointed as first lieutenant. For appointment as a captain, the basic requirements for first lieutenant are needed plus a bachelor's degree from an accredited college or university, with the major field in nursing and seven years' experience including two years' teaching, supervising, or administration; or, a master's degree from an accredited college or university, with the major field in nursing, allied medical science, or personnel field, and six years' experience, including two years' supervision or administration; or, current certification by the American Association of Nurse Anesthetists and seven years of anesthesia practice, terminating not more than twenty-four months prior to the appointment.*

The Navy Nurse Corps

Today, Navy nurses serve in the United States and abroad. Nurses in this military

---

*Young people interested in Army nurse experience and information should apply to the Army Nurse Corps Counselor's Office, Headquarters Fifth Avenue, 1660 East Hyde Park Blvd., Chicago 60615, Illinois, or the Surgeon General, Department of the Army, Washington 20315, D. C.

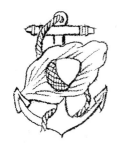

Navy Nurse Corps insignia

branch have an opportunity to practice all phases of nursing care for men and women of the Navy and Marine Corps and their families. All initial appointments are made by the Nurse Corps, United States Naval Reserve. The basic qualifications for commission require that the young women be: graduates of schools of nursing whose educational and professional standards are approved by the Surgeon General, United States Navy; currently registered at least in one state or the District of Columbia; high school graduate; a native-born or naturalized citizen of the United States; between the ages of 21 and 40 years; either single or married, but with no dependents under the age of 18 years; and physically qualified by the standards set up by the naval officers. Appointments are made in grades of ensign through lieutenant, senior grade, depending upon age and qualifications.

The functions of the Navy nurse are to give bedside care to patients, to instruct hospital corpsmen, and to help in the management and supervision of wards and clinics. In addition to the officers, the men and women of the Armed Forces and the families of the Armed Forces are also given care. As in the Army, there is an extensive in-service educational program in all Navy hospitals. Members of the Nurse Corps may be assigned to attend educational programs in colleges and universities. All nurses are encouraged to continue their education.

In keeping with the development of educational programs, both in civilian and in military groups, the Navy nurse postwar educational program was established in 1946. Navy nurses were assigned to schools for training in physiotherapy, anesthesiology, occupational therapy, dietetics, and ward administration. In 1947 the Army Nurse Act established the Nurse Corps as a permanent staff corps of the United States Navy. Captain DeWitt became the first director of the permanent corps.

The Korean emergency of 1950 necessitated a recall of reserve nurses to help care for Korean casualties. In 1955 continued education for the Navy nurse was stimulated by Public Law 20, called "The Career Incentive Act," which provided incentives in increased pay and allowances. Later in the same year an educational program was instituted that allowed a limited number of Hospital Corps Waves to enroll in approved collegiate schools of nursing with the expenses borne by the Navy. Upon the satisfactory completion of this program these students are commissioned as ensigns in the Navy Corps Reserve.

During 1957 and 1958 educational programs were continued, and increases in salary and promotions resulted. In 1957 the Navy Nurse Corps Cadet Program permitted qualified students in approved collegiate schools of nursing to enlist during their final year in the school of nursing. Educational expenses are paid by the Navy, and upon graduation from the school of nursing, the nurses are commissioned as ensigns in the Navy Nurse Corps Reserve.

In May of 1958 the Nurse Corps proudly celebrated its golden anniversary, having established for itself, as other branches of the military have, an honored place in the military history of America.

The Air Force Nurse Corps

Until 1949 Army medical personnel had been assigned to duty with the Air Force. Since that date, however, the Air Force Medical Service has become an entity distinct from the Army Medical Service. Since World

War I, Air Force medicine had been concerned with such problems as lack of oxygen at high altitude, the forces and strains to which the human being is subjected because of great rates of speed, quick changes in temperature, and other areas now included in aviation medicine.

The United States Air Force Medical Service is composed of six groups of medical personnel: medical, veterinary, medical service, dental, women's medical specialist corps (dietitians, physiotherapists, and occupational therapists) and the Air Force Nurse Corps, which includes both the flight nurses and the Air Force nurses serving on the ground in Air Force hospitals.

During World War II, official air evacuation was begun in 1942 when an Air Ambulance Battalion was organized at Fort Benning, Georgia. This was moved to Beaumont Field, Kentucky, later in the year, and training for flight nurses in air evacuation squadrons began. Flight teams consisting of one flight medical technician and one flight nurse were organized. The Flight Nurse School is now located at the Gunter Branch of the Aviation School of Medicine, Gunter Air Force Base, Montgomery, Alabama.

Nurses entering the Air Force Nurse Corps today must be graduates of a nursing school acceptable to the Surgeon General, United States Air Force; have active registration in any state, territory, or District of Columbia, and be physically and professionally qualified; be between the ages of 21 and 45 years, either married or single; and be female citizens of the United States, with high moral standards. Appointments are made from second lieutenant to major, depending upon age, professional experience, and educational equipment. The minimum tour of active duty is two years. Training programs and in-service education are an important part of the program.

The course of study includes such subjects as aviation physiology, psychology, nursing procedures for the in-flight care of patients, and the newest development in

therapeutics. The course is difficult but responsibilities as a flight nurse are great, and when the nurse has satisfactorily completed the course, she may wear her silver wings with an "N" superimposed upon them.

In addition to bedside nursing and the instruction and supervision of nonprofessional workers, a nurse may be assigned to many clinical specialties such as; head nurse, supervisor, chief nurse, or administrative director. She may also go into one of the specialized fields—operating room supervision, nurse anesthetist, psychiatric nursing, or flight nursing. Personnel policies make it possible for both regular Air Force and reserve nurses to become eligible for retirement benefits. Regular Air Force nurses may retire after twenty years; retirement pay is determined by length of service and grade held. Reserve Air Force nurses may apply for retirement benefits after the age of 60 years, having completed twenty years of satisfactory active and/or reserve service. A number of regular and reserve Air Force personnel nurses are given university education leading to a degree, during which time they receive full pay and allowances. Other educational opportunities are made available through the United States Armed Forces Institute and the United States Air Force Extension Institute. The Air Force Nurse Corps, as true of other military branches, provides for health supervision and medical care. Physical examination is given at the time of appointment and repeated annually. Nurses receive immunization regularly, and hospitalization and sick leave are provided when required.

Aerospace nursing

A relatively new specialty developing within the Air Force Nurse Corps is Aerospace Nursing. An intensive 52 week course was initiated in 1965 at Patrick Air Force Base, Cape Kennedy, to equip nurses to function as part of the Bioastronautic Operational Support Unit. BOSU is engaged in intensive research on the effects of all forms

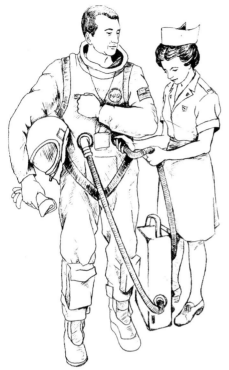

One of the most exciting fields in modern life, the space program, presents new opportunities for the nurse and her special skills.

of stress on healthy human beings. This research reveals new knowledge which can be applied here on earth as well as in space. Nurses working in BOSU are concerned not only with the care of the astronauts but also with preparation for disaster on the test range.

The Veterans Administration

A great variety of nursing positions, from the staff nurse to chief of nursing service, is available to properly qualified graduate nurses.* Nurses are appointed to the Department of Medicine and Surgery of the Veterans Administration by a Nurse Professional

---

*Information concerning employment in the Veterans Administration can be obtained from the nearest Veterans Administration Hospital or by writing directly to Veterans Administration Headquarters, Washington 20420, D. C.

Standards Board composed entirely of nurses. Qualifications include being:
1. A citizen of the United States.
2. A graduate of a senior high school and school of nursing acceptable to the Administrator of the Veterans Administration.
3. Currently registered as a graduate nurse in a state, territory, or the District of Columbia.
4. Under 40 years of age unless applicant possesses outstanding qualifications. (There is provision for a special type of appointment, not to exceed three years, for nurses over the 40-year age limit who meet all other basic requirements. The appointment of nurses under this provision is dependent upon the recruitment needs of individual hospitals.)
5. Physically qualified by standards set for appointment in the Department of Medicine and Surgery.

Promotions are based on daily performance and educational and professional background.

Nursing service in the Veterans Administration has continued on a very high plane because of the careful selection of all nurses on the staff and a continued and expanding educational program. There are now 174 Veterans Administration hospitals and 52 regional office clinics in the United States. The nursing staff is comprised of over 15,000 professional nurses and over 20,000 trained practical nurses and hospital aides.

Since patients in the Veterans Administration hospitals and clinics represent every medical specialty, planned programs are worked out in each hospital and regional office clinic to meet the nursing needs of their patients. Inservice education for the nurse aims to prepare her for administration, teaching, and supervision, as well as to improve her ability to give nursing care. The elaborate in-service program includes preservice information, orientation, supplementary instruction and experience, and continuing in-service education. In addition, nurses are encouraged to study part or full time in college or university programs of nursing. Nurses wishing to participate in this continued education may be granted a maximum of 280 days' leave of absence, including salary and other benefits.

The training of practical nurses and hospital aids has been continued by expansion of on-the-job instruction. This instruction includes approximately 498 hours of planned theory and supervised practice. This instruction is given to improve the worker's nursing ability in meeting such specific nursing problems as those presented by psychotic, tubercular, geriatric, paraplegic, or neurologic patients.

The Peace Corps

The Peace Corps presents that great opportunity for "people to help people" directly in providing economic, social, or educational assistance. The cause of peace is thus advanced through mutual understanding, personal love and affection, and by sharing.

The Corps came into being on March 1, 1961, when President Kennedy issued an executive order establishing the Corps on a provisional basis. Congress established the Peace Corps permanently on September 21, 1961. Objectives defined by the Act for the Peace Corps are to promote world peace and friendship by making available to interested countries Americans who will:

1. Help the people of these countries meet their needs for trained manpower.
2. Help promote a better understanding of the American people on the part of the peoples served.
3. Help promote a better understanding of other peoples on the part of the American people.

Registered nurses are one of the desired groups required by the Peace Corps, and any registered nurse or student nurse in her last year of nursing school, regardless of age, who is a United States citizen may apply for service as a Peace Corps Volunteer. Volunteers must be in excellent physical and mental health. After an intensive Peace Corps training designed to prepare volunteers for effective service overseas, a nurse will be sent to any one of twenty countries in Latin America, Africa, the Near East, South East, Asia, or South West Asia.*

---

*To apply, write to the Professional and Technical Division, Peace Corps, Washington 20325, D. C.

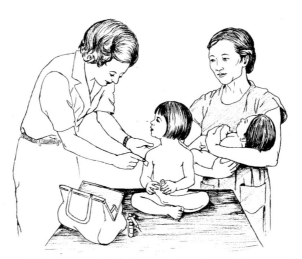

The Peace Corps volunteer nurse is called upon to practice a wide range of nursing skills.

MEN IN NURSING

According to the 1958-1960 census figures there were 440,355 nurses in the United States. Of this total, men nurses comprise 1%; this made them the smallest subprofessional group in the health field in the United States. The history of men in nursing extends back through the history of the Christian era. It reached its height during the time of the Crusades when the flowering of European manhood were members of the various military religious orders whose essential work was nursing and hospital administration. Their many hospitals and holdings dotted the countryside of Europe. Some remnants of these orders still remain, but for the most part, the role of men in modern nursing in the United States began about 1888 when the first school of nursing for men was established at Bellevue Hospital in New York City. It was named the Mills School, after Ogden Mills who had en-

dowed the school. Except for the war years, this school has been in operation continuously. Many other schools of nursing for men have since developed. It is, however, only recently that men have been admitted into regular schools of nursing in any large numbers. The percentage of men in nursing schools, particularly in the Associate Degree programs, is much higher than the 1% of nursing practitioners from this group would indicate.

ECONOMIC SECURITY

The years of 1964, 1965 and 1966 were ones of ferment and turmoil for nursing. All over the country, courageous nurses banded together for the first time in history to act as a cohesive social force in a battle to win improved working conditions and increased economic security.

The first major victory, which received national attention from the public, was won

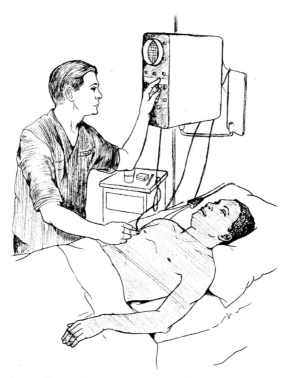

Nursing is becoming an increasingly popular occupation for men as it expands in scope.

by over 3,500 nurses employed in the New York City Department of Hospitals. Negotiations begun in May, 1965 were concluded one year later, just five days before the nurses' resignations would have become effective. National news was also made by nurses who resigned, or threatened to resign, in Chicago, San Francisco, and Los Angeles. It was not just in the giant metropolises that these actions occurred, however. The ANA Economic Security Unit reported over 140 "situations" all over the country in the first six months of 1966.

The public's support was behind nursing when they learned that the resignations, "slow downs," and "strikes" were not only over salaries but also because of hospital conditions which made adequate patient care impossible. Major contractual concessions included establishment of committees to examine nursing and non-nursing duties and release time and reimbursement for attending professional meetings and workshops.

The most significant gain, however, has been substantial salary increases across the country. At the biennial convention of the American Nurses' Association in 1966, the House of Delegates adopted a resolution calling for a minimum base salary of $6,500. In a nationwide press conference about this salary goal, Jo Eleanor Elliott, ANA President, said, "If quality care is to be assured to all persons, salaries of nurses must be more attractive. Today's salaries discourage the recruitment of qualified young people. We know, too, that many married nurses with young children cannot aford to practice their profession; the salaries they can earn are not enough to compensate them for costs of child care. Substantial increases in salaries are required to regain the services of many nurses."

CONCLUSION

In a dynamic society, any fundamental function such as nursing, is bound to change if it is to meet the needs of the society.

Nursing functions today range from uncomplicated activities such as those dealing mainly with personal hygiene or assisting with and carrying out relatively simple procedures to very complex ones demanding not only expert skill, judgment, and technical experience but also knowledge in such fields as sociology, psychology, social work, and other health, social, and welfare areas.

The very nature of nursing and the wide range of functions from the relatively simple to the complex have resulted in the need for more than one kind of nurse.

The educational programs for preparation of nurses today are changing to meet the changing demands made on the profession. Conditions are progressing so rapidly that changes may be made in the program during a student's own experience in school.

In such fields as industrial nursing, anesthesiology, office nursing, nursing in various health agencies, and such administrative positions as those with state and national nursing organizations, we find ever-growing specialization, resulting in constantly increasing job opportunities.

Many married nurses continue nursing, either part or full time. Although there was a traditional attitude against married nurses, and particularly against any student's getting married, during World War II and the

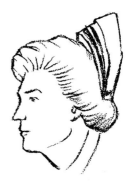

**University Hospital of
Good Shepherd graduate nurse**

following years this attitude has changed as has the situation: the number of married women in all industries has increased steadily.

It is becoming more and more important for nurses to take an active part in community activities, in addition to belonging to professional organizations. Until relatively recent times all professional nurses except the few in public health nursing lived highly institutionalized lives and even after graduation continued to live in the nurses' residence, with very little opportunity or wish for outside activities.

Chapter 28

Organizational changes—American Nurses' Association and National League for Nursing

In planning for the future it is fitting that consideration be given to the type of organization that will function best. The organization of nurses is of vital importance if plans and programs for the future are to be carried out satisfactorily.

In 1939 the question arose of uniting more closely the three oldest nursing organizations: the National League of Nursing Education, the National Organization for Public Health Nursing, and the American Nurses' Association. World War II both helped and hindered this movement. It was not until 1944 that definite plans for these three organizations could be considered. In 1945 the National Association of Colored Graduate Nurses, the American Association of Industrial Nurses, and the Association of Collegiate Schools of Nursing were added to the committee.

THE RICH REPORT

The National Nursing Council for War Service, Inc., prepared a comprehensive program for postwar nursing, which appeared in *The American Journal of Nursing,* September, 1945, under the title "A Comprehensive Program for Nationwide Action." Many doubts were revealed about the ex-

isting structures of the national nursing organizations, and it was believed that these doubts could be resolved only by a complete study. Consequently the Raymond Rich Associates were empowered to make this study, hereafter referred to as the Structure Study.

At the Biennial Convention in 1946, the Rich Report was discussed and studied. The study was continued during the greater part of 1946 and the spring and summer of 1947 through the National and State Structure Study Committees. In September, 1947, the House of Delegates of the American Nurses' Association held a special meeting to study the Rich Report. At that session the delegates of the American Nurses' Association were given the right to express opinions and to vote on the Structure Committee as other delegates had from the beginning. At this time, the average nurse showed more interest in the organization of the profession than ever before. The Rich Report actually gave the nurses and lay people a new interest and knowledge about nursing. They asked, "Why is a new organization necessary?" "Why should all types of nursing care be organized under one head?" or "Should they?" "Can the industrial nurse join with

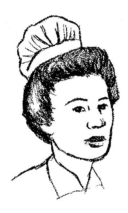

**Columbia, South Carolina,
Hospital graduate nurse**

the staff nurses and have specialized needs in organization recognized?" "Should the Negro nurses be given the added help that will be found in a larger organization of all nurses or will these nurses become a minority group without voice?"

In the 1947 plan, called a Tentative Plan, there was to be one organization, to be known as the American Nursing Organization, with nurse members grouped into sections of interest and composing the House of Delegates and the Board of Governors. In addition, this single association was to have divisions, which were to have nonnurse, agency, and school members as well as nurse members. Only nurse members of the divisions were to be eligible for election as division representatives in the House of Delegates and Board of Governors, but all types of members were to elect the division representatives.

This organization was not considered adequate by the National Organization for Public Health Nursing and the National League of Nursing Education who had had very great support and help from their lay members. They believed that the lay members should have equal consideration in an organization if they were to continue to take an active interest in that organization.

Then the question of membership in the International Council of Nurses arose. Could an organization with active lay participation still remain a member of the International Council of Nurses? The International Council of Nurses' rules state that the member organization from any country must be of and controlled by nurses. After extensive study there seemed no way to have a single organization with free lay participation and continued membership in the International Council of Nurses.

Revised plans in 1949 provided for the establishment of two organizations. This plan was based upon an effort to increase more democratic participation in the work of the organization, both by every registered graduate nurse and by the lay public interested in nursing service. The inclusion of the lay member in a professional nurses' organization is a controversial subject. If a nurse believes that active lay participation is necessary for the furtherance of nursing service, this nurse will believe that it should be provided for in the organization. However, there are nurses who have never worked with cooperative lay members and who fear the idea of the lay persons' taking an active voting part in the organization's work.

Basically the Structure Study was an effort of the six national nursing organizations to coordinate their work and to make it more effective in service to nurses as they tried to meet the nation's constantly increasing demand for nursing services.

It was the Structure Study Committee's assigned to task to bring to the profession a recommendation of the organizational structure most favorable to the best development of nursing. In pursuing this primary objective, more has been learned about organizational life of professional nursing than ever before.

At the biennial convention in Atlantic City in 1952, nurses voted to have two national organizations: the American Nurses' Association and the National League for Nursing.

The original joint statement of purposes and functions follows.

THE AMERICAN NURSES' ASSOCIATION AND THE NATIONAL LEAGUE FOR NURSING

A Joint Statement on Purposes and Functions*

The American Nurses' Association and the National League for Nursing are separate organizations with a common objective—to provide the best possible nursing care for the American people.

Each organization has distinct purposes and functions.

Purposes

Through ANA, nurses work for the continuing improvement of professional practice, the economic and general welfare of nurses and the health needs of the American public.

In the NLN, nurses and friends of nursing of all races, creeds and national origins act together to provide the people of their communities with the best possible nursing services and to assure good nursing education.

Functions and serivces

ANA	NLN
Defines functions and promotes standards of professional nurse practice	Defines standards for organized nursing services and education
Defines qualifications for practitioners of nursing, including those in various nursing specialties	Stimulates and assists communities, nursing services and educational institutions in achieving these standards through effective distribution, organization, administration and utilization of personnel
Promotes legislation and speaks for nurses regarding legislative action for general health and welfare programs	Promotes continual study and adjustments in nursing services and educational curricula to meet changing needs
Surveys periodically the nurse resources of the nation	Assists with or conducts community nursing surveys
Promotes the economic and general welfare of nurses and works to eliminate discrimination against minority-group nurses in job opportunities	Provides consultation, publications, cost analysis methods and data, and other services to individuals, nursing services, schools and communities
Provides professional counseling service to individual nurses and to employers in regard to employment opportunities and available personnel	Conducts a national student nurse recruitment program cosponsored by the ANA, the American Hospital Association, the American Medical Association
Finances studies of nursing functions	Carries out and promotes studies and research related to organized nursing services and educational programs
Represents and serves as national spokesman for nurses with allied professional and governmental groups and with the public	Represents nursing services and nursing education units with allied professional, governmental and international groups and with the public
Implements the international exchange of nurses program and assists displaced persons who are nurses	Accredits educational programs in nursing
Serves as the official representative of American nurses in the International Council of Nurses	Offers comprehensive testing and guidance services to institutions with practical, basic or advanced nursing education programs
Works closely with the various State Boards of Nursing in the interpretation of nurse practice acts and the facilitation of interstate licensure by endorsement.	Provides, in cooperation with state licensing authorities, examinations and related services for use in licensing professional and practical nurses

---

*Pamphlet published by the American Nurses' Association and the National League for Nursing, 10 Columbus Circle, New York, N. Y.

Membership

All ANA members are professional registered nurses, representing every occupational field of nursing. There are two types of members: Active and Associate (retired or inactive nurses).

NLN members are professional and practical nurses, men and women in allied professions, other people interested in good nursing, nursing service agencies—hospitals and public health —and institutions offering educational programs in nursing

Constituent groups

The ANA is a federation of 53 constituent associations including the [48] states, the District of Columbia, Puerto Rico, the Panama Canal Zone, Alaska and Hawaii. State Nurses Associations, in turn, usually are composed of constituent District Associations. ANA membership also is divided into district, state and national sections according to occupational specialties within nursing.

As of April, 1954, NLN counted as affiliates 45 state Leagues for Nursing, the District of Columbia, Hawaii, and Puerto Rico. Many state Leagues are organizing constituents known as local Leagues for Nursing. A Council of State Leagues for Nursing, comprised of the president or alternate of each state League, NLN's officers and the ANA's president, coordinates state programs and purposes with those of the National League for nursing

Operating plan

Members of state sections elect representatives to the ANA House of Delegates who, in turn, vote for the Board of Directors. ANA section executive committees are elected by section members attending the biennial conventions. Programs and policies of ANA are determined by the House of Delegates. The work of the ANA between conventions is furthered through the activities of standing and special communities and the Board of Directors. A national headquarters with an administrative staff is maintained.

Every NLN member has a voice in the organization's policies and programs. The Board of Directors is elected by direct vote of all members. Four departments represent major fields of interest in nursing service and education. A steering committee, elected by department members, guides the staff in carrying out each department's program. Each department also has a Council of its Member Agencies. Interdivisional councils and committees represent cross-sections of special interest groups.

History

ANA

ANA was organized in 1896 as the Nurses' Associated Alumnae of the United States and Canada. When the Association was incorporated in New York in 1901, it was no longer possible for Canadian nurses to be affiliated. The present name was adopted ten years later. In 1951 the National Association of Colored Graduate Nurses became integrated with ANA. A year later, in the structure reorganization of nursing groups, ANA took over some of the work (definition of functions and qualifications of individual practitioners) formerly carried by the National League of Nursing Education and the National Organization for Public Health Nursing, which were combined into NLN.

NLN

The NLN was formed in 1952 when three national nursing organizations and four national committees combined their programs and resources. National League of Nursing Education (founded 1893), National Organization for Public Health Nursing (1912), Association of Collegiate Schools of Nursing (1933); Joint Committee on Practical Nurses and Auxiliary Workers in Nursing Services (1945), Joint Committee on Careers in Nursing (1948), National Committee for the Improvement of Nursing Services (1949), and National Nursing Accrediting Service (1949)

Continued.

During the 16 years since nursing voted for two national groups many organizational difficulties have arisen between the two structures. Perhaps the grand ideals embodied in the original concepts were too global, too complex. Perhaps the professional organization felt it had relinquished some of its vital prerogatives to a "lay" group. Thus, in 1958 the ANA House of Delegates called for one national organization. This call proved to be unobtainable for a variety of reasons. However, since this action the two organizations have improved relationships noticeably and have issued joint statements clarifying their functions. Two of the statements follow:

Working relationships between The American Nurses' Association and National League for Nursing*

The American Nurses' Association and the National League for Nursing as cooperating organizations in the field of nursing have the need to examine periodically the fundamental premises on which they will work together and serve society. While they are totally different organizations in both responsibilities and structure, they are complementary in purpose and function.

---

*Approved by ANA and NLN Boards of Directors, January, 1966.

The American Nurses' Association, as the professional organization, is moving to fulfill those functions of standard setting for education, practice and organized services traditionally carried by professional organizations. In the development and modification of such standards, ANA secures consultation and advice from NLN and elsewhere, but retains responsibility for deciding the final content. Normally, standards are in advance of current practice. They are authoritative, based on the expertise of the profession. ANA works through its members and its constituencies, with NLN and with a variety of organizations and governmental bodies to implement these standards.

The National League for Nursing, composed of individuals, educational institutions, and nursing service agencies, is the organization to which the profession and the public look for services to promote and to improve nursing education programs and organized nursing services. These activities of NLN include among others accreditation, consultation, and involvement of educational programs and service agencies in programs of self-improvement. In planning and conducting such services, NLN involves its appropriate membership in the development of criteria for the purpose of evaluation. Such criteria and related guides must reflect the broad standards enunciated by ANA and their goals of the profession. NLN studies the application of criteria and their implications for standards and practice for education and for organized nursing services. These findings are shared with ANA. In these ways the two organizations are complementary, each with distinctive responsibilities and both necessary in meeting society's needs for nursing service.

The needs of the profession and the needs of the public for nursing service are different in 1966 from those of 1952 when a design for function and structure of both organizations was adopted. Change in the demands upon both organizations has caused each to examine its own functions and structure, and its relationship with the other. It is essential that ANA and NLN work cooperatively in areas of common concern as each builds its program in full recognition of the role of the other.

The American Nurses' Association and the National League for Nursing joint statement on community planning for nursing education

In recognition of the many changes taking place in the health field and the need for appropriate education for nursing personnel to meet present and future requirements, both in quantity and quality of nursing services, the American Nurses' Association and the National League for Nursing believe that sound community planning for nursing education is essential and should be begun or accelerated promptly.

The overriding concern of both organizations is that the nation receive the best possible nursing care. This will require increasing numbers of nursing personnel with quality preparation to meet the changing health care needs of the community and to fill the needs of institutions and agencies providing nursing services.

Both organizations have recently taken official positions on the future of nursing education. The American Nurses' Association in December 1965 issued a position paper stating that all nursing personnel should be prepared within the general system of education. The statement advocates baccalaureate preparation as the minimum education for professional nursing practice, associate degree preparation as the minimum for technical nursing practice, and vocational school preparation for nursing assistants. The National League for Nursing in May 1965 passed a resolution advocating community planning to implement the orderly transition of nursing education into institutions of higher education in such a way that the flow of nurses into the community will not be interrupted.

As was pointed out in the Report of the Surgeon General's Consultant Group on Nursing, "If new and expanded programs of nursing education are to be established in places where they are needed and in educational settings where they will thrive, it is essential that they be intelligently planned. Such planning . . . must consider needs

for cooperation among adjoining geographic areas. . . . Cooperation within and among states in the planning of nursing education programs is desirable both to prevent needless duplication of effort and as a basis for pooling of . . . resources."

Today when major changes are taking place in the type and placement of nursing education programs, it cannot be left to chance that the right number of nurses with the appropriate level of education can or will be produced.

The ANA and NLN both believe that guaranteeing the continuity and character of the nursing supply transcends the nursing profession itself. Educational, health, and welfare authorities, professional and volunteer groups in the health field and community planning bodies must plan and work cooperatively with nursing to insure an adequate nursing supply. Careful planning on the community level should precede any action to transfer or to develop new or different programs. Depending upon the social and demographic complexion of the area, planning may be undertaken for a local community, for several communities together, for a state, or for a region.

Communities are urged to base their decision as to the types of nursing education programs to be retained, revised, or newly developed taking into account:

1. What are the nursing care needs of the community? What kinds of nursing personnel are required to meet these needs?
2. What are the physical resources now available or planned in the community for educating nursing personnel? What junior and senior colleges, universities and clinical laboratory facilities are available for educational excellence?
3. Are qualified faculty available?
4. What financial resources are available which can be utilized for nursing education?
5. How can available resources be channelled into a new design of education for nursing personnel to meet the current and anticipated needs of the community?

Only through such planning and studying of the total situation is it possible to assure that nurses will be prepared in accordance with the needs of society and to assure the most effective use of available resources.

ACTIVITIES OF THE AMERICAN NURSES' ASSOCIATION

The American Nurses' Association has continued its twofold purpose of providing better nursing service and of helping the graduate nurse in every way possible. Through its programs, better personnel policies have been worked out through state and local nursing organizations, and much closer contact is developing between local and national groups as representatives from national headquarters go into local areas to help with special problems in nursing.

Since 1950 the ANA has been actively sponsoring a research program. Nurses have actively supported this program both through voluntary subscription and through dues. The ANA now has a Technical Committee on Studies of Nursing Functions and a Research and Statistics Unit. Studies are being made in the changing role of the professional nurse, and a fact-finding and research service is available for ANA members. In addition to compiling *Facts About Nursing* annually, and the inventories of professional nurses periodically, these committees help staff members and other committees conduct research.

The ANA Special Groups Section was organized in 1952. The main purpose of this section is to bring together nurses whose occupations place them in specialized groups too small to qualify for section status. Some of the interests represented are; the Executive Secretaries of the American Nurses' Association and district nurse associations, recruitment, nurses in the Armed Services, registrars, some Red Cross nurses, nurses in public relations, nurse editors, nurse anesthetists, physical therapists, and occupational therapists. The second purpose for this section is to give these groups a place to discuss their problems until the groups are large enough to form new sections. The ANA by-laws at present provide that a new national section may be established if at least one-third of the state nurses' associations have such a section.

During the 1962 Convention in Detroit two new conference groups were organized: one on Geriatric Nursing Practice with sixty-seven nurses from twenty-seven states as

members, and one on Medical-Surgical Nursing with one hundred forty-four nurses as members.

After years of study, discussion and deliberation by the Study Committee on the functions of ANA, the House of Delegates in San Francisco voted for sweeping organizational changes in the structure.

Nursing expertise was regrouped into Divions on Practice and Commissions. The Divisions on Practice that held their organizational meetings at the 1968 ANA Convention in Dallas are: Community Health Nursing, Geriatric Nursing, Maternal and Child Health Nursing, Medical-Surgical Nursing, and Psychiatric and Mental Health Nursing.

The new commissions are Economic Security and General Welfare, Education, and Nursing Services.

To encourage constant improvement for the practitioner, the new structure provides the mechanism for the recognition of excellence by the profession—an Academy of Nursing.

AMERICAN NURSES' ASSOCIATION PROFESSIONAL COUNSELING AND PLACEMENT SERVICE, INC.

The American Nurses' Association Professional Counseling and Placement Service, Inc., is one of the important activities of the American Nurses' Association and has developed as a nonprofit activity that provides counseling and placement service without charge. Service is given to American Nurses' Association members. The Professional Counseling and Placement Service was established in 1945. It is owned by the American Nurses' Association, and twenty-three of the state associations now have established counseling and placement services also. More than 105,000 nurses had their professional records on file as of December, 1963. ANA PC&PS and twenty-three cooperating state PC&PS offices held more than 14,266 interviews with nurses and employers during the period 1961-1963.

Counciling assists nurses to evaluate their aptitudes and skills, to learn about the types of positions for which they are best suited, and to make long-range plans. For this purpose the PC&PS keeps confidential credentials on file and will forward them to any other professional Counseling and Placement Service office or to an employer at the request of the nurse. This organization operates on a national, state, and district basis.

NATIONAL LEAGUE FOR NURSING

The National League for Nursing maintains close relationships with such allied organizations as the American Hospital Association, the American Medical Association, the American Public Health Association, the National Association for Practical Nurse Education, and the National Federation of Licensed Practical Nurses. The NLN carries out its work through extensive correspondence, national and regional conferences, workshops and institutes, consultation services, staff visits to local communities, manuals and handbooks, tests and guides, printed bulletins, and leaflets. Vital problems for the National League for Nursing are: better utilization of all nursing personnel, professional and nonprofessional; better and more extensive in-service education; and the development of teamwork among all nursing personnel, and with medical and nonprofessional nursing groups in the hospital and in the community. Through the Department of Public Health Nursing of the National League for Nursing, ways of helping communities to meet expanding needs for nursing service in the home are being studied.

This year (1969) marks the sixteenth year of the new organization. Membership has increased significantly. Although the individual membership has not shown such a marked increase, there is evidence that with a better knowledge of its program, League membership remarkably increased.

In the continuing studies of structure of the National League for Nursing, the Committee on Constitutions and Bylaws presented the following major amendment which was adopted at the 1963 Convention, held in Atlantic City.

ARTICLE V. OFFICERS

Section 2. Qualifications for Officers. Any individual member except honorary members shall be eligible to hold any of the elected positions specified in Section 1 of this article. The treasurer shall be an individual who is especially skilled and experienced in handling financial matters. No person shall be eligible for position as an elected officer or as a member of the Board of Directors of the American Nurses' Association.*

This important amendment removed the restriction that the president and first vice president of the National League for Nursing must be registered professional nurses as a qualification for those offices.

During the NLN convention in New York City in 1967, following several years of study, the membership voted for an entirely new structure giving more flexibility, freedom, and voice to the local membership.

The League continues to have both individual and agency members. Its 23,000 individual members are professional and practical nurses, nursing aides, doctors, hospital administrators, educators, social workers, therapists, and interested citizens. Agency members, numbering more than 1,800, include hospitals and other institutions providing nursing services, public health nursing agencies, and schools and colleges offering educational programs in nursing.

Today one of the main functions of the National League for Nursing is the accrediting services for the various types of educational programs in nursing. They are administered and conducted through four departmental units of the organization's national headquarters: The Department of Baccalaureate and Higher Degree Programs, the Department of Associate Degree Programs,

---

*Nursing Outlook 11:272, April, 1963. Reprinted with permission.

the Department of Diploma Programs, and the Department of Practical Nursing Programs.

PURPOSES OF ACCREDITATION

The purposes of accrediting programs in nursing education have been stated by the NLN as follows:

1. To stimulate continuous improvement of nursing education throughout the United States and thus to promote improvement of nursing services.
2. To offer assistance to educational units in nursing in the continuous process of self-evaluation and self-improvement of their programs.
3. To describe the essential and distinctive characteristics that each type of education program should have in order to make its appropriate contribution to society.
4. To publish periodically lists of programs currently accredited as meeting the accepted criteria for the designated type of program.*

The lists that are published serve as guides for prospective students in their choice of educational programs in nursing. They assist secondary schools, colleges, and universities in advising students in their choice of educational programs in nursing; assist employers of nurses in judging the qualifications of candidates for various types of positions; and aid interinstitutional relationships such as transfer of students and admission to graduate programs.

Accreditation is conducted under the principles adopted in 1956 for the League's total program of accrediting.

1. Accreditation in nursing is conceived as a program in which the educational units themselves play a vital part. In the process, every effort is made to involve as large a number as possible of the administrative and teaching staff of each educational unit in nursing in its own self-evaluation and thus to encourage self-development.
2. Criteria for accreditation must change as the profession itself evolves and as the society

which it serves makes changing demands. The continuing development of these criteria is a responsibility of the NLN agency members. The function rests with the appropriate councils. (For associate degree programs, this is the Council of Associate Degree Programs.)
3. The individuality of institutions and their special contributions are of paramount importance. Therefore, provided that there is basic conformity to the standards generally accepted by the profession and by society as essential for the functioning of the graduate of an institution at the level and in the field for which the institution purports to train, emphasis is placed upon the evaluation of the total program and its general excellence as well as upon its achievement with regard to particular aspects. Furthermore, the dynamic quality of a program and the rapidity with which it is moving toward clearly defined and desirable goals are recognized. This implies that there will be flexibility in accrediting procedures.*

The National League for Nursing is recognized by the National Commission on Accrediting for the accreditation of baccalaureate and higher degree programs in professional nursing, and as an auxiliary accrediting association at the associate degree level.

NATIONAL STUDENT NURSE ASSOCIATION

The National Student Nurses' Association was organized during the convention of the National League for Nursing in 1953, in Cleveland. Since 1924 student nurses had attended national nursing conventions. Now, students have conventions of their own. In 1950, meetings of student nurses were scheduled and sponsored by graduate nurses. In Atlantic City in June, 1952, the students met and began to talk about forming a national organization. Since the next national convention was to be held in Cleveland in 1953, the job of setting up the constitution and by-laws for a national student organization was delegated to the Ohio stu-

*Policies and procedures of accreditation of the department of associate degree programs, NLN, New York, 1967.

*Policies and procedures of accreditation of the department of associate degree programs, NLN, New York, 1967.

dent nurses. The by-laws were formally adopted and the first slate of officers was elected in 1953 at the meeting held in conjunction with the NLN Convention in Cleveland. Student nurse conventions are now held in conjunction with the alternating biennial conventions of the American Nurses' Association and the National League for Nursing. Most of the time, attendance exceeds 4,000 members.

The National Student Nurses' Association, Inc. (NSNA) consists of individual members in the 51 constituent associations in 49 states, the District of Columbia, and Puerto Rico. There are, in addition, about 240 district or local associations.

The purpose of the student organization as defined in the by-laws is, "to aid in the preparation of student nurses for the assumption of professional responsibilities."

The organization serves as spokesman for students by taking a stand on issues of importance to nursing students. The NSNA serves as a voice for students and as a source of direction and information. NSNA has taken official action in recent years in support of economic security, changes in education for nurses, a broad range of legislation, American Nurses' Association Code for Professional Nurses, and the student's right to educational experience rather than being expected to provide nursing service.

PRACTICAL NURSES

Qualified practical nurses are eligible for membership in the NLN as voted at the National League for Nursing's first convention in 1953. After this convention it was also voted unanimously to authorize the NLN Board of Directors to provide for a Department of Practical Nurse Education if advisable before the next biennial in 1955. A Council on Practical Nursing was created at the annual convention in 1957.

The National Association for Practical Nurse Education was organized in 1941 and is concerned chiefly with education. Membership is offered to both practical and professional nurses as well as to other persons engaged in activities to further the objects of the association. One of the most important activities of this organization has been to survey and to accredit educational programs for practical nurses. Any practical nurse is eligible for NLN membership if he or she is licensed as a practical nurse or by an equivalent title in a state that provides for such licensure, or if she is a graduate of an approved school of practical nursing if the state or states within which she practices or resides do not provide for licensing.

During the 1963 Convention of the National League for Nursing, the Department of Practical Nursing Programs' Council of Member Agencies took one more step towards the development of criteria for evaluating schools of practical nursing when they met and discussed tentative statements presented by the Committee to Study Criteria for Evaluation of Practical Nursing Programs.

OTHER NURSING ORGANIZATIONS

When the American Nurses' Association and the National League for Nursing were reorganized in 1953, not all of the existing nursing organizations were incorporated within the frameworks of these two major associations of nursing. Some of the better-known nursing organizations that have retained their identity are described.

The American Association of Industrial Nurses was organized in 1942. Their official publication is the *American Association of Industrial Nurses Journal*. The aims of the association follow:

1. To formulate and develop principles and standards of industrial nursing practice in order that the nurse in industry may more fully utilize her professional knowledge and training in her service to workers and management—and to the community.
2. To promote, by means of publications, conferences, institutes, and symposia, both formal and informal pro-

grams of education designed specifically for the nurse in industry.

3. To identify the rightful place of nursing in the industrial health program and to encourage cooperation among all groups engaged in protecting the health and welfare of the workers.

4. To impress upon management, physicians, and allied groups the importance of integrating into the activities of industry the services of the industrial nurse.

In 1960 there were approximately 5,000 members of the American Association of Industrial Nurses.

The American College of Nurse-Midwifery was organized in 1955 since none of the existing organizations met the professional needs of this unique specialization in nursing. Representatives of the college have participated in meetings of the International Confederation of Midwives. They publish the *Bulletin of the American College of Nurse-Midwifery*.

The American Association for Nurse Anesthetists was organized in 1931 under the leadership of Agatha Hodgins. Under this association's sponsorship, minimum standards for competent practice were established, and a program of school accreditation was begun in 1952. By 1960 there were 123 accredited schools for nurse anesthetists in the United States. Their official bimonthly publication is *The Journal of the American Association of Nurse Anesthetists*.

The Association of Operating Room Nurses was organized in 1957 and currently has over 4,000 members. They hold a national four-day congress annually and sponsor two-day institutes all over the country. The official journal, *O.R. Nursing,* is published bimonthly.

CONCLUSION

One of the achievements of professional nursing after World War II was the completion of the plans for the reorganization of the structure of professional nursing,

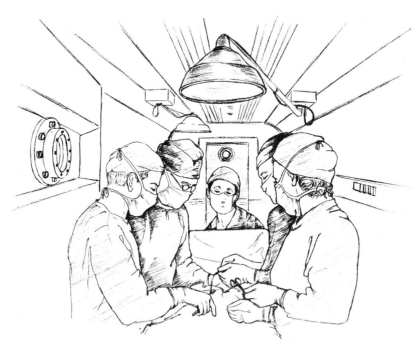

The surgical nurse is a vital part of the many exciting innovations in surgery, such as operating in a hyperbaric chamber.

which resulted in two major national organizations. One organization of, by, and for professional nurses, to have the full responsibility for those functions which the members of any profession should perform for themselves, is the American Nurses' Association. The second organization, the National League for Nursing brought together the National League of Nursing Education, the American Association of Collegiate Schools of Nursing, and the National Organization for Public Health Nursing. It provided, for the first time in nursing history, that all nurses from every occupational field would be able to plan jointly with allied professional workers and agencies for the best utilization, distribution, and financial support of nursing services and nursing education.

Miss McIver* in her article "Nursing Moves Forward" stated the principles that will influence nursing development in the future.

1. The supply of womanpower is limited; therefore, nursing personnel must be utilized for those functions that require nursing skill and judgment. Functions that do not require nursing skill or knowledge should be delegated to other types of workers trained for these functions. Auxiliary workers can be trained on the job, the professional nurse being by education and experience a team leader.
2. A second important principle is that be-

cause womanpower is limited, all schools must select students carefully. Educational programs and conditions of undergraduate experience should be such that desirable students not only come to the school but also stay there.
3. Another basic principle is that nursing schools in organization, administration, and support become integral parts of the total educational program and that the administration of nursing education be vested in educational institutions.
4. The fourth principle is based on the theory that demands for nursing services are likely to increase more rapidly than supply. Thus, demands for nursing are increasing as the types of fields expand tremendously, and the type of work and responsibility change rapidly as general medicine, science, and health change.
5. Every qualified member of a profession has the right and responsibility to participate in such professional activities as (a) defining the functions of a particular occupational group, (b) determining desirable qualifications for practice, (c) establishing employment standards, (d) conducting studies that will improve individual practice, and (e) promoting legislative action that will improve nursing standards and benefit nursing.

The American Nurses' Association is the organization through which the nurse will carry out these responsibilities. The National League for Nursing, on the other hand, will provide the opportunity for nurses and allied professional personnel and the public to work together to provide the amount and kind of nursing service and education needed in this country.

*McIver, Pearl: Nursing moves forward, Fifty-eighth Annual Report of the NLN, New York, 1953, pp. 181-187.

Chapter 29

Studies and programs

At the end of World War II there was no indication that professional nursing was going to settle back into any kind of complacency for a long, long time. As soon as hostilities ceased, all of the national nursing organizations set up planning committees. The National Nursing Council for War Service, Inc., initiated a domestic postwar planning group, which in 1944 developed into the National Nursing Planning Committee. This committee was composed of presidents, executive secretaries, and other representatives of national nursing organizations. It outlined objectives and defined areas in which programs for study should be developed. The results of its deliberations are to be found in "A Comprehensive Program for a Nationwide Action in the Field of Nursing."* In general, the areas for study and action were (1) the improvement of nursing services, (2) the total program of nursing education, practical as well as professional, (3) the distribution of nursing services, (4) the study of standards and the improvement of public relations, and (5) general information about nursing.

*A comprehensive program for a nationwide action in the field of nursing, American Journal of Nursing, September, 1945.

THE BROWN REPORT—NURSING FOR THE FUTURE

The National Nursing Council for War Service, Inc., might have abruptly ceased its activities at the end of World War II. However, members of this committee believed that a comprehensive study of nursing education was indicated. At their request, financial support for the study was obtained from the Carnegie Corporation of New York. Dr. Esther Lucile Brown, Director of the Department of Studies in Professions of the Russell Sage Foundation, served as the director of the study. This study was published in 1948 and is known either as the Brown Report or *Nursing for the Future*. In this study Dr. Brown approached the problem of what provisions should be made for the nursing and health needs of society. Programs for the future of nursing education could be worked out only in the light of meeting these needs. Few reports have had such a tumultuous reception as the Brown Report. Nurses, hospital administrators, and doctors have been loud in their approval or disapproval of it. The report has been made, and, from the findings, programs and plans for the future are being studied.

Important findings of the Brown Report

The Brown Report recommended that the term "professional" when applied to nurses should be used only for those who have studied in a school designated as "an accredited professional school." The education, financial support, and legislation for the training of practical nurses were discussed and recommended. This report also pointed out that schools of nursing should be nationally classified and accredited; that faculty standards, such as those formulated by the Association of Collegiate Schools of Nursing, be accepted in all schools; and that the nursing courses as given in the hospital school should be both shortened and improved, particularly as central schools of nursing in connection with teaching resources of colleges and universities were better utilized. It pointed out that the rapidly expanding demands of the nursing function could be satisfactorily met only when the nurse had made a place for herself on the health team, or with allied professional groups, such as physicians, health officers, social workers, and teachers. It pointed out that nursing education needs financial support from both private and public sources. It recommended that state and regional planning for nursing service and nursing education should be started immediately so that plans for the future could be worked out on the basis of need.

Two major changes suggested by Dr. Brown's recommendations were that schools of nursing should have affiliation with universities and have separate school budgets. Since about 800 schools of nursing in this country are still hospital schools, and many of these have very little if any affiliation with any educational institution, far-reaching changes were indicated. Dr. Brown pointed out that the inadequacy of nursing service in most hospitals exists because nurses have been poorly trained in schools of nursing that are inadequate for participation in any educational program. There has been a great deal of criticism about this report by nurses, particularly about the recommendation made that professional nurses be college-trained and that in order to relieve the nursing shortage two-year courses in practical nursing be established. Many registered nurses have believed that if this program were carried out, many of them would be demoted to the status of a practical nurse.

Tangible results of the Brown Report

One very important and constructive result of this report has been that nurses, doctors, hospital administrators, and the lay public have studied the whole question of nursing service and nursing education with a thoroughness seldom seen before. In order to stimulate thinking about the situation, the National Nursing Council for War Service, Inc., sponsored three regional conferences in 1948 in connection with the study. The results have been published in a book, *1000 Think Together.* The bringing together of nurses, doctors, hospital administrators, and interested lay people was most constructive. Incidentally, the technic of group dynamics was used, and to many in the nursing field this was a first experience with a new technic in conducting conferences.

The National Nursing Council for War Service, Inc., which had stimulated this study, *Nursing for the Future,* later changed its name to National Committee for the Improvement of Nursing Service.

NATIONAL COMMITTEE FOR THE IMPROVEMENT OF NURSING SERVICE

In 1951 the National Committee for the Improvement of Nursing Service was enlarged to include forty members, representing education, medicine, and general citizen groups. At this time, a *Newsletter* was published to keep the state nursing organizations informed and to help them organize state committees for the improvement of nursing service. Also published was the book *Nursing Schools at the Mid-Century.* When the interim classification of schools of nursing was made, schools were promised that the second study would be made within two years. However, it developed that a program of temporary accreditation seemed to be more helpful to schools in working toward full accreditation than a second classification would be. Funds were granted by the Rockefeller and Commonwealth Foundation and the National Foundation for Infantile Paralysis to support the program of temporary accreditation for a three-year period. This accrediting program was carried out by the National Nursing Accrediting Service, which had been organized early in 1949 under the auspices of the six national nursing organizations.

A subcommittee on the Improvement of Nursing Service had also been developing its program during this period. Institutes on Nursing Service Administration for both nursing administrators and hospital administrators were held by the National Committee for the Improvement of Nursing Service and the American Hospital Association.

In June, 1952, when the structure of the six national nursing organizations changed, the work and staff of the National Committee for the Improvement of Nursing Service were absorbed into the Division of Nursing Services of the National League for Nursing.

COMMUNITY COLLEGE EDUCATION FOR NURSING RESEARCH

The first programs in nursing within the framework of community colleges followed the publication of Dr. Mildred Montag's doctoral thesis, *Education of Nursing Technicians,* 1951. In 1952 a national research project was started to determine the feasibility of developing this new type of nursing education. The project, the Cooperative Research Project in Junior and Community College Education for Nursing, was under the direction of Dr. Montag. One purpose of the project was to develop and test this new type of program preparing young men and women for those functions commonly associated with the registered nurse. Before

the five-year project with the geographically selected schools was completed, the concept had more or less mushroomed; programs in community colleges were developed from coast to coast, and there are now over 330 programs. The curriculum is generally offered in a two-year academic period, in accordance with college policy and regulations of the various state licensing agencies. The Surgeon General's report, "Towards Quality in Nursing—Needs and Goals," anticipates a 445% increase in the number of graduates from Associate Degree programs by 1970.

The characteristics of Associate Degree nursing programs are described in a set of *Guiding Principles for the Establishment of Programs in Nursing in Junior and Community Colleges* as follows:

1. It is desirable that only junior colleges that are accredited by the appropriate regional educational associations establish associate degree programs in nursing.
2. The junior college assumes the same responsibility for the nursing program as it does for other programs; that is, it has complete control of the program and is wholly responsible for its quality.
3. The structure and organization of the junior college are such as to make possible the effective performance of its total function and to permit inclusion of nursing education as part of that function.
4. The administrative leadership in the junior college fosters a democratic environment throughout the entire institution, providing opportunities for the faculty and students of the nursing department to participate in the affairs and life of the college in the same way as do members of other departments.
5. The junior college provides competent leadership for the nursing program, selecting a qualified nurse educator as head of the nursing department and a qualified faculty in nursing.
6. The administration of the junior college takes the initiative in the organization of such lay advisory committees as may be deemed essential to assist the nursing department to achieve a quality program.
7. The junior college provides appropriate resources and facilities for the nursing program.

8. When a junior college makes arrangements with a hospital or other cooperating agencies for the use of facilities in which the college provides instruction for its students, there is an established formal relationship.
   a. This relationship is entered into only after the groups involved have thoroughly studied and reached agreement on the ways in which the facilities are to be used and the conditions governing their use.
   b. This relationship is clearly defined in a written statement approved by the appropriate boards of control.
   c. The junior college sees to it that the policies established and the mutual obligations specified in the formal agreement are implemented.
9. The junior college assumes full financial responsibility for providing a quality educational program in nursing and has the financial resources to meet such commitments.
   a. The student in nursing is not expected to bear any greater portion of the direct and indirect cost of the program than is required of any other student in the junior college.
   b. The junior college has a sound budgetary procedure for its nursing program as well as for all other programs.
   c. There is opportunity for the nursing faculty and administrative staff to participate with others in the preparation of the budget and in other financial matters.*

TESTING SERVICES

The volume of the testing service had become so great that a regular department of the National League of Nursing Education was created in 1946. In addition to the State Board examinations, a national test for prenursing and guidance was worked out. State Board Pool tests are now used in all of the states, District of Columbia, and several provinces in Canada.

Mrs. R. Louise McManus, Chairman and Director of the Division of Nursing Education, Teachers College, Columbia University, was responsible for setting up the State Board Pool which became a source for examinations and for the scoring of tests for State Boards throughout the country. To a certain extent, this was a development of World War II when State Boards of nurse examiners were being swamped with the work of testing and scoring State Board tests; many graduates were being delayed because they could not obtain results from their examinations quickly enough. After two years, Mrs. McManus had acquired a staff of thirty full-time workers in her testing service, and after the war the old system of State Boards was not resumed, but the National League for Nursing continued this testing service.

Staff workers are constantly developing better technics in testing and are closely associated with nurse educators from different parts of the United States representing both diploma and degree programs. The plan now worked out is that two nurse teachers in each of the major clinical areas of the basic programs spend one week at headquarters, deciding the general scope of material and developing test questions to be included in the examinations. In addition, the Evaluation and Guidance Service creates qualifying examinations for the graduate nurse. This examination is used by many colleges and universities.

RESEARCH IN NURSING

One sign of the maturity of any profession lies in its interest in, and the value of, research it sponsors and carries on. The American Nurses' Association voted in 1950 to finance more research than it ever had carried out in the past. A list of some of these studies follow on p. 216. Much valuable research also appears in the theses of graduate students working toward their master's and doctor's degrees.

Many foundations have been interested in providing money to support research in nursing, beginning with the Rockefeller Grant in 1919, which resulted in the publi-

*Committee of the National League for Nursing and the American Association of Junior Colleges: Guiding principles for junior colleges participating in nursing education, New York, 1961, National League for Nursing.

cation of the book *Nursing and Nurse Education in the United States.* The Commonwealth Fund, The Russell Sage Foundation, the Kellogg Foundation and other organizations are today supporting valuable studies in many areas of significance to nursing. Universities, particularly their social science departments, are participating with nurses in research.

Both the American Nurses' Association and the National League for Nursing have sponsored and carried out an increasing number of studies and research projects since World War II. This is very important as the profession matures. One of the most significant books, *Twenty Thousand Nurses Tell Their Story,** is the report on the studies of nursing functions sponsored by the American Nurses' Association, as decided by the House of Delegates of the American Nurses' Association in 1950.

The American Nurses' Foundation was established by the American Nurses' Association in 1955 to support research and studies in nursing and to sponsor special projects. The Foundation plans, guides, and coordinates nursing research and disseminates research findings. Supported in part by funds from the ANA, the Foundation receives contributions from individuals and from other foundations. A list of their recent projects follows:

AMERICAN NURSES' FOUNDATION, INC.
Research Grants

1. Nurses at work, Edwin A. Christ, University of Missouri
2. The private duty nurse, her role in the hospital environment of Washington, D. C., Barbara J. Suttell, Ph.D., Shirley S. Pumroy, American Institute for Research, Washington, D. C.
3. Patterns of psychiatric nursing, Harry W. Martin, Ida Harper Simpson, University of North Carolina

---

*Hughes, Everett C., Hughes, Helen MacGill, and Deutscher, Irwin: Twenty thousand nurses tell their story, Philadelphia and Montreal 1958, J. B. Lippincott Co.

4. A study of the registered nurse in a metropolitan community, Community Studies, Inc., Kansas City, Missouri
5. Nurse-patient relationship and the healing process, J. Frank Whiting, Ph.D. V.A. Hospital, Rutland Heights, Massachusetts, V.A. Hospital, Leech Farm Road, Pittsburgh, Pennsylvania, University of Pittsburgh
6. The role of the nurse in the outpatient department, Kenneth D. Benne, Ph.D., Warren Bennis, Ph.D., Boston University
7. The industrial nurse, Wendell T. Smith, Ph.D., Bucknell University
8. The adjustment of student nurses to a psychiatric affiliation, Raymond Forer, Ph.D., Mrs. Dorothy M. Douglas, R.N., Mrs. Helen A. McClafferty, R.N., Connecticut State Department of Mental Health
9. A study of the problems of bowel and bladder incontinence in geriatric patients, Barbara Williams Madden, M.S., R.N., Rancho Los Amigos Hospital, Downey, California
10. A program to identify and develop a research attitude in student nurses, Mrs. Frances G. Macgregor, M.A., Cornell University-New York Hospital School of Nursing
11. Premature infant nursing study of the effects of handling upon the behavior of prematurely born infants, Eileen Hasselmeyer, M.A., R.N., New York University
12. Expectations of administrators, staff members and patients in four nursing homes in King County, Washington, Mrs. Margaret Fenn, Ph.D., Washington State Health Department
13. Temporal parameters of aging as biologic basis for nursing intervention, Owen Jones Stephens, Ph.D., University of Minnesota, University of California
14. Admission of surgical patients, Mrs. Roslyn Elms, M.S.N., R.N., Yale University School of Nursing
15. Support of women in labor, Barbara Bender, M.S.N., R.N., Yale University School of Nursing, West Virginia University School of Nursing
16. Bacterial ecology of the perineum during labor, Frances Reiter, N.A., R.N., Graduate School of Nursing, New York Medical College
17. Absorption of insulin I 131 from the subcutaneous tissue, Martha Pitel, Ph.D., R.N., University of Rochester, University of Kansas Medical Center, New York University
18. A study of the effects of vestibular stimulation on infants' developmental behavior,

Mary Neal, N. Litt., R.N., New York University

19. A study of selected physiological responses to breathing exercise practice in patients with chronic obstructive pulmonary disease, Evelyn Elwood, M.A., R.N. New York University

20. Separation anxiety in hospitalized children; comparison study of three conditions of separation from mothering, Ellamae Branstetter, M.P.H., R.N., University of Chicago

21. Nursing and pain: a clinical experiment, Mrs. Mary A. B. McBride, M.S.N., R.N. Yale University School of Nursing

22. University of Utah research conference on architectural psychology, Calvin W. Taylor, Ph.D., Roger Bailey, Mildred Quinn, M.S., R.N., University of Utah

23. Study of vigilance decrement in nurse-patient monitoring, Major Lois Johns, M. Sc. Educational Psychology, R.N., University of Utah

24. Living open system, reciprocal adaptation and the life process, Gean M. Mathwig, M.A., R.N., New York University

25. Development of instruments for use in solving covert problems: a learning experience for nursing service, Mrs. Doris Citron, M.A., R.N., Mount Sinai Hospital, New York

26. Conflict, legitimation, and forms of protest, Rita M. Braito, M.S., M.A., R.N., University of Washington

27. Heart rate changes in adults related to the introduction of auditory stimuli, Mrs. Audrey L. Burgess, M.A., R.N., State University of New York at Buffalo

28. The making of modern nursing: a study of forces which have created the modern profession of nursing, Muriel Uprichard, Ph.D., University of California, School of Nursing, Los Angeles

29. Enculturation and popular health culture, Agnes M. Aamodt, M.A., R.N., University of Washington

30. An investigation into the aggressive postoperative play responses of hospitalized preschool children, Donna L. Vredevoe, Ph.D., University of California, School of Nursing, Los Angeles

31. The effect upon the palmar sweat index of hormonal changes related to the menstrual cycle, Mrs. Patsy Snyder Yoder, M.S., R.N., Wayne State University

Questions and study projects for unit seven

1. Discuss the shortage of all health and hospital personnel and show how nursing service and education are both affected by this shortage.
2. From the discussion in this unit and from your readings, list major trends affecting (a) nursing service and (b) nursing education. Show how these trends are linked to the general social and economic picture in our country.
3. If you are a student in a collegiate program, are there any major differences between your program and that of other undergraduate students in professional programs? Be prepared to discuss the differences and similarities in the programs.
4. If you are a student in a hospital school of nursing, are you aware of the differences between nursing service and nursing education? Discuss with your instructors, both in the hospital and in the school of nursing, the differences and similarities between the two programs.
5. Study an organizational chart of (a) your school of nursing and (b) nursing service in the hospital or hospitals in which you receive clinical experience. Be prepared to discuss these organizational charts in class.
6. Describe the current concept of profession in the United States. Does nursing qualify?
7. Make an annotated bibliography of recent articles appearing in *The American Journal of Nursing, Nursing Outlook, Nursing Research,* and any other journals available in your library relating to the discussion in this unit.
8. Name some postwar trends affecting nursing service and nursing education.
9. Discuss the Rich Report.
10. Why was the study, *Nursing for the Future,* made?
11. Evaluate the comments for and against the Brown Report.
12. In what ways is there evidence of joint action in professional nursing today?
13. Compare the findings and recommendations of the following studies and reports in nursing: The Goldmark Report, those of the Grading Committee, and the Brown Report.
14. What was the purpose of the Structure Study? What circumstances and studies brought it about, and what was the result of this study?
15. Discuss the practical nurse and the subsidiary worker in (a) nursing service and (b) nursing education.
16. What is the direct result of Dr. Mildred Montag's doctoral thesis, *Education of Nursing Technicians?*
17. List six characteristics of Associate Degree nursing programs.
18. How do these characteristics differ from the program you are now enrolled in?
19. Make an annotated bibliography of recent articles appearing in *The American Journal of Nursing, Nursing Outlook, Nursing Research,* and any other journals available in your library relating to the discussion in this unit.

References for unit seven

ANA facts about nursing, New York, published yearly by American Nurses' Association.

ANA standards for organized nursing services, American Journal of Nursing **65**:76, March, 1965.

Andreoli, Kathleen G., and Stead, Jr., Eugene A.: Training physicians assistants at Duke, American Journal of Nursing **67**:1442-1443, July, 1967.

Aynes, Edith A.: Medicare: bonanza or mirage?, Nursing Outlook **14**:57, June, 1966.

Barron, Nancy J.: A ride in the human centrifuge, American Journal of Nursing **67**:1653-4, August, 1967.

Berry, Elizabeth J.: Hope docks in guinea, American Journal of Nursing **66**:2238-42, October, 1966.

Bixler, G. K., and Bixler, R. W.: The professional status of nursing, American Journal of Nursing **45**:730-735, September, 1945.

Bloom, Samuel W.: The doctor and his patient—a sociological interpretation, New York, 1963, Russell Sage Foundation.

Breckenridge, Sophonisba P.: Women in the twentieth century, New York, 1933, McGraw-Hill Book Company.

Bridgman, Margaret: On types of programs, American Journal of Nursing **60**:1465-1468, October, 1960.

Brown, Esther Lucile: Nursing as a profession, ed. 2, New York, 1940, Russell Sage Foundation.

Brown, Esther Lucile: Nursing for the future (Brown report), New York, 1948, Russell Sage Foundation.

Brown, Esther Lucile: Newer dimensions of patient care, Part I, New York, 1961, Russell Sage Foundation.

Brown, Esther Lucile: Newer dimensions of patient care, Part II, New York, 1962, Russell Sage Foundation.

Carter, Barbara: Medicine's forgotten women, Reporter **26**:35-37, March 1, 1962.

Conlon, Alice Y.: Convincing the legislature, American Journal of Nursing **66**:545-8, March, 1966.

Edelstein, Ruth R.: Automation: its effect on the nurse, American Journal of Nursing **66**:2194-8, October, 1966.

Ellerbrock, Sister Mary Coralita: About Christian commitment to education for nursing, Nursing Outlook **15**:38, March, 1967.

Erickson, Roberta: Visiting wide neighborhoods, Nursing Outlook **14**:34, October, 1966.

Erne, Sister Mary Julie: Implications of trends in nursing education, Nursing Outlook **14**:36, September, 1966.

Fagin, Claire M.: The clinical specialist as supervisor, Nursing Outlook **15**:34, January, 1967.

Fritz, Edna: Baccalaureate nursing education—what is its job?, American Journal of Nursing **66**:1312-6, June, 1966.

Gelber, Ida: Family planning in a growing world, American Journal of Nursing **64**:98-103, August, 1964.

George, Joyce Holmes: Electronic monitoring of vital signs, American Journal of Nursing **65**:68, February, 1965.

Ginzberg, Eli: Nursing and manpower realities, Nursing Outlook **15**:26, November, 1967.

Ginzberg, Eli: The hospital and the nurse, American Journal of Nursing, **63**:16, November, 1963.

Goodnow, Minnie: Nursing history, ed. 8, Philadelphia, 1948, W. B. Saunders Company.

Goodnow, Minnie: Nursing history in brief, ed. 3, Philadelphia, 1950, W. B. Saunders Company.

Goodson, Max R.: Professional education, American Journal of Nursing **66**:798-801, April, 1966.

Griffin, Gerald J.: and others, New dimensions for the improvement of clinical nursing, Nursing Research, **15**:292-302, Fall, 1966.

Griffin, G. J., and others: Clinical nursing instruction by television, New York, 1965, Columbia University Press.

Hammerly, Aloha B.: "The Army's public health nurses," American Journal of Nursing **66**:765-7, April, 1966.

Hassenplug, Lulu Wolf: "Going on for a bachelor's degree," American Journal of Nursing **66**:83-85, January, 1966.

Jahoda, Marie: Nursing as a profession, American Journal of Nursing **61**:52-56, July, 1961.

Jamieson, Elizabeth M., and Sewall, Mary: Trends in nursing history, ed. 4, Philadelphia, 1954, W. B. Saunders Company.

Johnson, Dorothy, Wilcox, Joan, and Moidel, Harriet: The clinical specialist as a practitioner, American Journal of Nursing **67**:2298-2303, November, 1967.

Johnson, R. Winifred: Practical nursing—a part of MDTA, Nursing Outlook **15**:55, November, 1967.

Kelly, Dorothy N.: Equating the nurse's economic rewards with the service given, American Journal of Nursing **67**:1642-1645, August, 1967.

Killam, Lee: In good faith, American Journal of Nursing **67**:1883-1885, September, 1967.

King, Stanley H.: Perceptions of illness and medical practice, New York, 1962, Russell Sage Foundation.

Kriegel, Julia. Are we earning our salaries?, Nursing Outlook **15**:60, December, 1967.

Lewis, Edith P.: Scutari, U.S.A., American Journal of Nursing **65**:100, March, 1965.

Lewis, Edith P.: The Fairview story, American Journal of Nursing **66**:64-70, January, 1966.

Mahoney, Anne B.: Convincing the membership, American Journal of Nursing **66**:554, March, 1966.

Makin, Mildred C.: Phasing out a diploma program need not be a 'death watch', Nursing Outlook **15**:31, October, 1967.

Mechner, Francis: Learning by doing through programmed instruction, American Journal of Nursing **65**:98, May, 1965.

Mereness, Dorothy: Freedom and responsibility for nursing students, American Journal of Nursing **67**:69-71, January, 1967.

Mittman, Benand Bumganer, Beatrice: What happened in San Francisco, American Journal of Nursing **67**:80-84, January, 1967.

Moses, Evelyn: Nursing economic plight, American Journal of Nursing **65**:68, January, 1965.

Myers, Emily, and Pott, Ella: An internship for new graduates, American Journal of Nursing **68**:96-98, January, 1968.

Newton, Mildred E.: Nurses caps and bachelors gowns, American Journal of Nursing **64**:73-77, May, 1964.

Novotny, Dorothy R.: Suited for space life, American Journal of Nursing **67**:1655-1657, August, 1967.

Nuckolis, Katherine B.: Tenderness and technique via TV, American Journal of Nursing **66**:2690, December, 1966.

Nurses are making it happen, American Journal of Nursing **67**:285-288, February, 1967.

Nursing aides train at Job Corps center, American Journal of Nursing **15**:35, August, 1967.

Operating room nursing—is it professional nursing?, American Journal of Nursing **65**:58, August, 1965.

Pope, Irene: Medicare—impetus for change, Nursing Outlook **16**:34, January, 1968.

Porter, Elizabeth K.: What it means to be a professional nurse, American Journal of Nursing **53**:948-950, August, 1953.

Price, Elimina: Data processing: present and potential, American Journal of Nursing **67**:2558-2564, December, 1967.

Reiter, Frances: The nurse clinician, American Journal of Nursing **66**:274-280, February, 1966.

Ro, Kong Kyun, and Anderson, Odin W.: The cost of health, American Journal of Nursing **63**:21, November, 1963.

Roberts, Mary M.: American nursing: history and interpretation, New York, 1954, The Macmillan Company.

Rosenberg, Mervin, and Carriker, Delores: Automating nurses notes, American Journal of Nursing **66**:1021-23, May, 1966.

Rothberg, June S.: Why nursing diagnosis?, American Journal of Nursing **67**:1040-1042, May, 1967.

Rowan, Robert L.: Automation: its effect on the hospital, American Journal of Nursing **66**:2199, October, 1966.

Rutherford, Ruby: What bothers staff nurses, American Journal of Nursing **67**:315-318, February, 1967.

Sandve, Wanyce C.: Diploma programs need scrutiny, American Journal of Nursing **65**:103, February, 1965.

Scott, William C., and others: The long shadow, American Journal of Nursing **66**:538-43, March, 1966.

Silver, Henry, and Ford, Loretta: The pediatric nurse practitioner at Colorado, American Journal of Nursing **67**:1443-1444, July, 1967.

Stokes, Joseph: More physicians, more highly trained nurses, or a new health worker?, American Journal of Nursing **67**:1441-2, July, 1967.

Tarrant, Betty Jane: Automation: its effect on the patient, American Journal of Nursing **66**:2190-3, October, 1966.

Tate, Barbara, and Knopf, Lucille: Nursing students—who are they?, American Journal of Nursing **65**:99, September, 1965.

The Army nurse, American Journal of Nursing **66**:290-292, February, 1966.

The division of nursing, USPHS, American Journal of Nursing **65**:82, July, 1965.

The stars beckon, American Journal of Nursing **67**:1650-1652, August, 1967.

The Surgeon General looks at nursing, American Journal of Nursing **67**:64-67, January, 1967.

Transition in nursing education, American Journal of Nursing **67**:1211-1223, June, 1967.

Two-organization structure, American Journal of Nursing **50**:741, 1950.

United States Department of Health, Education, and Welfare, Public Health Service: Toward quality in nursing: needs and goals, Report of Surgeon General's Consultant Group on Nursing, Public Health Service pub. no. 992, Washington, D. C., 1963, United States Government Printing Office.

Whitaker, Judith G.: The nurse as a professional person, Nursing Outlook **9**:217-219, April, 1961.

Woolley, Alma S.: The "now" generation in nursing, Nursing Outlook **16**:26, March, 1968.

Yost, Edna: American women of nursing, Philadelphia, 1948, J. B. Lippincott Co.

Associate degree nursing references

Aasterud, Margaret, and Guthrie, Katheryn: What can be expected of the graduate with an A.D.?, Nursing Outlook **12**:52-53, August, 1964.

ANA. A position paper: educational preparation for nurse practitioners and assistants to nurses, New York, ANA, 1965.

Anderson, Bernice E.: Nursing education in community junior colleges, Philadelphia, 1966, J. B. Lippincott Co.

Butler, Jean: Nursing service director in an Associate in Arts Program, Nursing Outlook **7**: 19-20, January, 1959.

DeChow, Georgeen H.: Accreditation of Associate Degree Nursing Program, Journal of Nursing Education **4**:27-32, August, 1965.

Forest, Betty: The utilization of associate degree nursing graduates in general hospitals, The League Exchange Number 82, National League for Nursing, 1968.

Hallinan, Bernadene, and Aldrich, Martha: Teaching nursing care in a community college Associate Degree Program, Journal of Nursing Education **6**:13-8+, January, 1967.

Harris, Norman C.: Technical education—problem for the present, promise for the future, American Journal of Nursing **63**:95-9, May, 1963.

Harty, Margaret B.: Team teaching, Nursing Outlook **11**:59-61, January, 1963.

Heller, Melvin P., and King, Imogene: Team teaching: values and advantages, Nursing Outlook **13**:50+, October, 1965.

Ingwersen, Ina J.: Teaching mental health and mental illness in an associate degree nursing program, Nursing Outlook **15**:33-4, February, 1967.

Kinsinger, Robert E.: A core curriculum for the health field, Nursing Outlook **15**:28-29, February, 1967.

McCandless, Mary R.: Preparing the community for associate degree education in nursing and the planning year: a consultant's point of view, Nursing Science **2**:199-205, June, 1964.

Montag, Mildred L.: The education of nursing technicians, New York, 1951, G. P. Putnam's Sons.

Montag, Mildred L.: Nursing programs in junior and community colleges, Yearbook of Modern Nursing, New York, 1956, G. P. Putnam's Sons.

Montag, Mildred L.: Technical education in nursing?, American Journal of Nursing **63**:100-3, May, 1963.

Montag, Mildred L.: Utilization of graduates of associate degree nursing programs, Journal of Nursing Education **5**:5-9, April, 1966.

Montag, Mildred L.: Nursing curriculum and facilities, Proceedings Associate Degree Workshop, July 25-29, Boulder, University of Colorado, 1966.

Montag, Mildred L., and Gorkin, Lasser G.: Community college education for nursing, New York, 1960, McGraw-Hill Book Company.

NLN: Department of Associate Degree Programs, criteria for the evaluation of educational programs in nursing leading to an associate degree, New York, NLN, 1966.

NLN: Policies and procedures of accreditation of the department of associate degree programs, New York, NLN, 1967.

Sister Juliana: An Experience in Transition in Nursing Education, Hospital Progress **48**:67+, February, 1967.

The associate degree program, American Journal of Nursing **64**:78-79, May, 1964.

Transition in nursing education, American Journal of Nursing **67**:1211-16, June, 1967. (Discussion of Response to N. Y. State's *BLUEPRINT*.

Vosloh, Lillian: Public relations for a new nursing program, Nursing Outlook **5**:230-2, April, 1957.

Wiggins, Virginia L.: The teaching team, American Journal of Nursing **56**:764-6, June, 1956.

Worledge, Clara B.: Teaching nursing by television, Journal of Nursing Education **5**:33-37, April, 1966.

Zimmerman, Esther D.: Associate degree graduate in nursing service, Journal of Nursing Education **2**:11-164, April, 1966.

Unit eight

*Legal aspects**

Elwyn L. Cady, Jr., J.D., B.S.Med.

"The administration of justice is a practical affair, an invention for the adjustment of the rights of individuals and not a technical and accurate science, but an applied science, adjusting itself to work out justice in all the protean shapes the dealings of mankind assume."[†]

---

*Originally written by the late John F. Spaulding, LL.B.
[†]The Honorable Henry Lamm, Justice, Supreme Court of Missouri, 1904-1914.

Chapter 30

Introduction to the law and lobbying

Regardless of background, training, or accomplishments, each person is an individual with a specific identity in the eyes of the law. If a person has had special training and experience in a profession, additional duties and legal responsibilities are thus acquired. The legal status of the nurse in a professional capacity is generally outlined in this unit.

BASIC CONCEPTS

First, one may wonder about the necessity of such legal study. When it is realized that in law, as in disease and accident, prevention is far better than cure, it becomes evident that basic legal knowledge is to help one avoid rather than to become involved in legal difficulties.

Second, one is often confused by newspaper reports, rumors, or doubtful tales regarding certain legal matters ranging from criminal and lurid divorce proceedings to the more routine acts of executing a property deed or will. It must be remembered that the source of such information is often people who have misformed concepts of the law.

Finally, nurses are particularly concerned with the law that deals with their day-to-day professional life. Most professional actions taken by the nurse have substantial legal significance. This is not to say that lawsuits will arise out of every action, but as a citizen of the community the nurse has a continuing duty to "follow the law."

Now, just what is "the law"? Many authorities on jurisprudence (legal philosophy) have devoted extended attention to the matter of definition. Recognizing the limitations of any brief definition, we merely quote the following:

1. A law is a sequence of events: if one occurrence, called the condition, takes place, another occurrence, called the consequence, follows.
2. [In positive law] The connection is not causal but what has been called normative and is expressed by the word "ought," i.e., if somebody does this, then somebody else ought to do that.
3. [Blackstone defined state law (positive law)] "A rule of civil conduct prescribed by the supreme power in a state, commanding what is right and prohibiting what is wrong." A better definition is "the aggregate of those rules and principles of conduct which the governing power in a community recognizes as those which it will enforce or sanction."*

Note, then, that law has to do with rules of conduct. To enforce compliance with those rules, the government has established

---

*Snyder, Orvall C.: Preface to jurisprudence, Indianapolis, 1954, The Bobbs-Merrill Co., Inc., pp. 71-73.

agencies of law enforcement. The most obvious agency is the local police force. A system of courts organized to adjudicate disputes is also a vital part of the machinery of justice. Then, too, there are numerous other regulatory agencies acting with the force of law.

The importance of knowing that the rules of law are binding along with some understanding of the particular rules applicable to nurses can best be stated in the historical maxim that ignorance of the law is no excuse. Of course, this does not mean that everyone is expected to carry around a memorized listing of laws in his head but merely indicates that he may not plead ignorance of the law as a legal defense when he is before the court. Otherwise, violators of the rules could escape sanctions of the law that have been established for the common welfare.

Incidentally, lawyers themselves are not trained to memorize innumerable rules. They are primarily trained in the analysis of legal situations and in how to "look up the law." This involves what the scientist would call a minor research project in that counsel must do a certain amount of research whenever he is asked to render a legal opinion. It becomes a major research project when complications arise, claims are presented, suits filed, and briefs written. For day-to-day guidance it is usually best to select a personal lawyer much as one would select a personal physician. Through his services the nurse can preserve the investment in his or her profession and often can prevent unpleasant legal complications.

DIVISIONS OF LAW

In general there are two legal systems extant in the world today, the Anglo-American "common law" system and the "civil law" system. It is perhaps a surprise to realize that most areas are under the latter system rather than the common law system that applies in the United States except for Louisiana. Further discussion in this unit will be oriented toward the common law system although most principles will hold also for nurses in Louisiana.

In practice there are two primary sources of law, case decisions (precedents) and statutes. The case method is the distinctive approach of the Anglo-American system. Each case decided at the appellate level and reported in the law reports becomes an "authority" for the adjudication of future cases. This is expressed in the term *stare decisis,* meaning "to stand by decided cases."

Statutory law is written and includes enactments of legislatures, local laws, and ordinances of counties and municipalities, and rules and regulations of administrative agencies such as boards of nursing examiners.

In American procedure judges finally determine what the law is in particular controversies. Lawyers, as advocates or "paid champions" of their clients, are duty-bound to plead their clients' causes before judges and juries, as partisans. Lawyers are also under a duty, as officers of the court, to assist judges in determining the correct applicable rules of law, whether derived from the body of common law precedents or to be found in the statute books.

In jury-tried cases, a jury's function is to make "findings of fact" or decisions based upon its findings of fact and the instructions of the judge as to what rules of law apply.

Provision for keeping the law up to date is made under the Anglo-American system by (1) the fact that courts may, and often do, overrule previous decisions in determining a lawsuit and (2) amendments and revisions of the various state and Federal statutes by legislative bodies from time to time.

THE LEGISLATIVE LOBBY

Recognizing the importance of statutory law as a dynamic force in keeping legal concepts up to date, we will briefly delve into lobbying to demonstrate how statutory law is often made and changed.

Under Federal regulatory definitions lobbying refers to any direct communication with members of Congress with the object of procuring passage or defeat of pending legislation.

One state statute defined it to be any personal solicitation of a member of a legislative body by means and appliances not addressed solely to the judgment. Thus, a dubious quality is sometimes attached to the concept of lobbying.

On the other hand, a popular image of the lobbyist as one who performs a genuine public service is desirable. The Canon of Ethics that governs lawyers who lobby is in this spirit:

A lawyer openly, and in his true character may render professional services before legislative or other bodies, regarding proposed legislation and in advocacy of claims before departments of government, upon the same principles of ethics which justify his appearance before the Courts; but it is unprofessional for a lawyer so engaged to conceal his attorneyship, or to employ secret personal solicitations, or to use means other than those addressed to the reason and understanding, to influence action.

Writing to or conversing with your representative regarding specific bills or proposed legislation is lobbying in the general sense although it may be done without pay and with idealistic intent. If in a letter or conversation one can put forth salient facts or other information to a legislator, positive public service can be rendered to both the legislator and the public. However, by the use of distorted data or statements the lobbyist can become a public menace instead of a public servant.

The importance of lobbying in today's democracy is based upon two considerations: (1) it is a fundamental right of the people to express themselves to a legislative body or administrative agency and (2) a modern legislator cannot thoroughly consider all legislative issues without assistance. Lobbyists, then, become a significant source of technical assistance to the harried legislator.

ROUTE OF A BILL

Assume that a nursing group is interested in legislation to license convalescent homes in your state, in which no license requirements presently exist. Assume further that your reasons are adequate and proper. The group should first outline in written form what is believed to be proper standards for operation of such a home, for example, maintenance, management, equipment, and other essentials. After this written outline is completed, an attorney should ordinarily be consulted. Consultation about drafting the proposed legislation, including advice about what agency should regulate or enforce such legislation if it becomes law, can usually be obtained through a legislator. Congress and nearly all state legislatures have a staff of experts on legislative drafting to aid them in this phase. A specific legislator may be unfriendly to such legislation —therefore the group should interview several members of a legislative body before submitting ideas and requesting help.

Assume that the group has found a legislator who is interested in such legislation and that the proposed idea has been drafted in the terminology necessary in the form of a bill. The bill must be introduced by one or more members of one of the houses of the legislature. The basic route of a bill is as follows:

1. The bill is introduced in either House or Senate by the sponsor or author of the bill who must be a member of the legislative chamber in which it is introduced.

2. Many states and Congress vary in the requirements at this time as to reading the bill, entering it into record, and so forth; therefore, only the basic steps will be outlined here. The second part of the bill's journey is its referral to a legislative committee. The legislative body usually has certain standing com-

mittees made up of members of the legislative body. Subject matter of a bill determines to which committee it is referred. Usually legislative bodies have a standing (meaning permanent) committee on health and welfare. If we assume that the basic intent of your proposed bill is to ensure better care for patients in convalescent homes, this may be the logical committee to study the bill.

3. The committee, having received the bill, has the power to report on it to the legislative house as a whole after the committee has made its study. This study involves hearings at which the nurse group representatives are heard. Anyone opposing it or desiring to change it is also heard. This is the most important stage of the bill.

Assume that the committee finds the bill meritorious and reports it back to the house with a recommendation to pass it. Legislatures differ about how a committee must act in this instance. Some require that it must be reported out of committee with a recommendation one way or the other. Other states require that if it is reported out it may or may not have an accompanying recommendation. In others a bill does not have to be reported out at all and therefore can be allowed to languish and die in committee. To break this down geographically, state by state, would serve little use here because the rules of legislative conduct are subject to change and they are best determined by inquiry directed to a specific legislator.

Assume that the committee, after hearing the nurse group's selected representative, finds the bill to be desirous and reports it back to the house.

4. The bill now goes before the house as a whole. It is entered upon the calendar or docket to be called up in order or at a time agreed upon by the sponsor or author and the officer presiding over that house. When called up for consid-

eration by the house body as a whole, the bill is subject to debate and amendment by the members. If it meets little objection or if all objection is overcome and it is passed by said house, the bill then is sent to the other legislative house. In this instance assume that the bill was introduced in the House of Representatives. It thereupon is sent to the Senate and passes through the same procedure. If the Senate acts upon the bill favorably and without amendment, it then is sent to the President of the United States, or the governor, in the case of a state, for his action.

Having reviewed the basic steps in the route of a bill, we are now ready to follow this same journey in studying the common technics of lobbying.

FUNDAMENTAL LOBBY METHODS

The means used by lobbyists are myriad, and each day brings new ingenuity into this field. Underlying this vast differential are certain similarities.

The lobbyist must be thoroughly grounded in his subject and alert and adaptable to constant changes. He or the group as a lobby must assemble all salient data on the subject involved with a proposed bill. It may be exceedingly helpful to outline this material in brief written form for the use of legislators as in a research brief.

Thorough education of the members of the nurse group is necessary to prevent division within the group itself at the time of legislative hearings.

One begins to realize that there are many tasks to be performed long before actual introduction of a bill. These tasks must be begun and many completed even before the legislative sessions begin. The true lobbyist or group lobby must be coordinating these matters constantly.

Undivided group support is first necessary before a group lobby can start enlisting the support of other groups in similar fields and of the populace generally. Assume that the nurse group is educated about the subject of a proposed bill and no longer has any serious objectors. The next task is the enlistment of popular and organized support. It is well to remember that in the original preparation of the bill other groups might be involved pro or con. These interests, if in favor of the proposals, should be consulted for their views and experience. As certain interests will probably object to the proposals and no common ground may be possible, it is absolutely necessary to know the adversaries and their arguments.

Long-range planning and long-range contacts go hand in hand. Well-planned lobbying begins contact with legislative members when these members are campaigning for office. Some groups use written questionnaires to determine whether a candidate favors their proposals. Many other groups having membership in practically all districts arrange for members who reside in a district to interview personally the various candidates and to obtain their views as definitely as possible. Quite often the result of these interviews, by whom, and with whom, is compiled centrally by the coordinator of the lobby for future reference when needed. This helps in being able to catalogue within limits the general views of the successful candidate in addition to having the very important facts as to the constituents who actually talked to the elected member in his home district. If a survey were taken to name the single most powerful influence factor in legislation, the most recurring force mentioned would be contact of an elected member by one or more of his constituents, with the contact being made in the home district if possible. Second in order would, no doubt, be contact by letter or other means from the home district voters.

Popular support is the next factor in the lobbyist's campaign and requires marshalling of various media—booklets, leaflets, newspaper, and editorial support. Purchase of television and radio time may be advisable, depending upon the issue and the lobby treasury.

The next step is the very important decision about which member of the legislative body should introduce the bill. For various reasons, depending upon alignment of legislative groups geographically, economically, or even politically, it may be valuable to determine in which house of a legislative body it would be best to begin. Determination of who should introduce the bill may thus be narrowed.

In any instance the member who introduces the bill should be one definitely favorable to it. A legislator who is also a member of a standing committee that would usually hear such legislation is an important possibility. The legislator should also be one who is thoroughly grounded in the facts behind the bill or at least be one who is willing to be briefed and will work at such preparation. An important point to be remembered is whether the member has the ability and time to devote to your bill or whether he has too many irons already in the fire.

Preferably the legislator should be a member of the majority party. In referring to the majority party, it should be noted that a cardinal principle of the lobby is to avoid political alignments or factions. Not to do so might well mean ostracism after the next election. Personal ties, social contacts, and other forms of association are to be encouraged, but the political connection is to be avoided unless your lobby is political.

After introduction of the bill and its reference to a committee has occurred, the committee hearings are in order. Here is the most important phase of the entire journey of the bill.

Plans, contacts, and work done one or two years previously must now produce results. If the bill has no opposition the chairman of the committee may believe a hearing is not necessary, but usually a nominal hearing is held, if requested, although no known opposition exists. If the bill has some opposition, the chairman may be requested to hold a hearing by the opposition and the nurse group lobby as well. This presents the opportunity to air the differing views. If the spadework of previous months has been done effectively, the results will appear, in marshalling popular support and favorable votes of members of the legislative committee. The lobby should present its views through a few members of its group who preferably have diversity in their fields and geography, but who possess the ability to express themselves succinctly and briefly and are not easily ruffed or befuddled. The general duty nurse who speaks sincerely and accurately on a health or nursing bill may be far more effective than a team of research experts and a thousand pages of testimony.

During the time of the hearing and about one or two days before the legislative committee votes on the issue, mail from the home district voters can be highly effective. The intent behind the use of form letters, postcards, or wires is extremely obvious from the recipient's view and has little or no effect. Methods for contacting members of the nurse group in order to signal the time for them to write to their legislators should be worked out well in advance of the time of the hearing. Along with the method of communication, members should be taught to write their own sincere letters rather than to follow some set form. Threats to the legislator are rude and deserve neither answer nor heed.

If the bill is voted upon favorably by the legislative committee to which it was assigned, it is sent to the floor of the house for consideration. Here the bill is debated, and amendments introduced, some of which are sponsored by the opposition to cripple or to make ineffective the proposed legislation.

It is at this stage that the lobby must enlist influential speakers and furnish data and, if requested, speech texts. Again it is seen that previous planning and compilation of data are necessary.

At this time it may again be necessary to have the members of the nurse group write, wire, or telephone their respective legislators to consider the bill favorably. If the bill passes, it then is sent to the other legislative house for the same processing although the hearings and debate may be more limited since the issues involved are usually more thoroughly aired in the house of introduction.

THE ADMINISTRATIVE LOBBY

The administrative lobby is a force that is often forgotten or underplayed. The influence of the administrative lobby is extremely important and in connection with a proposed bill begins long before the actual legislative session and continues long after the session ends. The administrative lobby has four important stages, best listed here in chronological order as related to the legislative lobby.

First, long before the legislative session begins and at the time of preparation of a proposed bill, it is important both to seek the counsel and to avoid the enmity of the administrative officials that may be connected with the proposals. Certain administrative agencies may have jurisdiction in the field your proposed bill will affect. Since the legislative committee may call upon some of these administrative officials for data or expert testimony, it is important to interview them to determine whether or not they have any views that would be contrary to your proposals and to obtain data that their departments might have easily at hand. Quite often early interviews with these officials may avoid opposition to the proposed bill, and occasionally their aid may be enlisted. The help of administrative agencies cannot be minimized. The data in their files are usually unbiased, and their contacts with the members of the legislative body may be better than can be marshalled by your own group.

Second, if the administrative agencies related to your proposals are friendly to your ideas, such agencies may use their work force to complete or to obtain additional data or more modern data than presently exists. The experts in the administrative agency may be called upon to testify before a legislative committee when the hearing is held. Their presentation can be a powerful factor since they are speaking both as experts and as members of the administrative branch who make the policy of the government.

Third, in addition to presentation of data from an unbiased and expert view, the administrative agency may actively lobby with various legislators who belong to the same party or are known to be friendly to the causes of that particular administrative department. This can result in having a second and seemingly unrelated lobby force that is extremely helpful without the nurse group lobby becoming involved in a political imbroglio.

Fourth, the cooperation and friendliness of the agency, acquired early in the lobby campaign, will avoid undesired interpretations by that agency after the bill becomes law. Many lobbies believe their job to be accomplished when the bill is passed by both houses and has the signature of the President or governor, as the case may be. Actually, unfavorable administrative rulings can hamstring the basic purposes of the entire lobbying effort!

Additional appropriations of money may be needed before an agency can enforce or administer the new law. If the agency does not like the new law it, in league with the opposition to such a law, may not push for the money needed to carry it out. What may be needed dollarwise to implement the law must be estimated in the original preparation of the bill and must be part of the data compiled to support the argument of the nurse group lobby.

Assume that additional appropriations are not needed by the administrative agency. The agency can and does have certain discretion as to the allocation of its funds. Many of us can remember excellent bills that became law, only to be defeated by the stratagem of diverting funds.

A last resort used by opposition to the bill, now law, is judicial interpretation. This is often brought out quickly by a test case. If the administrative agency is friendly to the nurse cause, the agency interpretation will be upheld and represented by the government's legal counsel, and an ally exists for the nurse lobby. If the agency is unfriendly, the agency interpretation of the law will be against the nurse lobby interests and possibly in favor of the opposition. The lobby group must then become the instigator of the test case and then will be on the uphill side of the legal battle. The nurse group will not have the government lawyers advocating their cause but will face the legal talent of the government and the lawyers of the opposition.

Chapter 31

Professional status of nursing

Thus far only certain basic concepts of the law and the basic methods of the lobby have been reviewed. The nurse in a professional capacity must now be considered.

The courts recognize that nurses are especially equipped to render professional services at a high professional level. As a New York court proclaimed, "They are grouped with doctors and lawyers rather than with cooks and chambermaids."*

Before discussing specific legal situations, it is necessary to consider the status of the nurse in relation to the physician. Rapid expansion of health services in recent years has resulted in modifications in traditional interrelations of these professions.

One of the characteristics of a profession is provision for licensure. During the early years of the twentieth century nursing groups and others interested in the health field worked toward legislation regarding licensure for nursing. Some of the first acts were experiments and, although helpful at the time of passage, soon became outmoded by the rapid advancement of new technics, drugs, and changing attitudes toward nursing and its component services.

The first and primary purpose of licensure laws, then and now, is protection of the public and the safeguarding of the health of the public. Requirements for licensure, renewal of licenses, and powers regarding revocation of licenses are for the public welfare and not for the creation of an organized profession. Admittedly, the practical tendency is to create the latter as an indirect outcome, but this very result serves to protect the public and aids the profession by separating unqualified from qualified practitioners.

ADMINISTRATION OF LICENSE LAWS

Administrative boards are established to carry out licensure laws. In most instances the board has an autonomous nature and appointments to the board are made by the governor of the state. Board members usually serve staggered terms to ensure continuity despite the possibility of sweeping changes in the political complexion of the state administration.

Some state have boards or governing agencies in connection with the Health Department or similar divisions that perform the same functions.

The basic function of the State Board of Nursing is governing the profession in such a manner that the public will know that a currently licensed practitioner is qualified

*In Re Renouf, 254 N.Y. 349, 173 N.E. 218 (1930).

to perform duties normally expected of that professional position.

To do this the board has the following basic duties:

1. Conducting and grading the examination of applicants who have met basic requirements.
2. Renewal of licenses of those already admitted to practice.
3. Enforcement of proper practice standards by appropriate investigations.
4. Revocation of licenses for unprofessional conduct of members.
5. Surveying schools of nursing in conjunction with their licensure and accreditation.
6. Maintaining a central office for the conduct of board business.
7. Making administrative rules to carry out the purposes of the Practice Act.

Under the influence of the American Nurses' Association, the constituent state nurses' associations have vigorously pressed adoption of new legislation in respect to the nursing profession in each state. No national or federal licensure exists because this subject matter is reserved to the states under the Federal Constitution. As a result, there is a lack of uniformity among the laws of the various states. In order to learn specifically and correctly the requirements of a given state at a particular time, one should contact the State Board of that state at that time.

RELATIONS OF MEDICAL AND NURSING PRACTICE ACTS

As we have pointed out, the various states by statute have undertaken legal control of the professions through provisions for licensure. This type of law ordinarily deals with four major problems: (1) definition, (2) monopoly, (3) administration, and (4) criminal penalties.

Definition

An effort is made both to distinguish professional nursing by registered nurses from practical nursing and to prevent encroachment upon the practice of medicine. This is not to say, however, that there is no overlap in the kinds of actions permitted under the law. For example, it might well be possible under statute to administer an anesthetic to a patient as a physician, as a registered nurse, or as a practical nurse. Thus, a particular act is not necessarily forbidden to one group merely because another is also authorized to perform it. To illustrate, the definitions provided in the New York law are as follows:

> *Medical Practice.*—The practice of medicine is defined as follows: A person practices medicine within the meaning of this article, except as hereinafter stated, who holds himself out as being able to diagnose, treat, operate or prescribe for any human disease, pain, injury, deformity or physical condition, and who either shall offer or undertake, by any means or method, to diagnose, treat, operate or prescribe for any human disease, pain, injury, deformity or physical condition.*
>
> *Nursing Practice.*—The practice of nursing is defined as follows:
>
> a. A person practices nursing as a registered professional nurse within the meaning of this article who for compensation or personal profit performs any professional service requiring the application of principles of nursing based on biological, physical and social sciences, such as responsible supervision of a patient requiring skill in observation of symptoms and reactions and the accurate recording of the facts, and carrying out of treatments and medications as prescribed by a licensed physician or by a licensed dentist and the application of such nursing procedures as involves understanding of cause and effect in order to safeguard life and health of the patient and others.
>
> b. A person practices nursing as a licensed practical nurse who for compensation or personal profit performs such duties as are required in the physical care of a patient and in carrying out of medical orders as prescribed by a licensed physician or by a licensed dentist requiring an understanding of nursing but not requiring the professional service as outlined in paragraph a.†

---

*New York Education Law §6501, par. 4.
†New York Education Law §6901, par. 2.

Monopoly

Licensing laws usually contemplate that the group licensed has an exclusive right to act in a certain type of endeavor. Because of the overlap of the kinds of activities carried on by the allied healing professions, the courts emphasize the right to hold oneself out to the public as engaged in a particular profession. In many cases it is this "holding out" that is reserved to the licensed group rather than a complete monopoly on performing particular professional acts.

Administration

Administration was discussed on p. 230.

Criminal penalties

We have emphasized earlier in the general definition of "positive law" that it comprises rules of conduct that the government will *enforce*. Accordingly, enforcement of licensing laws is accomplished through criminal sanctions. Thus, in New York, there is this provision:

Penalties.—1. It shall be a misdemeanor for any person to (a) sell or fraudulently obtain or furnish any nursing diploma, license, record, or registration or aid or abet therein, or (b) practice nursing as defined by this article under cover of any diploma, license, record or registration illegally or fraudulently obtained or signed or executed unlawfully or under fraudulent representation or mistake of fact in a material regard, or (c) practice nursing as defined by this article unless duly licensed to do so under the provisions of this article, or (d) use in connection with his or her name any designation tending to imply that he or she is a registered professional nurse or a licensed practical nurse unless duly licensed to so practice under the provisions of this article, or (e) practice nursing during the time his or her licensed issued under the provisions of this article shall be suspended or revoked, or (f) otherwise violate any of the provisions of this article.
2. Such misdemeanor shall be punishable by a fine of not more than five thousand dollars or by imprisonment for not more than one year or by both such fine and imprisonment. Subsequent violation shall be punishable by both such fine and imprisonment.*

*New York Education Law §6910.

A misdemeanor is a minor crime, as distinct from the more serious "felony," and punishment by imprisonment cannot ordinarily extend beyond one year. Provisions for fines are also commonly included, as in the New York law.

THE SEVEN AREAS OF PROFESSIONAL NURSING

Lesnik and Anderson, in their excellent authoritative text, have analyzed legal patterns of definition and performance regarding professional nurses.

Nursing functions

Considering independent functions, Lesnik and Anderson have made the following statements.

. . . (T)he overwhelming number of functions and the majority of areas of control involve obligations of performance independent of medical orders. The study of judicial decisions indicates that the preponderance of functions determined by the courts in the first 6 areas of control involve independent functions.
(1) The supervision of a patient involving the whole management of care, requiring the application of principles based upon the biologic, the physical and the social sciences.
(2) The observation of symptoms and reactions, including symptomatology of physical and mental conditions and needs, requiring evaluation or application of principles based upon the biologic, the physical and the social sciences.
(3) The accurate recording and reporting of facts, including evaluation of the whole care of the patient.
(4) The supervision of others, except physicians, contributing to the care of the patient.
(5) The application and the execution of nursing procedures and technics.
(6) The direction and the education to secure physical and mental care.*

Lesnik and Anderson list one area that may be termed *dependent* rather than *independent*.

*Lesnik, Milton J., and Anderson, Bernice E.: Nursing practice and the law, ed. 2, Philadelphia, 1955 (with revisions, 1962), J. B. Lippincott Co., pp. 259-261.

(7) The application and execution of legal orders of physicians concerning treatments and medications, with an understanding of cause and effect thereof.*

When a physician does direct the activities of the nurse, he does not relieve himself of the legal duties of the physician-patient relationship. In fact, he may acquire additional duties in respect to the instruction and warning of nurses about particular problems or possible complications in a given case under treatment.

In the event that a nurse is charged with the crime of practicing medicine without a license or becomes involved in other legal difficulty, concerning the performance of independent or dependent nursing functions, the courts will be prone to give great weight to the official pronouncements of the American Nurses' Association. Thus, the Association's *Statements of Functions, Standards, and Qualifications* should be read by all nurses in the light of the Lesnik and Anderson formulation.

The Association, in commenting upon its model definition of nursing practice, states:

In order that the interests of the public and the practitioner both be protected, the definition of nursing practice in the licensing law must clearly differentiate between those acts which are independent nursing functions and those which are dependent upon the prescription of the physician or the dentist.

The statements of functions prepared and approved by the sections of the American Nurses' Association are the principal authority for this legal definition of nursing practice. The definition reflects the essential and, for the most part, common elements of nursing practice described in the definitions of nursing functions adopted by the occupational groups represented in the sections of the professional organization.

Delegation by medical authority is provided for the circumscribed area of nursing practice where such delegation is required, namely for the administration of medications and treatments. For clarity, the definition includes a prohibition of acts of diagnosis and prescription of therapeutic or corrective measures.*

The *independent-dependent* distinction is expressly set out in the Private Duty Nurses' Section statement of Functions and Standards:

III. Executes independent nursing procedures
  a. Adapts nursing procedures and techniques in relation to the individual needs of the patient in order to promote his comfort and hygiene
  b. Performs those independent nursing procedures (for example, elevate the head of the bed of a cardiac patient who becomes dyspneic, give oxygen in case of sudden cyanosis, et cetera) which may be used to meet emergencies, with the knowledge of the doctor's and/or hospital's emergency procedures

IV. Executes dependent nursing procedures and techniques under the direction or supervision of a licensed physician
  a. Complies with the laws governing medical and nursing practice in the particular state in which the nurse practices
  b. Administers drugs and medicines in compliance with the physician's written orders and fulfills other therapeutic measures as prescribed by him and which the nurse understands will not have a deleterious effect on the patient
  c. Verbal orders may be executed in an emergency. These orders should be written and as soon as possible countersigned by the physician.†

---

*American Nurses' Association: Functions, standards, and qualifications for practice, New York, Rev. 1963, p. 48.
†American Nurses' Association: Functions, standards and qualifications for practice, New York, Rev. 1963, p. 35.

---

*Lesnik, Milton J., and Anderson, Bernice E.: Nursing practice and the law, ed. 2, Philadelphia, 1955 (with revisions, 1962), J. B. Lippincott Co., pp. 259-261.

Chapter 32

Contracts

WHAT IS A CONTRACT?

A contract is defined as an agreement between two or more persons, comprising a promise or mutual promises enforceable by law.

Contracts are made daily by nearly everyone involved in any field of endeavor, including nursing. The importance of this realization is too often glossed over when one is busily engaged in professional practice. Preparation of a patient for treatment, observance of symptoms and general condition, application of nursing procedures, and other such acts of the nurse pertaining to the care of the patient do not lend an aura of contracts being made and completed.

A common misconception among nurses and others is the idea that a contract is always a written document. As a matter of fact most contracts are oral. By law, certain types of contracts must be in writing to be valid. It is often wise to reduce contracts to writing to prevent later entanglements and misunderstandings.

Legal components of contracts may be stated in five parts: (1) an offer by one or more parties, (2) an acceptance by another or other parties, (3) legal capacity of both parties to contract (4) to do or not to do a legal act for (5) a consideration (consideration meaning price in money or any item

or act having a value to the party receiving it for services performed).

OFFER AND ACCEPTANCE

In daily conversation the remark is often heard, "What were you offered for it?" This indicates one party made a money offer for a specific article belonging to another party. In shopping for clothing or even in the daily grocery marketing, contracts are constantly made. The grocer displays his wares and the price. The shopper in selecting an item and placing the item in the shopping bag has entered into a contract. Upon paying the grocer (the consideration) the contract is completed. A credit account is based upon contract. After certain grocery items are selected, the grocer enters the items and amounts in his records, and the parties have entered into a contract. The grocer has offered his wares for a price to be paid once a month. The shopper has accepted the offer and agreed to pay at the end of the month. Formal words, orally or in writing, were not involved; yet a contract was formed, and credit accounts are easily provable in court.

When a nurse indicates he or she is available for nursing care, that nurse is inviting offers for his or her services. In other words, when one is available but does not indicate a specific condition, this is an invitation to another party to make an offer. An example remark is "Shall we talk terms?" If, instead of indicating availability, the nurse indicates that the services are available for a specific sum, then a specific condition has been added, and the invitation becomes an offer. The patient accepting the offer becomes the other party to the contract, and a contract is made.

Actually an offer of nursing services is usually more detailed and involves additional consideration regarding meals, lodging, length of service, shift, laundry, and other privileges and conditions. The nurse may be offeror or acceptor; which the nurse is depends upon which party actually made the offer. In a large number of instances the nurse is the acceptor because the patient or institution usually seeks the nurse by stating the terms upon which the party will engage the nurse. Acceptance of such terms by the nurse makes the contract.

In the act of acceptance one cannot accept part of the terms and reject part. An acceptance is total or it does not exist and the contract is not made. Because nursing services are in a special category that often includes meals, lodging, and other privileges, this concept of totality of acceptance is important. In talking terms with the prospective recipient of nursing services, the nurse may not desire lodging and may prefer additional pay instead. This requested change in terms is two things, namely, a rejection of the original offer and a counteroffer. When this occurs the nurse then becomes the one making the offer; if the other party accepts the change in terms suggested by the counterofferor, then the contract is made.

Several cardinal points regarding offer and acceptance should be remembered. First, a face-to-face contact is not necessary to make a contract. Reverting momentarily to the grocery-shopping illustration, assume that the transaction of purchasing the groceries was conducted with the grocer's clerk. The contract was made as certainly as with the grocer personally. The clerk is his agent and is obviously empowered to accept payment for the groceries selected. In contracting for nursing services, face-to-face contact with the patient usually occurs after the contract for services has been made. The nurse is contacted initially on many occasions by a physician, registry, or a member of the patient's family. In institutional work the nurse nearly always deals with an agent of the hospital and not the owner.

Second, local custom may enter the picture in contracts. In stating terms one often does not mention certain aspects that are customary in that locality regarding nursing services. In private duty nursing the providing of meals is presumed, and if such is the custom locally, the actual mentioning of it is advisable but not necessary for it to be a condition of the contract. It becomes part of the contract under the law of custom.

Implied conditions are a third point to be considered. Every offer of personal services of a professional nature implies that the services will be performed with due care and within existing professional standards and ethics. Implied promises, like custom, operate upon both parties as a contract. Thus, the patient impliedly promises that he will not obstruct the nurse's performance of services.

The final point regarding relation between offer and acceptance is the timing factor. If an offer is made, when may it be withdrawn, and after receiving an offer how soon thereafter must the acceptance or rejection be communicated? The basic concept is the necessity that an acceptance must be communicated to the offeror. Unless the acceptance is clearly communicated, it is obvious that no contract exists because both parties have not agreed. An offer may be withdrawn at any time before acceptance or rejection is stated by the recipient of the offer. An acceptance must be given within a reasonable time after receipt of the offer or a presumption of rejection exists. What is a reasonable time is determined by several factors such as method of communication (telephone or mail), geographic area (within the same city or far distant), the emergent nature of the situation ("time is of the essence"), and other matters related to the parties offering and accepting. Acceptance does not have to be communicated in the same manner as the offer unless one of the terms of the offer is a stipulation as to manner of acceptance. This type of stipulation often occurs in the business field whereby the offeror uses a telegram to make an offer and stipulates that the answer be by wire. This also serves to indicate generally the time when the acceptance must be made, if made.

Because nursing services are frequently obtained by someone other than the patient, knowing the patient's agent and the apparent or implied powers of the agent is important. When a patient is in a condition that makes it physically impossible for him personally to obtain nursing services, the physician or registry is usually requested to obtain a nurse. In most instances in which the patient, although ill, is able to convey this authority to someone, little or no difficulty will arise, and information as to whether the agent has such authority is easily ascertained.

When a patient is legally incapable of requesting an agent to act for him, it is sometimes necessary to contract with a responsible member of the family who is of legal age and who agrees to pay for the nursing services if the patient does not. Failure to do this in cases in which the patient does not have the legal capacity to contract may result in loss of pay. The patient, upon gaining legal capacity, may disavow any contracted services, thus leaving the nurse to look to some other member of the patient's family or a friend, and if the nurse has not specifically agreed with someone other than the patient, her nursing

services become a gratuity to the recipient although involuntarily given.

LEGAL CAPACITY OF CONTRACTING PARTIES

Offer and acceptance make the agreement but without both parties having legal capacity to enter into such an agreement the contract is unenforceable.

Whether a party has legal capacity depends on four basic considerations. Historically a *married woman* had little or no right to contract with anyone. In the comparatively recent times of the middle and late 1800's the "Married Women's Acts" were put into effect. These statutes gave married women emancipation as to contracts, property, and other legal rights, which theretofore were dominated by the male spouse. Today a married woman can contract for nursing services for herself, and when the husband-patient is mentally incapable, the wife may contract for such services in her own right or bind her husband as hereafter explained.

The wife has the additional power to contract and bind the husband in the purchase or acquisition of necessaries.* In this capacity the wife does not necessarily contract in her own right but can bind the husband without his authorization or approval.

The second legal incapacity considered here is that of the *infant*. The legal term "infant" is far broader than the lay use of the term, covering all parties below a certain age. In nearly all states this age is 21 years although a few states have fixed the legal age of females at 18 years.

Agreements with infants in the majority of states are valid agreements but are voidable on the part of the infant. Therefore, the act of contracting with an infant is entered into with no recourse if the infant upon reaching majority disaffirms the con-

---

*The definition of necessaries includes clothes, food, heat, and medical assistance, which includes nursing.

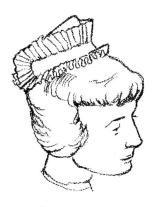

Philadelphia General graduate nurse

tract. The infant upon reaching the majority age must disaffirm a contract within a reasonable time. In most states misrepresentation of age by the infant does not prevent the infant from disaffirming the contract upon reaching the true majority age.

In the United States it is now generally held that the father of an infant is chargeable for necessaries furnished the child. Also, others who assume to stand *in loco parentis* (in place of a parent) may be liable.

Mental illness of a party is another category concerning legal incapacity. When a person is severely ill enough psychiatrically, the law throws a mantle of protection around him to prevent others from taking unfair advantage of the one so disabled. Difficulty arises, of course, in respect to determination of the extent of such illness which justifies judicial indulgence.

In general, it may be said that a contract entered into with one who is mentally incompetent is voidable. If an effort is made to contract with one who has been declared incompetent as a result of some type of legal adjudication, there is no contract. The attempted contract is void.

The mentally incompetent, however, is legally liable for necessaries. This is true even when they are furnished at the request of others. Assessment of the value of such necessaries is made by the court.

Fraud and undue influence is the fourth

and final part dealt with here in the question of legal capacity. During the time of entering into a contract one party may not have full comprehension of the seriousness or meaning of the conditions and when the other party, knowing this, uses such to obtain an advantage, the contract becomes unenforceable. The result of legally declaring the contract void is based upon fraud rather than legal capacity. This is mentioned here for the reason that when parties are standing on an unequal footing a case is often argued erroneously from the legal capacity standpoint rather than from the proper standpoint of misrepresentation or fraud. An example of this follows: P (patient), although elderly, is clear minded and contracts with N (nurse) for her services. P is confined to the home that is in a small community in which there are no other nurses. At the time of negotiating the contract, P asks N what the customary daily fee is of a private duty nurse for an eight-hour shift. N states that it is $25, rather than $15, which is customary in that area. N knows that P has no knowledge of the customary wage and has taken advantage of the situation, and P, having no other recourse at the moment, accepts the proposal or offer. Thus, although the parties had the legal capacity to contract, misrepresentation rendered the agreement unenforceable.

TO DO OR NOT TO DO A LEGAL ACT

In all contracts it is inherent that the parties thereto will do some act, even if only an act of forebearance. The act to be done or not done must be legal, that is, one not prohibited by law.

To allow anyone to recover for another's failure to perform an illegal act would violate basic ideas of justice.

In addition to illegal acts another type of act must be considered. Acts that are against "public policy" are not enforced in the courts. To define public policy is impossible, but to understand its connotation is not. Certain rights are inherent and inalienable to each individual, and although all of these rights are not spelled out specifically in our laws, they are nevertheless understood by all. For example, an attempt by a person to offer a large sum of money to another for his promise not to become a nurse would be against public policy, and such a contract is unenforceable. Whether the other party becomes a nurse or not, it is the sole right of that party to make that decision. Although these rights are not spelled out specifically in our laws, they are nevertheless understood by all. It is not illegal not to become a nurse, but the attempt to restrain the individual's right to make the choice is against "public policy."

CONSIDERATION

The final part of a valid contract, consideration, is generally that service, act, promise, or matter agreed to by the parties. Consideration is the all-encompassing term as to legal detriment or benefit: right, doing or forebearing to do an act, money, or other matters. An approved technical definition is given as "a benefit to the party promising, or a loss or detriment to the party to whom the promise is made."

Validity of a contract does not hinge upon the amount of the consideration. The value placed thereon is that which is agreed by both parties, and what or how those parties value a specific matter is their right. The value of consideration is upon occasion a factor in determining whether misrepresentations were made, but the review of consideration then is only to support or to deny a charge of misrepresentation.

Without consideration there is no contract. With consideration of any nature the contract will not be held unenforceable because of small amount or apparent valuelessness to others not party to the contract.

BREACH OF CONTRACT

Having reviewed the fundaments of making contracts, we now will discuss their breaking.

Breach of contract is failure to perform, and it is fundamentally covered by the following categories: (1) prevention, (2) repudiation, and (3) impossibility.

When one is prevented from performing a contracted act by the other party to the contract, a breach of contract occurs. The breach is made by the party's preventing performance. This type can and does occur in nursing when the patient resists nursing care that had been contracted for. Repudiation of a contract occurs after the contract is made but usually before any contractual act is begun. The party so repudiating is the one guilty of a breach although the other party may have not begun any contractual act either. Under repudiation as a form of breach, inconvenience can be considered one of the most oft-occurring reasons for repudiation. After a contract is entered into, the fact that the execution of it will cause inconvenience is no excuse, and the party inconvenienced must continue or be liable for breach of contract. Abandonment of a patient is a breach explained more fully later in this chapter.

Failure to perform because of some impossibility that was not foreseen at the time of contracting is treated differently in various states. An example of impossibility would be the occurrence of a transit strike if the party, such as a nurse, could not reach her destination by other means. In some states the patient could allege breach of contract on the part of the nurse and be upheld. These states believe that had proper precautions been arranged the nurse could have reached the patient and that impossibility of performance was not a defense to the charge of breach of contract. The event that causes impossibility of performance must, of course, be an event that is not under the control of either party.

Several other states recognize impossibility with such variances that it is impossible to categorize or draw clear lines of authority.

Although *assignment of contract* is not

usually a cause of breach of contract, it is to be noted that assignment of a contract for nursing services when the right of assignment is not provided in the contract is a breach. Because of the personal nature of nursing services, many nurses are retained not only as such but also as specific personalities. When a patient requests a registry to furnish a nurse, legal recognition of this request differs from that in the situation in which the patient specifically requests Miss X as a nurse. If Miss X accepts an offer in this respect, she cannot assign her contract or substitute anyone else without the consent of the patient.

DEFENSES

Breaches of contract that are defensible are categorized generally as (1) material misrepresentation, (2) impossibility, in some states, (3) Act of God, (4) sickness, and (5) death.

Material misrepresentation must be a misstatement regarding a vital matter that would have prevented the making of a contract between the parties had the true facts been known. A nurse who claims to be a licensed professional registered nurse and is in fact not such would be in a position of making a material misrepresentation if such fact were of vital importance to the patient or institution requesting the services. The correct reasoning in this situation is that a contract was never actually entered because the offer or the acceptance was not fully understood.

Impossibility is listed again because some states treat or accept it as a proper defense.

Forces or events that are not man-made are encompassed by the defense legally known as an "Act of God." Storms, floods, lightning, and other such phenomena are legally acceptable defenses if such events prevent the performance of a contract.

Sickness as a defense, in some states, is based upon the Act of God premise. In other states sickness is given independent stature. Of course sickness is not a defense unless it would prevent the execution of the contracted conditions. Sickness is important in contracts in which personal services must be rendered. Sickness would most certainly not be a defense when the sick party merely has to pay a specific sum or sign a deed.

Death is an obvious defense but in part is similar to sickness. When A, an administrator of a medical clinic, has hired N to work a certain shift, caring for and aiding patients confined therein, the death of A does not stop the operation of the contract. N's death would do so, though, because of the nature of the nurse's part of the contract, personal services. In private duty cases death of the patient always ends the contract because this is an implied condition to the offer and acceptance.

A final point that must be considered because of its ramifications both contracturally and from the standpoint of liability for negligence is abandonment. After caring for P for a short period, N abandons P. This obviously is a breach of contract because it is a failure to perform completely the conditions of the contract. Presume that P resisted the care of N, and this therefore became a defense to abandonment. N would not be held on the contract but may very well be held liable for negligence. N's liability would be based on tort, which is reviewed in a later chapter, and it is to be noted that under such a situation when N, although contractually correct, abandons P, P must not be left in a more serious condition than existed at the time N gave nursing care.

LEGAL REMEDIES

The remedies afforded to the injured party of a breached contract are in two basic forms: (1) money damages and (2) specific performance. Nearly all remedial judgments are in the form of dollar damages. Occasionally the damage due to a breach of contract is irreparable in terms of dollars, and the court therefore orders that the contract be specifically performed. An example often used in this respect is that A contracts to buy a piece of real estate owned by B; B later refuses to deed the land to A. Because there is no other land exactly like the particular parcel the court will order B to deed the property to A rather than to pay dollar damages. In contracts regarding personal services like nursing, the court cannot order specific performance because to do so would essentially place one in a position of slavery, which violates our Constitution. Here a compensatory dollar award is the usual remedy and in certain circumstances the court may add punitive damages. Punitive damages comprise an amount to be paid in addition to actual damages as a penalty for capricious conduct by the party breaching the contract.

In conclusion it must be added that the time limits for bringing suit to remedy a breach of contract are set by law in most states and delay in these matters can be fatal. Generally speaking a lawsuit on an unwritten contract should be brought within three years from the time the breach of contract occurred. Some states have a longer period, but none has a shorter period. On written contracts the period within which suit must be commenced is usually longer.

Negligence is one branch of the law of torts. A tort is fundamentally construed to be any wrongful act (not involving a breach of contract) for which a civil action will lie. In certain instances a breach of contract will also involve liability in tort such as negligence. If a nurse fails to sterilize certain instruments properly and if infection is the result of such carelessness, a breach of contract exists, because it is an implied condition of nursing services that due care will be used. The patient so affected may have the choice of suing the nurse for breach of contract or for negligence. There are many other acts that are classified legally as torts, and some of the other torts will be treated in Chapter 34.

A wrongful act in the law of negligence is usually an act improperly performed without criminal intent. Not all crimes require intent. In certain instances in which a crime is committed, both a criminal and a civil action will lie, and in this instance, one is not exclusive of the other as in the choice of suing for breach of contract or taking legal action on negligence.

There has been some confusion concerning use of the term *malpractice*. Probably it would be best to refrain from its use and to employ the designation *professional negligence* when describing negligence occurring in the course of professional activity. Actually, malpractice means only bad practice and so may be involved in criminal law (criminal malpractice), civil law (civil malpractice), or even in codes of professional ethics (ethical malpractice).

THE FIVE D'S

The specific elements of negligence cases can best be analyzed in terms of the so-called five "D's" (see diagram on p. 244).

DUTY

Duty in the law of negligence means that inherent imposition placed upon one to conduct himself and his property in a reasonable and prudent manner for the avoidance of injury to other people and other property. This duty exists inherently and does not require statutory enactment. In certain instances statutory enactment clearly defines standards of conduct; these specific limitations are in addition to the basic duty of reasonable and prudent conduct. Examples of specific enactment would be speed limits, traffic signals, and quarantine regulations.

When a legal duty is breached, negligence exists. Thus, a nurse who fails to answer the call of assigned patients within a reasonable time is guilty of negligence.

Because *legal duty* is fundamental in the

Plaintiff must prove:

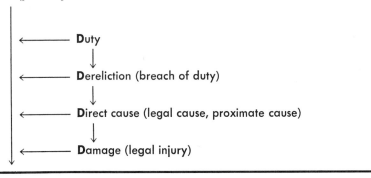

Duty

Dereliction (breach of duty)

Direct cause (legal cause, proximate cause)

Damage (legal injury)

Defenses — contributory negligence, assumption of risk, etc.

(Defendant must prove)

The five "D's"

(Courtesy Hubert W. Smith; from Gradwohl, R. B. H.: Legal medicine, St. Louis, 1954, The C. V. Mosby Co.)

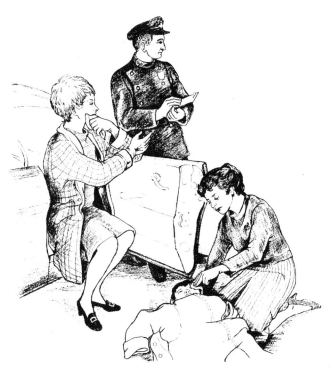

Nursing care volunteered at the scene of an accident may sometimes lead to legal problems for the nurse.

analysis of negligence suits brought against nurses, we will set out the various elements that enter into professional duties.

First of all we must consider how duty arises. Ordinarily, the nurse is employed under a contract. The duties toward a patient, however, are fixed by the law of torts and not by contract in the usual situation. In fact, the courts will hold contracts that attempt to absolve the nurse of responsibility for any negligence void as against public policy.

How does duty terminate? When the nurse is acting as an independent contractor (Chapter 35), termination of the nurse's duty would be analogous to termination of a physician's duty toward the patient. The courts have spelled out four ways in which such a relationship may be ended legally:

1. Death of the patient.
2. Discharge of the nurse by the patient.
3. Mutual agreement of patient and nurse to end the relationship.
4. Appointment of a qualified successor or the giving of notice to the patient in advance so that he will have ample time to secure a successor.

In general, the scope of a nurse's duty involves a continuing obligation to give the patient's case proper attention. Specific duties have been outlined in various cases, mostly involving physicians, but it is quite likely that the same types of duties are required of nurses.

1. Duty to bring certain qualities to the bedside.
    (a) Knowledge or learning based upon advanced training. The courts are not in agreement as to whether the fact that a person without an appropriate academic degree or registration, and so not licensed to practice, is in itself evidence of negligence. Some say that the failure to be licensed has no connection with the injury to the patient inasmuch as the act of licensing confers no additional skill upon the nurse. On the other hand, it is argued that the purpose of licensing nurses is to prevent unskilled persons from caring for the sick.
    (b) Reasonable skill, ordinary care, and ordinary diligence. These terms are used interchangeably by the courts in measuring performance of nurses. Obviously, there are no hard and fast rules as to just what is or is not proper care in all cases. Each case must be considered individually. It must be remembered, however, that the profession in a very real sense determines what this standard shall be. Thus, in the event that a professional negligence case is tried against a nurse, it is proper, and often necessary, that both sides place nurses on the witness stand as expert witnesses. When properly qualified, they are permitted to testify as to what the prevailing standard of ordinary and usual care, skill, and diligence actually is in the particular community or in like communities. The defendant-nurse's conduct is measured against this standard by the trier of fact—judge or jury, as the case may be.
    (c) Best judgment. Judges are wont sometimes to state that a professional practitioner is held to the standard of his best judgment. In contrast to the previous elements set out, this factor of "judgment" has more of a subjective tinge— the individual nurse's best judgment at the time in question and in view of all attendant circumstances in the case. Thus, if hindsight indicates that another course of action would have been preferable, this is not enough. The situation must be viewed through the

eyes of the nurse as of the time of decision.

2. Duty of exercising the above-named qualities. It is evident that the nurse must use knowledge, skill, care, diligence, and judgment. It is no defense to show merely that the individual *possesses* these qualities. The nurse must *use* them in the particular case in order to avoid liability.

3. Special duties of the nurse.

   (a) Fiduciary duties. The law recognizes that the relation of a patient to his nurse is one of trust and confidence. General rules of law as concerns the trust relationship are applicable. In particular, the following duties are of special importance:

      (1) Duty of utmost good faith. All transactions between a nurse and patient are carefully scrutinized by the courts lest the nurse's superior position be used to effect fraud or undue influence.

      (2) Duty of disclosure. There is a general duty applied to the physician to reveal all pertinent information to the patient or a close relative. Dicta in some of the cases would indicate that the nurse has the same duty. Perhaps there is a privilege to withhold diagnosis and other information if the patient's medical status would be adversely affected by disclosure. This is a knotty problem which the courts have not fully clarified.

      (3) Duty of nondisclosure to third parties. Although it seems that no case has found its way into the reports as regards nurses, it should be evident that nurses have at least a strong moral obligation to keep confidential such information as they may obtain in the nurse-patient relationship.

      (4) Duty to gain consent of patient for therapeutic measures undertaken. This, of course, is primarily a duty of the physician. When a nurse is delegated to carry out a specific procedure, particularly if it be somewhat unusual, at least implied consent should be gained from the patient. In other words, the competent adult patient has a perfect right to refuse treatment at any time, and invasion of his person without consent would amount to a battery.

      (5) Duty to keep abreast. All professional persons are held to keep abreast of the technical advances made in their particular field of endeavor. This does not mean that the nurse must adopt every new technique as it is discussed in the professional nursing journals, but it does require the abandonment of horse and buggy methods that have been supplanted by more modern and approved ones.

      (6) Duty to give instructions. A physician's obligation to give instructions as to the detailed aftercare of a patient is often delegated to nurses. They probably have an independent duty, over and above that of the physician, to see that a patient is properly instructed before he leaves the office or hospital.

LEGAL CAUSE AND DAMAGE

Even though a nurse be under a duty and that duty has been violated, there is still no tort liability unless the patient has suffered legal injury ("actual loss") as the proximate result of the nurse's negligence. Details of what amounts to "legal cause" and "legal damage" must be left to the scholars of the law inasmuch as the refinements of this subject become rather complicated. On the other hand, the nurse is entitled to use common sense ideas of "direct" as opposed to "remote" cause. Regardless of view of "cause", some learned judge somewhere is probably in agreement with the nurse! The same holds true concerning "legal injury."

DEFENSES

Two basic defenses exist in respect to negligence: assumption of risk and contributory negligence. The injured party may have assumed the risk or contributed negligence that helped cause the injury.

Assumption of risk has limited application since it amounts to a proposition that the plaintiff has consented to absolve the defendant from wrongful conduct toward him and agrees to "take his chances" of injury from a fully appreciated risk.

A case in which a patient refused to comply with a nurse's health instructions would be in point. Thus, if a nurse instructed a patient in muscle rehabilitation exercises and the patient suffered contractures because of his failure to carry out the exercises, suit by the patient against the nurse could be won by the nurse on the defense of assumption of risk.

Contributory negligence is widely employed as an affirmative defense. Patients who fail to cooperate with nursing care being rendered, even though that care was itself negligent, may find themselves "out of court" on the ground of contributory negligence.

Other defenses include the statute of limitations (the "time limits" discussed on p. 228) and such technical matters listed as release, *res judicata,* judgment for services, workmen's compensation, and written notice requirements. All of these possible defenses hinge on legal technicalities with which the individual nurse need not be familiar since the lawyer will explore them thoroughly if claim is made against the nurse.

SPECIAL PROBLEMS IN NEGLIGENCE

There are many special facets of negligence law that may involve a nurse from time to time. Two of the most important involve emergency situations and the problem of legal immunity of certain organizations.

EMERGENCIES

No new rule of law applies in emergencies. The nurse is required to act as a reasonably prudent nurse under the circumstances. In practice, of course, the courts recognize that skill and care may fall below that ordinarily applied under more leisurely conditions. Also, the nurse may have wide discretion to employ rather radical means that would ordinarily be within the province of a physician. Thus, in a cardiac arrest case in which no physician is immediately available, a nurse may properly open the chest and begin cardiac massage. It must be realized that in such cases, the nurse is employing skilled first aid rather than "practicing medicine." So, also, any layman with first-aid training is not in violation of law when he applies his skills in an emergency.

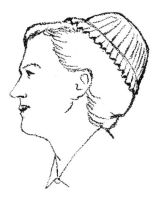

Bellevue Hospital graduate nurse

IMMUNITY

During the development of law in England, two special doctrines of tort immunity sprang up. The one, governmental immunity, was based on the once-prevailing notion that "the King could do no wrong." The other, "charitable immunity," arose as the result of two rather dubious court decisions that were shortly overruled.

Governmental immunity as a doctrine of law still holds sway in most of the individual states, but the Federal Government has waived a large portion of its immunity for tort liability.

Although the doctrine of charitable immunity was soon overruled by cases in England, in the first case in the United States, a suit against Massachusetts General Hospital, the Massachusetts judges called upon the authority of the then-overruled English cases to sustain the position of charitable immunity. Most of the states followed this Massachusetts decision, and it has been only in recent years that the trend of decision has definitely pointed in the other direction.

Current status of these immunity doctrines varies from state to state, so that for authoritative information reference should be made to the latest decisions of a particular state. The trend away from immunity has practical importance for nurses and other employees of governmental and institutional establishments. When immunity is the rule, an injured patient can look only to the individuals caring for him for monetary damages. Thus, a nurse or physician exposes his estate to substantial loss in the event of an adverse judgment. When immunity no longer prevails, it is much more likely that the plaintiff will seek recovery against the hospital or other institution having assets more easily collectible. Although an individual be joined as a party in such a suit, efforts to collect are ordinarily directed toward the governmental or corporate treasury.

Chapter 34

Other torts

Rather than attempt to discuss all torts, this chapter will deal with those other torts that would most likely occur in relation to nursing services, namely, assault and battery, false imprisonment, and slander and libel.

ASSAULT AND BATTERY

Assault and battery are generally treated together, because if a battery occurs, it is usually preceded by an assault. Legally, assault and battery are separate torts and may exist separately as shown by the following fundamental definitions.

An assault essentially is (1) a threat or attempt (2) made with an ability (apparent to the one threatened) to commit the threat or attempt (3) which causes the one threatened immediately to fear an offensive or harmful contact, (4) which is intended by the assaultor and (5) is not wanted by the one threatened—which is legally termed consent—nor is privileged as outlined under defenses of privilege.

It is a fundamental precept that no one may threaten or endeavor to touch another's person unless a defense of consent or privilege exists. A threat may be made by action or words or both. The slightest effort in the manner of a threat is sufficient to establish assault legally.

The ability to commit the threat or at-

tempt need only be apparent to the one threatened. The fact that the assaultor had no intent to carry out the threat is of no importance, and the fact that the threat could not have been carried out is of no avail as a defense. If the one threatened thought or believed that the assaultor had the ability to commit the threatened act, the threat was an assault. The oft-used example of the hand in the pocket simulating a hidden gun is an excellent illustration of this point.

Fear of offensive or harmful contact must exist. The manner of threat is unimportant provided the manner would cause fear in the mind of the one threatened. In this connection one most often thinks of a gun, knife, club, fist, or foot, but other methods are included as long as such methods would cause fear or offensiveness.

Legal delineation between immediate fear and a threat that would be performed at some future time must be remembered. A nurse tells a troublesome but sane patient, "If you don't stay in bed I will strap you down"; any fear caused would be immediate. If the statement were "If you don't stay in bed today, I will strap you down tomorrow," the immediacy factor would not exist; therefore, no assault exists. This latter threat, even if serious or harmful fear is the result, is not assault in the legal sense.

Intent is necessary as shown by point 4

of the definition, so an objective standard of intent is adopted for all pactical purposes in law. Thus, it is presumed that everyone intends the results of one's actions. A person's actual subjective intent is disregarded. Consequently, to admit one's action and to state that it was done only in fun is no defense. Assume that an innocent bystander is injured; the intent still exists in that the assaultor did intend the acts set in motion although not the specific results nor the results to a disinterested third party.

The elements of consent and privilege, being defenses, will be outlined following a review of battery.

The usual coupling of assault and battery is easily understood when the definition of each is compared. Battery is the (1) execution of the threat or attempt of the assaultor, which (2) causes bodily contact (3) with intent and (4) without consent or privilege.

The slighest touching of another's person is battery if the contact is unlawful. This also includes any instrument used. Thus, any unconsented surgical procedure or, for that matter, any touching of the patient at all that is unconsented amounts to a battery. Of course, there must be legal damage to enable substantial monetary recovery for such a tort.

CONSENT AND PRIVILEGE

The defenses to these two torts are consent and privilege. Consent may be implied or expressed, depending upon the circumstances. Consent may be rendered by anyone who has sufficient understanding of the consequences. The hard and fast rules regarding age, as in contracts, are not controlling. Each instance will stand or fall depending on the specific circumstances. As a precaution parental consent should be obtained for procedures involving children. Not only will the parents then be obligated for services rendered under contract but also consent will serve to preclude liability for assault and battery.

Express consent reaches only as far as the expression given. Thus, consent to amputate the left hand is not a consent for loss of the right hand. Express consent is of no avail in instances involving an unlawful purpose so that consent to an illegal abortion is not recognized at law. In patient care the physician and nurse must on occasion go beyond express consent at times when it is impossible to obtain additional consent. The law sanctions such emergency care in appropriate cases.

Implied consent is the other fundamental form of consent and is easily recognized in most instances. When one requests certain services, usually of a personal nature, such as those of a beautician, masseur, barber, or shoe or clothing salesman, the request itself is evidence of consent in an implied form. In nursing services implied consent exists by the act of contracting for services, but this consent usually extends only to normal services of the nurse.

The defense of privilege is direct rather than dependent upon the other party as is consent. The privilege of self-defense and defense of others in peril is well known. The important factor in defense is that the defender has the right of defense limited to only the resistance necessary to defend. Excessive resistance is unlawful. Resisting with a club an unarmed child is obviously excessive.

The privilege of discipline of children by parents is another obvious instance. In some states the teacher has statutory protection in this respect as long as the discipline is not excessive.

There is a privilege to eject unlawful persons from one's property. This is limited to only the force necessary to eject, and any unnecessary injury is unprotected. On occasions the privilege of defense of others and property coexist because someone may be threatening your children or spouse while on your property. The existence of both defenses does not increase the resistance one may legally use.

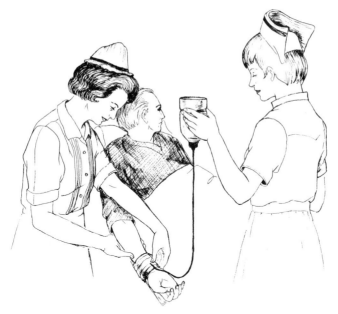

The laws governing the nurse's role in certain medical procedures, such as starting an intravenous infusion, vary from state to state.

FALSE IMPRISONMENT

False imprisonment is any act that (1) causes confinement (2) unlawfully and (3) with intent; also, (4) the confined person has knowledge of the confinement, and (5) there is no consent or privilege.

Confinement includes any means to restrain the freedom or movement of a person. A threat to a person that prevents him from leaving a room through fear is sufficient. The restraint must be complete to the extent that the execution of the threat is the only alternative. Confinement in a hospital for nonpayment of a bill can constitute false imprisonment.

The length of time of false imprisonment is not a factor other than to determine how aggravating or serious the confinement was. A restraint of only a few seconds is still restraint.

The necessity of intent again appears here, and it is treated in the same light as the intent of assault and battery.

The restrained or confined person must realize that he is being restrained. In this regard many believe that restraint of children or the mentally ill, in connection with nursing services, is protected because the child or mentally ill person does not understand or comprehend. This is not necessarily true, since the resistance of the child or the mentally ill to restraint may be evidence of enough comprehension to satisfy this element of false imprisonment. Of course, defenses of privilege or consent are usually more readily available for nurses in instances regarding children or the mentally ill.

Defenses of consent and privilege are available as in assault and battery cases. Two special problems of restraint with which nurses deal should be mentioned, however.

As regards confinement of the mentally ill, it was early held in this country that anyone was privileged to restrain such a person if it was evident that he was in danger of harming himself or others. This common-law privilege fell into disuse as modern hospitalization laws for the mentally ill developed. This privilege, however, should probably be utilized more often than it is.

In a recent *cause célèbre,* a patient in an outstanding psychiatric hospital signed out against medical advice. Apparently, hospital officials believed they were impotent to restrain him although his clinical record showed his assaultive tendencies. Within a matter of weeks he had killed another man with his bare hands.

Restraint for nonpayment of bill is another delicate matter. Hospitals have been known to threaten or actually to restrain patients from leaving until the bill was paid. If there is a matter of mistaken identity or other minor clerical problem, there may be privilege to restrain a patient until the matter is cleared. There is, however, no authority for a hospital to restrain a patient in any way because of nonpayment of bill.

Hotels, hospitals, or general merchants may restrain guests, within limit. If identity is unknown, a guest may be restrained until identity is established or a mistake of identity is corrected. Very brief detention, which is of reasonable length, may be upheld but even this is doubtful in some jurisdictions since the courts are extremely sensitive about allowing confinement, regardless of purpose.

SLANDER AND LIBEL

Slander is fundamentally defined as a malicious utterance to a person or persons, with intent, and without truth or privilege, by speaking defamatory words regarding another's reputation or profession, which would expose that person to contempt, ridicule, or public hatred.

Libel is identical in definition except that the utterance is published by writing in any form. Caricatures, signs, printing, handwriting, and any other form of a permanent nature are included.

Reviewing the definitive parts we find that malice in the legal sense is broader than in the lay sense. In addition to personal spite and nasty temperament, the definition of legal malice extends further and includes any wrongful act that is performed without good reason. It is possible to act with good intention and have the act, if wrongful, presumed malicious under the law.

The utterance itself is reviewed in the light of the locality, colloquialisms as understood locally, lay meaning of words, and the society in which stated. Prefacing defamatory statements with statements of admitted doubt, such as "I know it is hearsay, but did you hear about Miss Jones . . .," or "Have you heard the rumor about Dr. John Doe . . .," is of no effect in avoiding guilt.

The malicious utterance is not ordinarily slander or libel unless conveyed to a third person. The defamatory words must be understood by the party who hears or reads the defamatory statement. To say a defamatory statement in French to a gathering of people in a room who understand only English is not legally actionable.

The intent factor is the same as in assault and battery and false imprisonment. The fact that one does not believe the statement is no defense to the act of passing it on to someone else.

It is now necessary to consider what is meant by the phrase "actionable per se." This legal phrase means that the statement by itself is slanderous or libelous, and a legal action in the form of a lawsuit will lie. It is not necessary to show the situation and circumstances surrounding it, and damage exists "as a matter of law." The only question left is the degree of damage.

Certain classified statements are regarded as actionable per se. Accusations of the following things are so considered.

Crime: Accusation of the type of crime that would cause one to shun the presence of the accused is actionable per se. Charges that a nurse is not licensed or that a nurse has commited forgery, burglary, or murder are examples. Violation of traffic laws or a parking meter fine would not be such.

Disease: This includes certain diseases by virtue of their infectious, communicable, or moral nature, such as venereal disease, leprosy, or similar "heinous" conditions. Measles or chickenpox would not be such.

Unfitness: As to trade or profession one cannot call another a "butcher," "quack," "shyster," "ambulance chaser," "sadist," or similar terms implying unfitness for the practice of trade or profession. This type of statement affects the manner in which another makes his living. If such an accusation is untrue, it is actionable per se.

Immorality: Accusing one regarding unchastity is actionable per se. Charges of this nature may also come under the criminal prohibition. One cannot accuse another of committing adultery without striking both the criminal and civil rules. The indirect inference of pregnancy when the party is single imputes an immoral connotation and would be actionable per se under the rule of accusation of immorality.

DEFENSES

The defenses to libel and slander fall into two categories, truth and privilege. Truth in most states is an absolute defense, but when relying upon such a defense, the truth of the entire statement must be proved. In some states truth is only a partial defense because it is also necessary to prove that although true, the utterance was not made in malice and for deliberate injury.

Privilege exists under certain circumstances. For example, communications made under the special privileges under the rules of evidence, discussed in Chapter 38, would also be privileged under the law of libel and slander. Also, there is judicial privilege for statements made in court and legislative privilege for statements made in legislative chambers.

Privilege to make defamatory statements also exists between members of a household, provided the one making a statement believes such to be true. What constitutes members of household has been interpreted broadly and would include cousins, grandparents, aunts, uncles, and nephews. Whether or not they live under one roof has not been found to be any guide in this instance.

Another instance of privilege is that between former employer and prospective employer, provided that no malice exists, and the statement made is based upon the belief that it is true. This same privilege also is recognized between partners or associates in a business for the same obvious reasons.

Chapter 35

Independent contractor and employee

A key role is played by nurses in determining liability in tort cases by virtue of their "in-between" legal status. That is, a nurse is often an intermediary involved with patients, physicians, and hospitals. Technical legal status may vary, depending upon circumstances.

If by contractual negotiation a nurse enters into the relationship of employee with another party or institution, the historical legal rule of master-servant comes into effect. Then if that nurse negligently injures a third party or in other ways causes damage, the employer *also* is liable. The master is held for the acts of the servant. The legal term used is the Latin phrase *respondeat superior.* Let the superior respond—meaning let the employer pay or be responsible for the acts of the employee.

However, if the nurse is engaged on a case as an independent contractor, he or she *alone* would be held responsible for his or her own negligence. This becomes of practical importance inasmuch as it is more likely that a patient will look to a hospital or a physician for payment of damages than to an underpaid nurse with limited assets. Even in cases in which the employer is held, however, he ordinarily has a right of action against the employee if the injury was caused solely by that employee. As a practical matter, however, hospitals and physicians rarely seek such reimbursement from nurses.

It is therefore apparent why a determination of whether a nurse is an employee or an independent contractor can be of great significance in court. One status precludes the other. No one can be both at the same time, regarding the same act, to the same party.

Legal decision about which relationship exists in a particular situation is often difficult. The rules distinguishing the two are constantly changing.

Many scholars have listed rules or indicia of what determines the relationship. None of these are complete, and essentially they include only fundamental concepts; the facts of the given situation are usually controlling in a specific case.

The following questions should be considered when one is attempting to determine whether one is an independent contractor or an employee:

1. Who has reserved control over the manner in which the services are to be performed?
2. What amount of skill is required?
3. What is the method of payment?
4. Who supplies the instrumentalities, tools, and place of performance?

5. Are the services to be performed part of the employer's normal business?
6. What is the intent of the parties to the contract?

RESERVATION OF CONTROL

The most decisive element of those listed is the reservation of control. If a client engaged an attorney to defend him in a trial, it would be most unusual for the client to retain the power to determine how the trial should be conducted. In this instance the attorney undoubtedly retains control over the manner in which he will exercise his skills. Surgeon and patient, portrait artist and model, garage operator and auto owner are a few of the many instances in which we easily recognize retention of control and, therefore, the existence of the independent contractor. In nearly all instances the private duty nurse is an independent contractor for the same reason.

A nurse hired by an institution does not retain full control over his or her services and does not decide to whom the services shall be rendered. Consequently, the nurse is an employee.

An important analysis of control is *what, when,* and *how* certain acts are to be done. Hospital employment of a nurse implies *what, when,* and *how* will be dictated by the institution or by the staff physician. Although the physician does not contract with the institutional nurse, the employment contract of the nurse with the institution impliedly, if not specifically, includes the condition that control of any nursing services remains with the institution, and part of that reserved control is the right to assign the nurse to an area or a particular physician who may be using the facilities of the hospital.

Another doctrine, however, applies when the nurse is under the direct supervision of physicians and surgeons in the hospital. This is called the "loaned servant" or "borrowed servant" doctrine. Briefly, it provides for the situation in which the hospital is the principal or usual employer of the nurse. When the nurse is in the operating room, however, cases hold that the surgeon becomes the special or temporary principal while the nurse acts under his direction. Thus, for any negligent acts of a nurse while a loaned servant, there would be liability as against the nurse and surgeon, but not as against the hospital ordinarily.

SKILL REQUIRED

The second fundamental, although not as important legally, is often a mental stumbling block in the determination of status. The skill required to perform a task is a factor but is not an absolute test. Such skill is important only to differentiate between tasks that are obviously within the grasp of almost everyone, such as sweeping the corridors, and those tasks that require a certain level of ability and training to perform. Thus, in cases holding that a private duty nurse is an independent contractor, the courts have recognized that skilled performance requires independent professional judgment and that the nurse is not, as an employee, the mere servant of the patient.

MANNER OF PAYMENT

Manner of payment is a third fundamental regarding the independent contractor. When one is paid a weekly or monthly salary, which is based on the premise that one party will render forty hours a week of one's time to the other, an employee status is indicated. Independent contractors may work on a time basis, but they are paid for a completed job. A lawyer may thus determine his charge on an hourly basis, but the client usually pays by the job. The method of charge and method of payment are distinct concepts.

INSTRUMENTALITIES

The party furnishing the instrumentalities, tools, or place of work is also considered by courts when deciding whether a party is an independent contractor or employee. The difference between the institutional nurse and the private duty nurse is apparent in this respect, but again this is not absolute and is generally only a factor to be reviewed when the question of independent contractor or employee arises.

Consider the private surgeon, employed by a patient in the hospital, who uses the operating facilities furnished by a third party—the hospital. He is an independent contractor despite the fact that the instrumentalities, tools, and place of work are supplied by another.

NORMALITY OF SERVICES

Are the services performed part of the regular or normal business of the employer? The hospital contracting with a builder to construct an additional wing is obviously creating an independent contractor relationship. A difficult situation to assess is one wherein a hospital engages a nurse to do private duty nursing for a specific patient. When the hospital obtains a nurse and the nurse is to be paid by the patient, the hospital staff merely performs a courteous accommodation for the patient. The nurse is an independent contractor to the patient and has no relationship to the hospital. When the hospital goes further and obtains a nurse for this duty, pays the nurse, and bills the patients accordingly, a different relationship may occur, and the determination of whether this is a normal or regular part of

the operation of that particular hospital becomes an important factor in determining liability. Courts in each state may vary in borderline cases of this type. For this reason only fundamental factors are outlined in this chapter. Each case must be reviewed on the facts involved; a slight variance of the facts may result in a different decision although the over-all situation may seem very similar to a previously decided case.

INTENT

The sixth and final factor listed herein deals with the intent of the parties involved in the contractual relationship. This means actual mental intent. Merely calling or referring to the other party as an independent contractor is not sufficient. The law does not give great weight to nomenclature but looks almost solely to the factors previously listed and to the intent of the parties as shown by conversation, statements, written documents, or other indicia.

X may tell a friend, "I contracted to build a new home," when, in fact, X has only hired a carpenter to work under his supervision and direction. X has retained the power to decide upon each phase of woodwork as to how it is to be done and when it is to be done. The existence of an employer-employee relationship is apparent, and words will not change the relationship. The facts of the operation are usually the best criteria in establishing true intent.

Chapter 36

Wills

Technically, a will is a person's declaration of what is to be done after his death and usually deals with the disposition of his property. This declaration can be revoked during the person's lifetime and has no effect until his death. It is then applicable to the situation as it exists at the time of death.

Legal requirements for making a will are contained in the various state statutes. It is advisable for the nurse to discuss these requirements with a personal lawyer when his or her own will is drafted. Because a nurse is often requested to witness a will, some familiarity with general requirements for valid wills should be acquired.

A VALID WILL

Fundamentally, four elements must exist for a valid will. These are (1) the person making the will [testator, if male; testatrix, if female] must have testamentary capacity; (2) testator or testatrix must declare that the instrument is a will; (3) testator or testatrix must sign the will in the presence of the witnesses; and (4) there must be witnesses to the will, who cannot be beneficiaries, who sign the instrument in the presence of each other and the testator.

Testamentary capacity is similar to contractual capacity although some courts hold that a person who is mentally incompetent to contract in a business deal has enough grasp of the situation to execute a will. Mental competency here is usually measured in terms of the "understanding test." It is said that the testator must be able to understand the extent and value of his estate, his obligations to relatives and other "objects of his bounty," and the nature and effect of executing his will.

Next, the testator must declare to the witnesses that the instrument is his will and that he desires them to be witnesses to his signature. Witnesses do not have to know or read the contents of the will. The testator's declaration that the instrument is such is sufficient.

The signature must be affixed in the view and presence of the witnesses. If the party is disabled to the extent that he needs help to guide his hand in making his signature, such aid may be given, provided he knows that he is signing his will. This is important when a patient may dictate his will to an attorney who takes notes on the provisions and later drafts the will in his office. Upon the return of the attorney to the patient's bedside it is important that the testator know his own act of signing, especially if the patient has been given narcotic injections at periodic times or during the absence of the attorney, who may know of this fact. In the event the testator is illiterate, the nurse should have the testator draw an X as his mark, and then one of the witnesses must actually write the name of testator with the X in the middle and write the additional phrase "his mark" or "her mark."

If one is a beneficiary, this does not disqualify one as witness, but the witness-beneficiary loses any rights as a beneficiary under the will. The property provided for a witness-beneficiary goes into the estate to be divided under the laws of intestacy.

It is extremely important that the witnesses sign in the presence of each other and the testator and that the testator sign in the presence of all the witnesses. States vary as to the minimum number of witnesses required, either two or three. As a matter of caution many lawyers use three, regardless of state.

Wills may be challenged and set aside for any of three basic reasons: lack of certain legal requirements in the execution of the will, lack of testamentary capacity on the part of the testator, or undue influence upon the testator.

Such things as failure to have the testator and all witnesses present together while the will is being signed would invalidate the will if contested.

Lack of testamentary capacity is probably the most widely used ground upon which to base an attack upon validity of a will. This makes it doubly important that the nurse

---

WILL

I, JANE DOE, being of sound mind and disposing tendency, hereby declare this to be my last Will and Testament and hereby revoke all prior wills and codicils.

First, I direct that all my just debts and expenses of my last illness and funeral be paid.

Second, I hereby give and bequeath the sum of One Thousand Dollars ($1,000.00) to the Missouri League of Nursing.

Third, I hereby give and bequeath the sum of One Thousand Dollars ($1,000.00) to my son, John.

Fourth, I hereby give and bequeath my diamond ring and bracelet to my daughter, Cecilia.

Fifth, all the rest and residue of my estate that I now have or may later acquire I give, devise and bequeath to my beloved husband, John Doe, of St. Louis, Missouri.

Sixth, I hereby appoint John Doe, my beloved husband, executor of this my last Will and Testament, and I direct that bond be not required of him in any capacity in any jurisdiction.

IN WITNESS WHEREOF, I have hereunto set my hand this 29th day of May, 1969.

_____

This will, identified by the signature of testatrix, Jane Doe, was signed and declared to be her last Will and Testament, in the presence of us, who in her presence, at her request, in the presence of each other, all being present at the same time, have hereunder subscribed our names as witness.

_____   _____
Witness   Address

_____   _____
Witness   Address

_____   _____
Witness   Address

who is witnessing a will take particular note of the behavior and mental status of the testator. In fact, it has been urged that psychiatrists or psychologists be called to witness particularly important wills.

The law expects and does not prohibit influence of the testator by various relatives in the manner of consideration, care, and thoughtfulness. Undue influence comprehends the use of threats, fears, force, or unnatural means, to substitute one's volition for the "free agency" of the testator. An attorney tells a testator that he has evidence that will send the testator's daughter to jail unless the attorney inherits the bulk of the estate; a clergyman tells a testator that he has led a sinful life and will go to hell unless the estate is left to the Foreign Missions of his particular religion; or a physician threatens to expose an illegal abortion to which the testator was a party; all are examples of undue influence.

Whenever a will leaves even a small bequest to a physician, attorney, nurse, or clergyman, the matter is given extremely careful analysis because of the confidential relationship that always exists between such parties and the testator. Many courts "presume" under such circumstances that there has been undue influence. In this event, the nurse or other beneficiary must affirmatively prove that undue influence was *not* employed.

DRAFTING WILLS

Because of the complexities involved, it is not advisable for a nurse to prepare wills for patients. In addition, if the nurse were regularly to perform such a service, he or she may be prosecuted for practicing law without a license. One court made this comment in "throwing out" a will, which a nurse had drafted for a patient:

This practice for a nurse is unwise, and such excursions in the field of law should be discour-

aged. The relation between patient and nurse is highly confidential. Under such conditions the opportunity for fraud and undue influence is too great for safety. The old adage that "a shoemaker should stick to his last" still has its application. The drafting of wills had better be left to the legal profession.*

SPECIAL TYPES OF WILLS

Usually wills are in written form (see example of a simple will on p. 258). Provision is made, however, in a number of states for oral wills of personal property. These are designated "nuncupative wills." In states providing for this type of will, there are numerous restrictions so that the particular state law should be consulted.

Some states will recognize a holographic will. This is a document written out and signed in the handwriting of the testator but lacking the attestation of witnesses.

Special exceptions are made in most states for wills of "soldiers and sailors." It has been held that nurses called to service duty are within this category. Again, the states vary in their requirement but for the most part an oral will in such cases is held perfectly valid to dispose of the entire estate of the testator.

INTESTACY

If a person dies without leaving a will, then the laws of intestacy provide for disposition of the estate. The court appoints an administrator to take charge of such disposition. Often there is a substantial loss to the estate and heirs in terms of both administration expense and taxes. These considerations, as well as the fact that the decedent's wishes concerning disposal of his estate are negated, render it advisable for one to execute a will early in life and then to have it revised from time to time as circumstances demand.

*In re Stegman's Will, 133 Misc. Rep. 745, 234 N. Y. S. 239 (1929).

Chapter 37

Crimes

Although many crimes are of an evil or immoral nature, one cannot so classify all crimes. Those wrongs that are inimical to public safety and have been expressed to be criminal as such by the people through their state and federal legislatures comprise the subject matter of criminal law. It was previously noted that certain types of contracts would be void by virtue of being against public policy. Crimes are "public wrongs" in contrast to the "private wrongs" called torts. Thus, the state prosecutes criminal violations for and on behalf of the entire community. A criminal action is styled "The People of the State of _____ versus John Doe" or "The State of _____ versus Jane Doe." A private civil action is entitled "Jane Doe versus Richard Roe."

Criminal laws are constantly being changed to meet new conditions. As distinct professions became recognized in this country, licensure laws were established, as we have noted. Violation of such laws was made a criminal offense.

Both Congress and the state legislatures may have passed laws covering a particular matter so that a single act may be in violation of both state and Federal law. Thus, though we have a food, drug, and cosmetic law on a national level, many of

the states also have passed legislation in this area.

WHAT CONSTITUTES A CRIME

The commission of a crime requires violation of a law so designating such by an overt act with intent. Injury in any form is not a requisite. Violation of public standards is a wrong and is a crime if it has been so defined by the legislature. Thus, selling liquor to a minor has been made a crime although the child has made no use of the spirits to his detriment.

Successful commission of an overt act is not required. A mere attempt is a crime. To confine punishment to those who successfully commit a crime would not only be unrealistic but would also afford the public far less protection than now exists.

An overt act is that part of the definition that actually establishes the crime because intent normally is imputed by circumstances in the same manner it is imputed in contracts, agency, or torts.

Intent alone is not a crime. One can wish death to another, and although this is morally questionable, it is not a crime without an overt act. For an overt act the law looks to some act, whether of commission or omission, which indicates a realistic attempt and by which intent may be reasonably imputed.

A holdup in which the victim screams and the robber flees without successfully obtaining any goods is an attempted robbery and is a crime. The overt act of pointing a weapon and making known to the victim that the robber intends to take something is an overt act, and the intent is shown by the act. Even if the robber's victim does not resist and the robber finds that the victim has no money, there is still a crime. Attempt is a crime so long as it is based upon an act reasonably designed to commit a crime although it was shown that a completed crime was impossible.

Although intent is imputed, it nevertheless exists as a separate element of a crime or attempt. For this reason lack of intent is a defense that can be used effectively in criminal prosecutions. The defense is usually based upon a plea of insanity at the time of commission of the act. Because insanity is broadly defined as mental illness that negates the requisite *mens rea* (guilty mind), there has been a large volume of cases in the criminal courts in which this plea has been raised. In fact, this defense has perhaps prompted more medicolegal literature than any other single phase of the administration of justice.

All crimes are classed as either misdemeanors or felonies. Whether a crime is one or the other is determined by the seriousness with which it is regarded, and this seriousness is usually shown by the punishment provided. In general, the misdemeanor is punishable by fine and/or imprisonment for less than one year in jail. The felony is punishable at least by imprisonment in a state penal institution for a term not less than one year. Of course, probation may result in no actual confinement. At the other extreme is the death penalty.

Another point regarding classification of crimes—and this consideration is a factor in whether a crime is felonious—is the matter of moral turpitude. If the crime is of a nature that is seriously immoral, it is termed *malum in se*. Rape, murder, and many others are *mala in se*. Crimes that do not represent moral depravity, such as those involving licensing provisions, certain liquor violations, food grading, and others of similar nature, that are crimes because the law makes them so are *mala prohibita*.

PARTIES TO CRIMES

Before discussing specific crimes, it is necessary to consider the parties to a crime. Parties to a crime are treated in two categories, principal and accessory. The classification of accessory is divided into accessory before the fact and accessory after the fact. This difference of position is drawn only in the case of felonies. In misdemeanors all parties involved are principals.

The principal is the one who actually commits the criminal act, or is the one who assists or is in attendance, or is the one who causes the commission of the crime although an innocent person actually causes the act.

The accessory classification, used only in felonies, usually carries a less severe penalty. An accessory before the fact is anyone who in any way aids, assists, or contributes to the commission of a felony but is not present at the commission or is too far away to render any assistance at the actual commission. Some states do not recognize this classification of accessory and treat such parties as principals.

Accessory after the fact is anyone who aids, assists, or contributes to help one who has committed a crime to escape, avoid capture, or obstruct justice in any manner, such as destroying evidence. In most states parents or spouses are immune from such a charge provided the aid given is rendered only to their spouse or children.

SPECIFIC CRIMES

In regard to specific crimes this text will deal only with those of most significance to nurses.

Homicide

The first to command our attention is homicide—the killing of a human being. Homicide may be *justifiable* (legal execution or an officer's slaying of a prisoner trying to escape, etc.), *excusable* (unintentional killing of a patient by drugs, legal abortion, other surgery, etc.), or *felonious.*

Felonious homicide comprises murder and manslaughter. Each state may have variations, but in general it can be stated that murder is the unlawful killing of a human being with malice aforethought.

Murder

The judicial definition of "malice aforethought" is such that one of the leading authorities stated flatly that it comprehends neither "malice" (ill-will in the lay sense) nor "aforethought" (since the cases hold that sufficient time to "make up one's mind to kill" can "arise simultaneously with the act"). Many states recognize two degrees of murder, holding that first degree murder requires an actual intent to kill, with deliberation or premeditation, or that the killing was done in the perpetration of certain other felonies. All other murders would be second degree in type and result in lesser penalty.

Manslaughter

Manslaughter is defined as all other homicides not provided for in the above definitions. *Voluntary* manslaughter is an intentional homicide committed in sudden passion caused by reasonable provocation. The classic example is the killing by a husband of his wife or her paramour when he discovers them *flagrante delicto.*

Involuntary manslaughter is homicide committed unintentionally but without excuse. It may arise as the result of malfeasance, doing of a criminal act not amounting to a felony. For example, an attempt to procure an abortion in a manner such as would be calculated to cause serious injury or death would be murder; if the attempt were not made so as to inflict serious injury or

death, but death unexpectedly ensued, it would be involuntary manslaughter.

A second category involves misfeasance, doing of a lawful act in a grossly negligent manner. Thus, in the older cases there are numerous prosecutions of physicians and surgeons for deaths of patients allegedly caused by professional negligence of aggravated character. Situations in which a surgeon was intoxicated or in which he recklessly administered lethal overdoses of drugs often prompted criminal action. Today, prosecutions of this nature are rather rare in the United States. In other parts of the world, however, the criminal law in this regard is much more severe, and physicians are known to serve jail sentences for what we would think of as only ordinary professional negligence.

A third type of involuntary manslaughter involves nonfeasance, failure to act when under legal duty. One prime example is death of young children through failure of parents or others charged with their care to give them proper nourishment, shelter, and medical attention.

CRIMES REGARDING PROPERTY

The crimes regarding property are burglary, larceny, robbery, embezzlement, obtaining property under false pretense, and malicious mischief.

Although burglary would not ordinarily occur in connection with nursing, it is believed necessary to consider it because it is often confused with larceny, especially when so often the crimes are committed together.

Larceny is generally defined as the taking of another's property with the intention to deprive that person of it. Burglary, which so often goes hand in hand with larceny, means breaking and entering. The criminal who forcefully enters any type of establishment with the intent to commit larceny also commits burglary.

Robbery is larceny with force. The force may be in any form provided the victim understands or fears the force to the extent that he will release the property or money the robber desires.

Embezzlement is the taking of property when the one taking already has custody of it. When one gives custody of an article to another and that other party later converts it to his own use, embezzlement occurs. In nursing, one is entrusted almost daily with some form of valuables from the patient. Not only is the nurse obligated to use reasonable care in handling and storing the items, but conversion in any form is banned unless the patient specifically gives permission for the specific use.

Obtaining property under false pretense by misrepresentation and then converting said property to one's own use is a criminal act. Many schemes to defraud have been prosecuted under this heading. Persons who obtain hospital services of room, board, medicines, and the like through clever malingering with no intention of paying would fall in this category.

Malicious mischief is willful destruction of personal property based upon actual ill will against the owner. Perhaps of most concern to the nurse would be prosecutions resulting from the destruction of medical records, valuable medical treatises, and animals.

OTHER CRIMES

Assault and battery, false imprisonment, and defamation were discussed in the chapter dealing with torts. The same kinds of conduct, with some technical variations, give rise to crimes similarly labeled. Thus, it is apparent that one may be subject to prosecution by the state, with fines and imprisonment as penalties, and also be sued in tort for damages for a single wrongful act.

NARCOTICS

Laws for the regulation of narcotic drugs affect the nurse directly. Forty-seven states have adopted the Uniform Narcotic Law.

Its pertinent provisions (parts of sections 7 and 9) are reproduced.

7. *Professional Use of Narcotic Drugs.* (1) Physicians and Dentists. A physician or a dentist in good faith, and in the course of his professional practice only, may prescribe, administer, and dispense narcotic drugs, or he may cause the same to be administered by a nurse or interne under his direction and supervision.

(3) Return of Unused Drugs. Any person who has obtained from a physician, dentist, or veterinarian any narcotic drug for administration to a patient during the absence of such physician, dentist, or veterinarian shall return to such physician, dentist, or veterinarian any unused portion of such drug, when it is no longer required by the patient.

9. *Record to Be Kept.* (1) Physicians, Dentists, Veterinarians, and Other Authorized Persons. Every physician, dentist, veterinarian, or other person who is authorized to administer or professionally use narcotic drugs, shall keep a record of such drugs received by him, and a record of all such drugs administered, dispensed, or professionally used by him otherwise than by prescription. It shall, however, be deemed a sufficient compliance with this subsection if any such person using small quantities of solutions or other preparations of such drugs for local application, shall keep a record of the quantity, character, and potency of such solutions or other preparations purchased or made up by him, and of the dates when purchased or made up, without keeping a record of the amount of such solution or other preparation applied by him to individual patients.

Provided: That no record need be kept of narcotic drugs administered, dispensed or professionally used in the treatment of any one patient, when the amount administered, dispensed, or professionally used for that purpose does not exceed in any forty-eight consecutive hours, (a) four grains of opium, or (b) one-half of a grain of morphine or any of its salts, or (c) two grains of codeine or of any of its salts, or (d) one-fourth of a grain of heroin or any of its salts, or (e) a quantity of any other narcotic drug or any combination of narcotic drugs that does not exceed in pharmacologic potency any one of the drugs stated above in the quantity stated.

Chapter 38

Evidence

Throughout previous chapters we have been discussing rights and duties of nurses under the law. To establish rights and to impose duties it becomes necessary at times to seek court action.

In order to "prove a case," that is, convince a judge or jury, a process of evidence characteristic of the Anglo-American system is employed. Evidence signifies a relation between a proposition to be proved *(probandum)* and facts submitted to establish the proposition (evidentiary facts). The law of evidence has to do with legal rules which govern this process in courts.

Evidentiary facts are classed as follows:
1. Autoptic proference (real evidence) is the presentation of the *thing itself* in persuading the trier of fact. Included here are such things as the production in court of surgical instruments which were used to perform an abortion.
2. Presentation of an independent fact from which, by inference, the persuasion is to be produced:
   (a) Testimonial (direct) evidence. This is the testimony of a witness who states she saw the criminal abortion performed.
   (b) Circumstantial (indirect) evidence. This is "everything else." Thus, the chain of facts that a young lady had been previously pregnant—

that she was seen entering a particular house—that she thereafter was seen being carried from the house —and that later she was taken to a hospital and discovered to have recently aborted—would constitute a line of circumstantial evidence that a criminal abortion had been performed.

TESTIMONY

From this analysis it is seen how vital testimony is. Testimony would be necessary to establish the various propositions constituting the chain of circumstantial evidence. So also would some testimony, in the way of identification at least, be required when real evidence is being shown to the jury.

In the following material* the points are presented in brief form that are most important for the nurse to know.

TESTIMONY

Introduction: In trials of lawsuits, it is often necessary for one of the parties or even the court to call upon a . . . nurse to testify. She may be called as an "ordinary witness" to tell of certain

---

*Rapier, Dorothy K., Koch, Marianna J., Moran, Lois P., Geronsin, J. R., Cady, Elwyn L., Jr., and Jensen, Deborah MacL., editor: Practical nursing, ed. 2, St. Louis, 1962, The C. V. Mosby Co., pp. 583-584.

events which she has observed, such as a fall or other accident. In addition, a . . . nurse may on occasion be called upon to testify as an "opinion witness." A common example would be in a will contest where the . . . nurse who has "witnessed" the will may be called upon to give an opinion as to the state of mind of the patient when he executed his will.

EXAMINATION OF A WITNESS

Examination of a . . . nurse as a witness will usually consist of three stages after she has been "sworn."

Direct examination: The lawyer representing the party calling the . . . nurse will conduct this phase. Usually, it will consist of questions put to her by the lawyer, followed by her answers. In most instances, the lawyer will have consulted with the . . . nurse in advance to outline the questions he will ask, so that she will have in mind the pertinent facts or circumstances of importance to the lawsuit.

Cross-examination: Next, the opposing lawyer is given an opportunity to question the witness. At times, this intense interrogation will be most trying to the . . . nurse. She must realize, however, that a lawyer will often try to engender anger or other emotion in the witness in an effort to discredit the testimony. She should remain calm and collected, answer only when she clearly understands the question and has thought over the reply, and should let the judge and her own lawyer protect her from abusive tactics.

Redirect examination: Finally, under ordinary circumstances, the lawyer who conducted the direct examination will be allowed to ask further questions designed to clarify any misunderstandings which have cropped up during cross-examination.

At times, memoranda may be used to aid the . . . nurse in giving testimony. There are two technical doctrines which the law distinguishes here—memorandum to refresh memory and record of past recollection.

Memorandum to refresh memory: This recognized practice permits the lawyer to hand a witness a memorandum for the purpose of "refreshing her recollection." Once memory has been so revived, the witness is permitted to testify as to what she recollects about a given transaction. Even a record made by someone other than the witness can be used. For example, the lawyer might produce a hospital chart and ask if a patient was in pain at a particular time. After seeing the chart, the . . . nurse might well recall that the patient *was* in pain at that time.

Record of past recollection: In this situation, a memorandum itself is offered as evidence under certain technical safeguards. The writing may not bring back to memory the facts recorded, but the witness is willing to testify that the facts so recorded were true. Under this doctrine, the . . . nurse would either be the one actually making the record or would be present either at or near the time it was made. She would then vouch for the correctness of the record, although she could not remember the facts stated in the particular record.

The . . . nurse should arrange sufficient time to confer with the lawyer calling her to testify. He can then explain in detail these and other technical points that may be brought up in court. He will explain how the . . . nurse can best cooperate in the proper administration of justice, which in the words of Daniel Webster is the "chiefest interest of man."

PRIVILEGED COMMUNICATIONS

One of the least understood areas of evidence law has to do with privileged communications. It was early held that a lawyer could not be forced to divulge information from the witness stand that he had gained while in an attorney-client relationship with a client. The privilege belonged to the client so that if a client waived it, the attorney could be compelled to testify. It was readily recognized that lawyers could not properly represent their clients in court in the absence of full disclosure from them in preliminary conferences. Unless a privilege was recognized, the administration of justice would be thwarted. Clients would fear to tell "all" to their lawyers.

Some states have passed laws that established a somewhat similar privilege respecting the patient-physician relationship. It was believed that a patient would not give full disclosure to his physician if such information could be divulged in court; therefore, therapy would suffer. Over half of the states now have such a law. They are construed strictly. Thus, it has been held that the fact that a nurse overheard a physician-patient interview removed the aura of confidentiality and so removed the privilege.

In a few states, on the other hand, it has been held that communication to a nurse is also privileged. The nurse is advised to refer to a personal lawyer for advice concerning the status of the law in the individual's own state. It must be remembered that we are dealing with information being disclosed in the courtroom from the witness stand. This is separate and distinct from the duty of a nurse to refrain from disclosing secret information to third parties "over the back fence."

Questions and study projects for unit eight

1. Define these legal terms found in the unit:
   (a) consent, (b) direct examination, (c) *stare decisis,* (d) statute, and (e) tort.
   Use the Glossary in Cady's *Law and contemporary nursing,* if necessary.
2. What should the nurse know about a valid will?
3. How is the practice of nursing defined by the Nurse Practice Act in your state?
4. Discuss the legal capacity of contracting parties.
5. What conduct is suggested for the nurse undergoing cross-examination?
6. What is the purpose of licensure laws for nurses?
7. How are license laws administered in your state?
8. Make an annotated bibliography of recent articles appearing in *The American Journal of Nursing, Nursing Outlook, Nursing Research,* and any other journals available in your library relating to the discussion in this unit. Give particular attention to the series, "The law and the nurse," beginning with the February, 1962, issue of *The American Journal of Nursing.*

References for unit eight

Chapter 33

Blackstone, Sir William: Blackstone's commentaries, ed. 3, Albany, N. Y., 1890, Banks & Brothers, Law Publishers.

Cady, Elwyn L., Jr.: Law and contemporary nursing, Totowa, N. J., 1961, Littlefield, Adams & Co., Part I.

Creighton, Helen: Law every nurse should know, Philadelphia, 1957, W. B. Saunders Co., chap. 1.

Federal Legislation and the ANA, American Journal of Nursing **53**:942-944, August 1953.

Javits, Jacob K.: Dear Congressman, American Journal of Nursing **53**:554-555, May, 1953.

Lesnik, Milton J., and Anderson, Bernice E.: Nursing practice and the law, ed. 2, Philadelphia, 1955 (with revisions, 1962), J. B. Lippincott Co., chap. 1-3.

Snyder, Orvill C.: Preface to jurisprudence, Indianapolis, 1954, Bobbs-Merrill Co.

Stone, Ferdinand F.: Handbook of law study, Englewood Cliffs, N. J., 1952, Prentice-Hall, Inc.

Chapter 34

American Law Reports, Rochester, N. Y., The Lawyer's Cooperative Publishing Co., Annotations:
   Duty of physician or surgeon to warn or instruct nurse or attendant, 4 ALR 1527.
   Liability of operating surgeon for negligence of nurse assisting him, 12 ALR 3d 1017.

Barbee, Grace C.: When is the nurse held liable?, American Journal of Nursing **54**:1343, November, 1954.

Cady, Elwyn L., Jr.: Law and contemporary nursing, Totowa, N. J., 1961, Littlefield, Adams & Co., chap. 8.

Creighton, Helen: Law every nurse should know, Philadelphia, 1957, W. B. Saunders Co., chap. 2.

Lesnik, Milton J., and Anderson, Bernice E.: Nursing practice and the Law, ed. 2, Philadelphia, 1955 (with revisions, 1962), J. B. Lippincott Co., chap. 4; Appendix.

Nursing Practice Acts, Loan Folder, New York, September, 1954, American Nurses' Association.

Regan, Louis J.: Doctor and patient and the law, ed. 3, St. Louis, 1956, The C. V. Mosby Co., chap. 13.

Spaulding, John F.: Missouri law and the R. N., The Missouri Nurse, pp. 4-5, 29, November, 1953; pp. 6-7, 31, December, 1953.

Chapter 35

American Law Reports, Rochester, N. Y., The Lawyer's Cooperative Publishing Co., Annotation:
Remedies for breach of decedent's agreement to devise, bequeath, or leave property as compensation for services, 69 ALR 14; 106 ALR 742.

Cady, Elwyn L., Jr.: Law and contemporary nursing, Totowa, N. J., 1961, Littlefield, Adams & Co., chap. 11.

Creighton, Helen: Law every nurse should know, Philadelphia, 1957, W. B. Saunders Co., chap. 3-4.

Lesnik, Milton J., and Anderson, Bernice E.: Nursing practice and the law, ed. 2, Philadelphia, 1955 (with revisions, 1962), J. B. Lippincott Co., chap. 5.

Simpson, Laurence P.: Handbook of the law of contracts, St. Paul, 1954, West Publishing Co.

Chapter 36

American Law Institute: Restatement of the law of torts, ed. 2, St. Paul, 1965, American Law Institute Publishers.

American Law Reports, Rochester, N. Y., The Lawyer's Cooperative Publishing Co., Annotations:
Applicability, in action against nurse in her professional capacity, of statute of limitations applicable to malpractice, 8 ALR 3d 1336.
Liability of private, noncharitable hospital or sanitarium for improper care or treatment of patients—failure to hire special nurse—failure of nurse to give constant attendance, 22 ALR 341, 345, 353; suppl. 39 ALR 1431, 1433, 1434; suppl. 124 ALR 186, 190.
Liability of surgeon leaving sponge or other foreign matter in incision—reliance on custom of nurse's count, 65 ALR 1023, 1026; 10 ALR 3d.
Nurse's liability for her own negligence or malpractice, 51 ALR 2d 970.

Barbee, Grace C.: When is the nurse held liable?, American Journal of Nursing **54**:1343, November, 1954.

Cady, Elwyn L., Jr.: Law and contemporary nursing, Totowa, N. J., 1961, Littlefield, Adams & Co., chap. 5.

Cady, Elwyn L., Jr.: Medicolegal aspects of cardiac arrest and resuscitation. In Stephenson, Hugh E., Jr.: Cardiac arrest and resuscitation, ed. 2, St. Louis, 1964, The C. V. Mosby Co., pp. 329-352.

Cady, Elwyn L., Jr.: Law relating to medical practice: the doctor's diagnosis and treatment of patients. In Gradwohl, R. B. H., editor: Legal medicine, St. Louis, 1954, The C. V. Mosby Co., chap. 4.

Cady, Elwyn L., Jr.: Forensic medicine: technical defenses in professional liability cases, Postgraduate Medicine **32**:A-42, September, 1962.

Cahal, Mac F., and Cady, Elwyn L., Jr.: Medicolegal case studies: negligence and the standard of care, GP **25**:51, June, 1962.

Cahal, Mac F., and Cady, Elwyn L., Jr.: Medicolegal case studies: the specialist v. generalist standard of care, GP **26**:199, July, 1962.

Cahal, Mac F., and Cady, Elwyn L., Jr.: Medicolegal case studies: tort, not contract, GP **25**:169, May, 1962.

Creighton, Helen: Law every nurse should know, Philadelphia, 1957, W. B. Saunders Co., chap. 7.

Lesnik, Milton J., and Anderson, Bernice E.: Nursing practice and the law, ed. 2, Philadelphia, 1955 (with revisions, 1962), J. B. Lippincott Co., chap. 7-8.

Prosser, William L.: Handbook of the law of torts, ed. 3, St. Paul, 1964, West Publishing Co.

Chapter 37

American Law Reports, Rochester, N. Y., The Lawyer's Cooperative Publishing Co., Annotation:
Libel and slander: privilege of statements by physician, surgeon, or nurse concerning patient, 73 ALR 2d 325.

Cahal, Mac F., and Cady, Elwyn L., Jr.: Medicolegal case studies: assault and battery, GP **26**: 185, August, 1962.

Cahal, Mac F., and Cady, Elwyn L., Jr.: Medicolegal case studies: defamation (libel and slander), GP **27**:201, March, 1963.

Cahal, Mac F., and Cady, Elwyn L., Jr.: Medicolegal case studies: false imprisonment, GP **26**: 209, October, 1962.

Creighton, Helen: Law every nurse should know, Philadelphia, 1957, W. B. Saunders Co., chap. 8.

Lesnik, Milton J., and Anderson, Bernic E.: Nursing practice and the law, ed. 2, Philadelphia, 1955 (with revisions, 1962), J. B. Lippincott Co., chap. 9.

Chapter 38

American Law Reports, Rochester, N. Y., The Lawyer's Cooperative Publishing Co., Annotations:
Circumstances under which the existence of the relationship of employer and independent contractor is predictable, 19 ALR 1168, 1189.
Nurse as independent contractor or servant, 60 ALR 303.

Cady, Elwyn L. Jr.: Law and contemporary nursing, Totowa, N. J., 1961, Littlefield, Adams & Co., chap. 17.

Creighton, Helen: Law every nurse should know, Philadelphia, 1957, W. B. Saunders Co., chap. 5-6.

Lesnik, Milton J., and Anderson, Bernice E.: Nursing practice and the law, ed. 2, Philadelphia, 1955 (with revisions, 1962), J. B. Lippincott Co., chap. 6.

Chapter 39

Atkinson, Thomas E.: Handbook of the law of wills, ed. 2, St. Paul, 1953, West Publishing Co.

Cady, Elwyn L., Jr.: Law and contemporary nursing, Totowa, N. J., 1961, Littlefield, Adams & Co., chap. 12.

Creighton, Helen: Law every nurse should know, Philadelphia, 1957, W. B. Saunders Co., chap. 10, pp. 122-126.

Lesnik, Milton J., and Anderson, Bernice E.: Nursing practice and the law, ed. 2, Philadelphia, 1955 (with revisions, 1962), J. B. Lippincott Co., chap. 11.

Chapter 40

Cady, Elwyn L., Jr.: Law and contemporary nursing, Totowa, N. J., 1961, Littlefield, Adams & Co., chap. 6-7.

Cahal, Mac F., and Cady, Elwyn L., Jr.: Medicolegal case studies: criminal liability, GP **28:** 163, July, 1963.

Creighton, Helen: Law every nurse should know, Philadelphia, 1957, W. B. Saunders Co., chap. 9.

Lesnik, Milton J., and Anderson, Bernice E.: Nursing practice and the law, ed. 2, Philadelphia, 1955 (with revisions, 1962), J. B. Lippincott Co., chap. 10.

Perkins, Rollin M.: Criminal law, Brooklyn, N. Y., 1957, The Foundation Press, Inc.

Chapter 41

American Law Reports, Rochester, N. Y., The Lawyer's Cooperative Publishing Co., Annotations:
Admissibility of hospital chart or other hospital record, 75 ALR 378, 120 ALR 1124.
Privilege of communications by or to nurse or attendant, 47 ALR 2d 742.

Cady, Elwyn L., Jr.: Law and contemporary nursing, Totowa, N. J., 1961, Littlefield, Adams & Co., Part V.

McCormick, Charles T.: Handbook of the law of evidence, St. Paul, 1954, West Publishing Co.

International relationships

International code of nursing ethics*

"Professional nurses minister to the sick, assume responsibility for creating a physical, social and spiritual environment which will be conducive to recovery, and stress the prevention of illness and promotion of health by teaching and example. They render health service to the individual, the family, and the community, and coordinate their services with members of other health professions.

"Service to mankind is the primary function of nurses and the reason for the existence of the nursing profession. Need for nursing service is universal. Professional nursing service is therefore unrestricted by considerations of nationality, race, creed, color, politics, or social status.

"Inherent in the code is the fundamental concept that the nurse believes in the essential freedoms of mankind and in the preservation of human life.

"The profession recognizes that an international code cannot cover in detail all the activities and relationships of nurses, some of which are conditioned by personal philosophies and beliefs.

"1. The fundamental responsibility of

---

*Adopted by the International Council of Nurses, July, 1953; printed in American Journal of Nursing **53**:1070, September, 1953.

the nurse is threefold: to conserve life, to alleviate suffering, and to promote health.

"2. The nurse must maintain at all times the highest standards of nursing care and of professional conduct.

"3. The nurse must not only be well prepared to practice but must maintain her knowledge and skill at a consistently high level.

"4. The religious beliefs of a patient must be respected.

"5. Nurses hold in confidence all personal information entrusted to them.

"6. A nurse recognizes not only the responsibilities but the limitations of her or his professional functions; recommends or gives medical treatment without medical orders only in emergencies and reports such action to a physician at the earliest possible moment.

"7. The nurse is under an obligation to carry out the physician's orders intelligently and loyally and to refuse to participate in unethical procedures.

"8. The nurse sustains confidence in the physician and other members of the health team; incompetence or unethical conduct of associates should be exposed, but only to the proper authority.

"9. A nurse is entitled to just remuneration and accepts only such compensation as the contract, actual or implied, provides.

"10. Nurses do not permit their names to be used in connection with the advertisement of products or with any other forms of self-advertisement.

"11. The nurse cooperates with and maintains harmonious relationships with members of other professions and with her or his nursing colleagues.

"12. The nurse in private life adheres to standards of personal ethics which reflect credit upon the profession.

"13. In personal conduct nurses should not knowingly disregard the accepted patterns of behavior of the community in which they live and work.

"14. A nurse should participate and share responsibility with other citizens and other health professions in promoting efforts to meet the health needs of the public—local, state, national, and international."

Chapter 39

Some nursing activities on an international level

In preceding chapters we have seen the progression of the emancipation of women toward an international movement with the increasing professionalization of nursing as an important result. We shall now see how nursing in turn has become an international development advancing first nursing, then the larger sphere of feminism, and ultimately that of internationalism and good fellowship among the peoples.

THE INTERNATIONAL COUNCIL OF NURSES

About the turn of the century the aims of the leaders of nursing, especially in Great Britain and the United States, had become very similar. In 1899 Mrs. Bedford-Fenwick placed before the Women's Council of Great Britain the proposal that the prominent nurses from many countries who were attending the International Council of Women held in London be invited to join in an International Council of Nurses. The proposal was enthusiastically accepted, and a provisional committee was promptly formed by nurses from Great Britain, the United States, Canada, New Zealand, New South Wales, Victoria, Holland, Cape Colony, and Denmark, countries that we noted in the past as being in the vanguard of nursing education.

The committee promptly formulated a constitution that established the purpose of the organization: to unite and to organize nurses of all countries within one common bond in order that they may together attain complete professional freedom. Through the development of self-government they could establish the highest professional standards and serve society to the utmost of their ability. They were perfectly aware that such an organization would serve the greater cause of feminism and achieve for one group of women that which was considered at least part of the goal of all women. It was also apparent that when women from many lands met together, friendships and personal ties would be formed that could help to prevent the bloodshed of international conflict. Gradually, as we as individuals come to know personally more and more of our colleagues in other countries, we shall become less and less enthusiastic about going to war against them.

However premature the ultimate purposes may have seemed, the immediate plans met with absolute success. By 1900 the Council was organized with Mrs. Bedford-Fenwick as president, Miss Lavinia Dock as honorary secretary, and Miss Snively as honorary treasurer. The first International Congress of Nurses was called during the Pan-American Exposition in Buffalo, New York, in 1901. At this time, membership was individual, but it was soon decided that it should be by association. Thereby, the members could better accomplish their aim, for by admitting only organizations that were controlled by nurses and had official national standing, they excluded organizations controlled by persons other than nurses, thus achieving professional self-government.

In Germany the free sisters took advantage of this. In 1903 they organized the German Nurses' Association under the able leadership of Sister Agnes Karll. In 1904 when the International Council of Women met in Berlin, they became hosts to the International Council of Nurses. The principle of admission by association was officially established, and the Council was begun with three members: the National Council of Nurses of Great Britain, the American Nurses' Association, and the German Nurses' Association.

The influence of the International Council of Nurses in raising standards in many countries is on record. In order to become members, the national nurses' organization in a country must be self-governing. This has spurred the movement for increasing educational standards as well as obtaining recognition and support in each country.

Organization and development

Headquarters were established first in Geneva, Switzerland, later in London. At first *The American Journal of Nursing* and the *British Journal of Nursing* were the official organs for the Council; later it established its own journal, the *I.C.N.,* which in 1930 became the *International Nursing Review*. It is now a most colorful and fruitful source for all information pertaining to the progress of nursing in the various countries.

Meetings were held every few years. World War I, as well as World War II suspended such activities, but since 1922 the Council has met every three or four years on both sides of the Atlantic. At each meeting more countries were admitted, so that before World War II there were thirty-two active members. Representatives of countries in which nursing organizations had not yet reached necessary development were admitted to associate membership, thereby gaining the support of the greater organization in their struggle. The admittance of a new member was described by Miss Dock, who was actively associated with the movement from its beginning:

Those who attend the congresses of the International Council of Nurses are always moved by the ceremony of initiation of member countries when, preceded by her national flag and accompanied by her national anthem, the new representative is presented by one of the older members and formally welcomed into the International sisterhood. There is something very real behind all the pageantry and symbolism of these impressive occasions. . . . The I.C.N. is a bright example of Internationalism at its best.

Much of the success of the Council was due to Miss Christine Reimann, for many years its permanent secretary and editor of the *Journal.*

INTERNATIONAL POSTGRADUATE COURSES

It was soon realized that to become a potent force the Council had to do more than meet and wave the flag every few years. At the meeting in Cologne in 1912, it was suggested that an educational memorial to Florence Nightingale be established. However, World War I soon broke out and temporarily stopped international activities, but when the guns were silenced, the idea was again taken up, this time by the League of Red Cross Societies. In 1920 a postgraduate nursing course in public health was established in London at King's College, later at Bedford College, where it has since remained. In 1924 a second course, in administration and teaching, was established at the College of Nursing, and nurses from many lands met under a common roof for a common purpose.

THE FLORENCE NIGHTINGALE INTERNATIONAL FOUNDATION

After about ten years of successful operation the International Council of Nurses was invited to join in the undertaking, and at the recommendation of a committee headed by Mrs. Bedford-Fenwick, a partnership was established between the two bodies in July, 1934. The outcome was "The Florence Nightingale International Foundation." It was decided that its home should be in London for it is there that "Florence Nightingale's spirit still lives in fullest radiance." The Foundation is financed by an endowed trust administered by a "Grand Council," consisting of five representatives of the League of Red Cross Societies, five from the International Council of Nurses, and two from each component National Nursing Committee. The students are selected by the National Committees and may pay tuition or study under a scholarship. They are selected for scholastic standing and potential leadership qualities. It is obvious that aims of the International Council of Nurses could in no way be better furthered than by bringing together a group of promising young women from different countries under a common roof where they could receive the stimulus of varied and valuable contacts. To com-

plete the organization, the College of Nursing donated the use of the beautiful Florence Nightingale International House as a residence for the students during their stay in London.

After they finished their courses, most students joined "the old Internationals," which was founded in 1925 as an organization through which students could keep in touch with each other. The organization maintains a library, which should develop into a historical collection and out of developed an International History of Nursing Society. This society was discontinued in 1939 at the outbreak of World War II. After the war the international courses in London were not reestablished.

In 1948 it was recommended that the Florence Nightingale International Foundation function within the International Council of Nurses. Through its activities the Foundation is associated with the International Council of Nurses in developing wider educational programs and activities than were possible before. The invested trust fund of the Florence Nightingale International Foundation provides a small income, and the International Council of Nurses is responsible for financing the general administration and program. The over-all objective of the Foundation as defined by the Council may be stated as improving nursing throughout the world through the stimulation and improvement of education for nursing.

Although the Florence Nightingale Foundation is the most ambitious undertaking in which the International Council of Nursing has been engaged, it is not its sole activity. Through its publications and meetings it has constantly worked for improvement of nursing standards throughout the world. By making acceptance by the Council desirable, it has forced improvement in backward countries; it has constantly endeavored to better define the scope and purposes of nursing; it has encouraged research into nursing technics, and it has attempted to

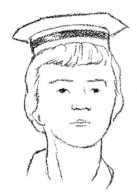

Hahnemann Hospital graduate nurse

apply modern scientific principles to nursing and modern teaching methods to the education of nurses. The Council has acted as a clearing house for the exchange of ideas and methods. In addition, it has endeavored to widen the scope of nursing by applying to it the widest possible definition: "Nursing is the safeguarding and building up of life forces in the individual and in the race." The hand of the public health educator is clearly seen in this definition.

Thus, it attempts, as far as possible, to recommend minimum requirements for a nursing curriculum, realizing, however, that such a guide must be influenced by the conditions of the land in which it is to be used. It does emphasize that nurses must receive a minimum of three years' consecutive training in a qualified school that is under the direction of a trained nurse and in which the curriculum comprises training in surgical, medical, and children's wards.

ACTIVITIES FOLLOWING
WORLD WAR II

Headquarters of the International Council of Nurses, which had been in London and Geneva, were moved to New Haven, Connecticut, from 1939 to 1944. Miss Effie J. Taylor, Dean of the School of Nursing at Yale University, had been elected president at the 1937 International Council of Nurses' meetings in London. At the end of the war, nurses in all European countries greatly needed not only books and educational tools but also uniforms, shoes, and food. A relief program was started, and the American Nurses' Association and the Canadian Nurses' Association did much to help their sister members in the International Council of Nurses. Gradually, in the years immediately after the World War II, contacts were reestablished, and conferences and meetings were planned.

In 1958 the following forty-six countries were members of the International Council of Nurses: Australia, Austria, Barbados, Belgium, Brazil, Canada, Ceylon, Chile, Colombia, Cuba, Denmark, Ethiopia, Finland, France, Germany, Great Britain, Greece, Haiti, Iceland, India, Iran, Ireland, Israel, Italy, Jamaica, Japan, Korea, Liberia, Luxembourg, Malaya, Netherlands, New Zealand, Northern Rhodesia, Norway, Pakistan, Panama, the Philippine Islands, South Africa, Southern Rhodesia, Sweden, Switzerland, Trinidad, Turkey, the United States of America, Uruguay, and Yugoslavia.

In 1961 the International Council of Nurses met in Melbourne, Australia. Thirteen new national nurses' associations were voted membership: Burma, British Guina, Egypt, Ghana, Jordan, Kenya, Mexico, Nigeria, Poland, Singapore, Thialand, Venezuela, and the Republic of China. These admissions brought to fifty-nine the number of national associations with full membership in the International Council of Nurses. At the same meeting, Mlle. Alice Clamageran of France was elected the new president of the International Council of Nurses, and Helen Nussbaum of Switzerland became the general secretary.

The International Council of Nurses has taken over the register of displaced nurses formerly maintained by the International Relief Organization and has assumed responsibility for it. In 1953 this register listed over 4,000 nurses who had had to leave their own countries for reasons beyond their control.

The International Council of Nurses is a member of the International Hospital Federation and the World Federation for Mental Health. Representatives from the International Council attend meetings of the World Medical Association. The Council also works with the nursing bureau of the League of Red Cross Societies.

The first postwar meeting was held in 1946, in Atlantic City when Miss Gerda Hojer was elected president. The second meeting followed in 1949 in Stockholm, Sweden. At the meeting in Stockholm in June, 1949, a very important step was taken when the Florence Nightingale International

Foundation was established within the International Council of Nurses as a legal entity. The Foundation has benefited by having the protection and strength of an older and larger organization. The Florence Nightingale International Foundation assumed the responsibility for the over-all educational activities of the International Council of Nurses.

ECONOMIC WELFARE OF NURSES

The Economic Welfare Committee of the International Council of Nurses was established in 1947. Its primary responsibility was outlined to be that of securing information about (1) professional recognition that has been granted to nurses and other aspects of professional and economic welfare and (2) economic conditions of nurses throughout the world in regard to salaries, pensions, and working conditions. The replies of twenty-one countries to a questionnaire were presented at the International Council of Nurses' conference in Brazil in 1952. Information from these questions covered such aspects as professional recognition and status, economic welfare, including machinery for the negotiation of economic conditions, salaries, pensions, hours of work, health protection, transfer, and promotion. The Economic Welfare Committee realized that the information contained in this report should be revised, corrected, and brought up to date during the next quadrennial period and that the work of the committee should be continued through the appointment of an economic correspondent in each country.

Because of the great difference in professional status, working conditions, general economic conditions, and many other aspects peculiar to each country, much work remains to be done, but a first step has been taken to study economic conditions under which professional nurses work all over the world.

Professional nurses are finding their places as world citizens not only through the International Council of Nurses but also through such international organizations as the World Health Organization in which they are cooperating with doctors and other health workers in improving the level of health for all people.

OTHER INTERNATIONAL PROGRAMS

In striving for improvement of international health standards, the International Council of Nurses does not stand alone. The World Health Organization (WHO), the League of Red Cross Societies, and the International Health Board of the Rockefeller Foundation have similar and supplementary aims. The total enterprise of advancing public health by international cooperation continues to make marvelous progress when world politics permit.

The activities of the International Council of Nurses are by far the most important international nursing activities, but there are others that must also be mentioned.

The International Unit of the American Nurses' Association supports the International Council of Nurses and the specialized agencies of the United Nations in the promotion of better understanding between nurses of all countries. The activities of this unit center about exchange programs for graduate nurses endorsed by the International Council of Nurses. Nurses from other countries come to the United States for observation, study, and experience, and nurses from this country go abroad for similar experiences.

INTERNATIONAL COOPERATION ADMINISTRATION

Many nurses are finding interesting foreign assignments in the Public Health Division of the International Cooperation Administration. The International Cooperation Administration is a unit of the Department of State and administers the technical cooperation (Point Four) program under the Mutual Security Program. Nurses wishing to participate in this program must have had several years of experience and have demonstrated competence in public health nursing, nursing education, or hospital nursing. Appointments are usually made for a two-year period. Assignments are made to nursing programs in Latin America, the Far East, South Asia, and Africa. Further information may be obtained from the regional office of the United States Civil Service Commission. Within the last seven years nurses have become a major factor in the achievements of the Peace Corps.

WORLD HEALTH ORGANIZATION

Through the International Council of Nurses the nursing profession's link with the World Health Organization has been represented at recent meetings of "WHO." Over 140 American nurses have gone to twenty-one different countries under this organization. They have helped teach school nursing, midwifery, and dispensary work, and they have taught people of backward areas to purify water, to prepare foods, and to grow vegetables and fruits.

One hundred thirty-four nurses of twenty-two nationalities are employed by the World Health Organization and are engaged in nursing projects in twenty-nine countries. The WHO publication, *Guide for National Studies of Nursing Resources,* is used by World Health Organization advisers. The assistance WHO gives in countries varies a great deal; sometimes it helps to establish good basic schools or assistance in curriculum planning, or the development of regional seminars and workshops. Sometimes nurses study and observe in fields of nursing education, clinical supervision, administration, public health nursing, and midwifery. The World Health Organization has been helpful in translating nursing texts and other literature into Spanish, particularly for use in Latin America. WHO is interested in building up professional nursing in different countries capable of participating in health and nursing activities and in giving leadership in those countries. The standards of the profession set up by the International Council of Nurses are promoted in these activities.

Questions and study projects for unit nine

1. What were the social and political backgrounds out of which the International Council of Nurses developed; how have changing international conditions shaped its course?
2. What is the Florence Nightingale International Foundation, and what are its contributions to nursing?
3. What are some other international activities that affect nurses and nursing?
4. Discuss the contributions of the following persons to nursing: Lavinia Dock, Mrs. Bedford-Fenwick, Sister Agnes Karll, and Christine Reimann.
5. Discuss the development and importance of international postgraduate courses for nurses.
6. Make an annotated bibliography of recent articles appearing in *The American Journal of Nursing, Nursing Outlook, Nursing Research,* and any other journals available in your library relating to the discussion in this unit.

References for unit nine

ANA and the United Nations, American Journal of Nursing **53**:1200, October, 1953.

A Nurse's U N, American Journal of Nursing **52**:1209, October, 1952.

Breay, Margaret, and Fenwick, Ethel Gordon: The history of the ICN, 1899-1925, Geneva, Switzerland, 1931, The International Council of Nurses.

Broe, Ellen: The Educational Division of the International Council of Nurses (Florence Nightingale International Foundation), International Nursing Bulletin **8**:10, 1952.

Calder, Ritchie: The lamp is lit—the story of the World Health Organization (pamphlet), Geneva, 1951, World Health Organization.

Chagas, Agnes: The work of WHO in Latin America, American Journal of Nursing **53**:410-411, April, 1953.

Convention report, Nursing Outlook **9**:372, June, 1961.

Disbrow, Mildred A.: A foreign student or a classmate? Nursing Outlook **11**:874-877, December, 1963.

Dock, Lavinia L.: Our international prospects, American Journal of Nursing **19**:781-782, August, 1919.

Editorial—Internationalism in nursing, American Journal of Nursing **22**:1, October, 1922.

Education and training of medical and public health personnel, Geneva, 1951, World Health Organization.

Fenwick, Ethel G.: The International Council of Nurses, American Journal of Nursing **1**:785-790, August, 1901.

Garesché, Rev. Edward F.: International Catholic Guild of Nurses, American Journal of Nursing **25**:188-190, March, 1925.

Goodman, Neville M.: Nursing and the World Health Organization, American Journal of Nursing **49**:134-136, March, 1949.

Goodrich, Annie W.: Florence Nightingale International Foundation, National League of Nursing Education, 1936, pp. 246-251.

International aspects of nursing education (a series of mimeographed addresses provided through the Annie W. Goodrich Lectureship Fund), New York, Teachers College, Columbia University.

Nursing and the League of Nations, American Journal of Nursing **31**:1283-1284, November, 1931.

Nursing on the world health front, American Journal of Nursing **50**:611, 1950.

Nursing service and nursing standards throughout

the world, American Journal of Nursing **53**: 1226-1228, October, 1953.

Patterson, Lillian B.: The Third World Health Assembly, American Journal of Nursing **50**: 760, 1950.

Petry, Lucile: Nursing on the world health front, American Journal of Nursing **50**:611, October, 1950.

Petry, Lucile: WHO and nursing, American Journal of Nursing **48**:611, October, 1948.

Rice, Donald T.: International crossroads of public health, Nursing Outlook **11**:836, December, 1963.

Schwarzenberg, Anna: Activities and program of the ICN, American Journal of Nursing **45**:718, September, 1945.

Steffen, Anna M.: Fourth World Health Assembly, American Journal of Nursing **51**:747, 1951.

Taylor, Effie J.: The International Council of Nurses, American Journal of Nursing **50**:615, 1950.

Taylor, Ruth G.: Fifth World Health Assembly, American Journal of Nursing **52**:1463, 1952.

The Florence Nightingale International Foundation inaugurated, American Journal of Nursing **34**:786-792, August, 1934.

The Florence Nightingale International Foundation, American Journal of Nursing **35**:452, May, 1935.

The Florence Nightingale International Foundation, American Journal of Nursing **36**:1001-1008, October, 1936.

The Florence Nightingale International Foundation, American Journal of Nursing, **38**:975-977, September, 1938.

Unit **ten**

Nursing in Canada

Mary B. Millman, B.A., R.N.

Canada may seem a country of comparatively small population but the health care
of its people has always been of great interest and nursing has been accepted since the
90's as one of the preferred professions for
young women of education and culture.

Chapter 40

History and present-day activities of nursing in Canada*

In the development of nursing in Canada, it is possible to distinguish influences from three countries. France provided an early influence, Great Britain provided the Nightingale system and the Victorian Order of Nurses, and the proximity of the United States provided a close relationship in more recent developments. There has been an exchange of ideas, close cooperation, and a resemblance in training and organization between Canada and the United States. Canada, with its large area, small population, rapidly growing industrial centers, and wide open spaces, has had unique problems in meeting its nursing needs.

THE FRENCH INFLUENCE

In the first half of the seventeenth century Duchesse d'Aiguillon, upon reading the Jesuits' *Relations* describing the difficult conditions of Canada, used her influence to obtain a grant of land in the City of Quebec for the purpose of erecting a hospital. The nursing staff was to consist of three Augustinian nuns. These nuns were joined by a small

group of Ursuline nuns under the leadership of Mère Marie de l'Incarnation and Mme. de la Paltrie who were going to Canada to act as teachers. They left Dieppe in May, 1639, and reached Quebec in August after an adventurous journey full of hardships. They were received with general celebrations. The Augustinian Sisters were conducted to the Jesuit mission at Sillery, where they found church, infirmary and mission house all behind palisades as protection against hostile Indians. They at once received the use of the infirmary for a hospital, and before they had a chance to recover from their journey, the sick crowded about them asking for help. Medical aid was practically unknown, and the need for nurses was out of proportion to what they could possibly provide. To make matters worse, the people of the region soon suffered from a violent outbreak of smallpox, which taxed their strength to the limit.

The Urusline Sisters were also soon involved with the smallpox epidemic, and instead of teaching, they found themselves confronted with the problem of nursing many more smallpox victims than the school building could accommodate. Fortunately no nuns were infected, but the epidemic severely tested their strength and delayed their plans for several months.

*The reviser of this chapter is indebted to the national and provincial associations, the university schools of nursing, the Canadian Red Cross Society, the Victorian Order of Nurses, and others for much of the material included.

283

Soon results of the good work, which had been so badly needed and was deeply appreciated, began to appear. The sick, white and Indian alike, crowded around the little building in Sillery. The Augustinian Sisters named their hospital "Hôtel Dieu" after its prototypes in Europe, and the work quickly expanded to a point at which a larger building was needed. In 1658 they had a new and larger Hôtel Dieu built under the immediate protection of the Fort of Quebec. The organization that they built there has endured to the present time.

After the epidemic the Ursuline Sisters returned to their original purpose of teaching, and by 1660 they had a fine stone convent, which still stands. Their part in the development of nursing henceforth became less important.

Jeanne Mance

About the same time another development took place which was profoundly to affect Montreal, then a most primitive settlement on an island in the St. Lawrence River. A young French woman, Mlle. Jeanne Mance, who had also read the Jesuits' *Relations,* learned of the Ursuline Sisters' going to Quebec. She became fired with their zeal and went to Paris to obtain the support of some wealthy women of her acquaintance. She was successful in her endeavor; Mme. de Bullion promised her that she would establish a hospital at Montreal.

Evidently the Jesuits' *Relations* was widely read. Others had the same idea. Jerome de la Dauversiére, tax collector in a small town on the Loire, became inspired to go to the island of Montreal to found a hospital and a nursing order. At the same time a young priest, Jean Jacques Olier, had a similar impulse, desiring to form a society of priests in the same place. The two men somehow got together (the legend says it was by a miracle) and they planned to organize their colonies with priests to govern, nuns to teach, and Sisters to nurse the sick. They organized their company and went to Rochelle in France ready to begin their journey. Here de la Dauversiére met Mlle. Mance by accident as they were leaving church, and she willingly joined the expedition, which seemed to promise her exactly what she was seeking.

The journey was difficult, and they did not reach Quebec until the fall of 1641, too late to travel up the river. However, when spring came, they reached the island. Deeply inspired and with appropriate ceremonies, they founded the colony of Montreal and devoted their services to the honor of God. In the summer their industry brought rewards; a settlement protected by palisades was built, and they were soon reinforced by new arrivals who also brought support to Mlle. Mance from Mme. de Bullion so that a hospital could be constructed. This was badly needed, because attacks from the savages constantly became more intense, and protection and care of the wounded had to take preference over the tilling of the soil. The hospital was completed in 1644 and was dedicated to St. Joseph. It was built of logs and was 60 feet long and 24 feet wide. It contained two "large" wards for patients, a kitchen, and rooms for Mlle. Mance and for the servants. Supplies were received from France, but there was no physician, so the responsibility for the care of the sick fell actually upon Mlle. Mance, who had to be guided, not by professional training, for she had none, but by common sense, endurance, and will power, of which she had plenty. Her kindness, even to the hostile Indians, seemed to overcome all obstacles, and although the hospital often was filled to overflowing, the little enterprise continued to prosper.

Mlle. Mance had, so to speak, to fight on two fronts: she had to maintain enthusiasm and support from home and at the same time keep the precarious enterprise going on the island. From Mme. Bullion she obtained further 24,000 pounds—demonstrating that it was not small change that the protectors of those days invested in such enterprises, for the money went entirely into the hospital, and it had greater purchasing power than now. Mlle. Mance was active not only in the hospital but also in all the affairs of the colonies. Several times she made the arduous journey back to France to gather new recruits and new funds. In 1659 she obtained three nurses of the Order of St. Joseph de la Fleche. One of them, Mere de Bresoles, became Mother Superior of the hospital. The difficulties in maintaining the colony continued to increase. The Indian attacks became more fierce, and the interest aroused by the Jesuits seemed to wane, so that home support was ever more difficult to obtain. The story is told about the necessity of patching the robes of the Sisters so extensively that the original material was no longer discernible and about snow drifting through chinks in the walls that had to be removed before any other ward work could begin. Food had to be thawed out in front of the fire before it could be eaten. Gradually, however, conditions improved, and when Mlle. Mance died in 1673, she left the colony well on its way. She had earned an enduring place in the hearts of all the citizens of Montreal. She never took the veil, for she thought she could do more good by not being thus restricted.

The Sisters had to pass through one more serious crisis. Government support gradually took the place of private contributors, but when Canada passed into the hands of the British, following the Seven Years' War, the Sisters found themselves deserted and facing complete poverty. It was then that one of the Sisters began baking as a source of income, which soon proved adequate, especially because it was later supplemented with the proceeds from a little soap factory, which they also organized. This is the early history of the Sisters of Hôtel Dieu of Montreal. They prospered, and now they possess one of the finest hospitals in the Dominion. It is an enduring monument to perseverance and zeal.

The French-speaking Sisters have con-tinued to conduct schools of nursing, but in recent years lay nurses have been appointed to senior administrative and teaching positions.

English-speaking Sisters also conduct schools of nursing throughout the Dominion.

BRITISH INFLUENCE

The subsequent nursing development in Canada is less romantic and more general. The British established municipal hospitals in all important places, but nursing soon sank to the same miserable level that we have recorded in England and in the United States in the later eighteenth century to early nineteenth century.

THE NIGHTINGALE INFLUENCE

When Miss Nightingale's efforts began to be influential, there was a movement in Canada to improve preparation for nursing, but it was difficult for this movement to gain a foothold. In 1864 the General and Marine Hospital of St. Catherines, Ontario, attempted to start a school by admitting one pupil nurse. This seemingly halfhearted attempt failed. A successful start was not made until ten years later when Dr. Theophilus Mack sent for two trained nurses and five probationers and organized the school that has since borne his name. About the same time Miss Nightingale sent, at the request of the Board of the Montreal General Hospital, a superintendent and four nurses. However, they encountered so much trouble that they returned home without accomplishing their purpose. After several more failures, Miss Norah Livingstone, superintendent of nurses at the New York Hospital, was induced to come to the Montreal General Hospital. She remained for twenty years and established an outstanding school, introducing into Canada both the preliminary term and the three-year course.

The second leading school in Canada, that of the Toronto General Hospital, was established by Miss Agnes Snively. She was a Canadian, trained at Bellevue Hospital in New York, and became one of the leaders of Canadian nursing, for she took an active part in the organization of the national and international nursing societies.

Another outstanding nurse of this period from Canada, Miss Anne Maxwell, established, in 1887, the nursing school at Winnipeg General Hospital. Later she became the head of the school at Montreal General, where she succeeded Miss Livingstone. Both of these schools prospered under her guidance and became outstanding in nursing education.

Once schools became properly established in Canada, they developed and multiplied, and nursing education soon reached the same level that had been achieved in England and the United States.

PUBLIC HEALTH NURSING

The success of the organization of the Queen's Jubilee Nurses led to the establishment of similar groups in the colonies. In 1897, the year of the Diamond Jubilee of Queen Victoria, Lady Aberdeen organized in Canada the Victorian Order of Nurses along these lines. The very geographical nature of this enormous country created a necessity for an organization of public health nurses of a high order. These nurses combined the pioneer spirit of the early French Sisters with a highly specialized training. Besides being graduate nurses, they were in the earlier years given a special course in various centers strategically located throughout the country. Here they learned to look after themselves and their charges of all ages from the cities in the east to the wilderness of the northwest, including the Indian Reservations. In fact, their training was so outstanding that many nurses from the United States sought it in preference to their own. With the organization of public health nursing courses in the universities, the need for the Victorian Order of Nurses to provide courses of its own has

ceased although it has continued to provide outstanding in-service education.

Not only was nursing supplied on a visit basis but also hospitals, such as the Lady Minot Hospitals, were established in newly settled communities and carried on until the community could assume the responsibility. As public health nursing progressed under official auspices, the Victorian Order of Nurses has turned over many phases of its work to public health departments, provincial or local.

Today, this is a national voluntary public health nursing organization with over one hundred branches established in centers across Canada in every province except Prince Edward Island.

Although its primary function is the provision of visiting nursing service, the program is adapted to meet the needs of a community. This has resulted in a variety of services being offered not only from branch to branch but from province to province. The program in any area is planned in consultation with local and provincial health authorities and is carried on in cooperation with hospitals and other health and social agencies. All branches of the Victorian Order accept the basic policies and standards of the national organization.

Over 750 nurses are employed by the Victorian Order; the majority of these have preparation in public health nursing. Within the past few years, male registered nurses have been employed in four large branches and registered nursing assistants are employed in nine branches. Other personnel that have been added are: physiotherapists, supervisors of housekeeping services, medical directors, and social workers on a part-time basis for home care plans.

To maintain standards of service, over-all supervision of the staff is carried out by regional directors employed by the national organization. The national professional staff is also available to all branches for consultant services.

A number of bursaries are offered each

year to assist nurses in obtaining public health preparation either at the basic or advanced level.

There has been increased interest in the development of home care programs in Canada. The Victorian Order has been an active participant, in both the planning and provision of services in these programs. At the present time ten Victorian Order branches are administering a home care program and three more are to initiate programs this year. A housekeeping service is being administered by the Victorian Order in five areas.

In many areas hospital referral programs have been established with the Victorian Order nurse spending a regular period in the hospital making ward rounds and planning with doctors and head nurses for continuing care for patients being discharged from hospital.

All branches of the Victorian Order assist in the education of nurses both in their basic and post-basic preparation when observation and experience in visiting nursing is provided. In centers where there are medical schools, these students also receive some observation in the home.

Since public health nursing has been recognized increasingly as a public responsibility, it has been organized within the responsibility of the provinces. The British North America Act placed the authority upon the provinces in regard to both education and health. The Department of National Health and Welfare, is responsible for international quarantine and for health services to veterans, Eskimo and Indians, and all residents of the unorganized areas of the Yukon and Northwest Territories. In recent years it has appointed a group of nursing consultants, upon whom the provincial health departments or private agencies may call for advice.

The medical findings regarding the recruits of World War I (1914-1918) demonstrated the need for a rapid increase in public health services Even with the stresses of war and the need to supply nursing care for the armed forces, definite developments already begun in the early years of the century were given impetus. One of the early and outstanding public health services was organized in 1912 in Toronto, Ontario, by two great pioneers, Dr. C. J. O. Hastings and Miss Eunice Dyke. In 1917, by the amalgamation of the school services with those of maternal and child care and communicable disease control, it set a generalized pattern that has been copied or adapted not only in Ontario but also throughout most of Canada and in many other countries.

Following World War I, the need for post-basic preparation for the nursing staff in both official and voluntary agencies was realized. With financial help for a three-year period from the Canadian Red Cross Society, one-year courses in public health nursing were organized in the fall of 1920 in five universities across the Dominion. Most of these courses were continued by the universities at the end of the three-year period, and other courses were organized in several more universities by 1940.

The federal government also realized the need for further education of public health nurses and allowed the gratuities of the military Nursing Sisters to be used for fees and maintenance in a public health nursing course. It is worth noting that the Department of Public Health of the City of Toronto added eleven of the university-prepared nurses to its staff in the fall of 1921, and at that date, recognizing the value of such preparation, decided that all new appointees must have this minimum qualification. This qualification later became a requirement in all Ontario official public health agencies. Other provinces have followed suit, as prepared public health nurses have become available. Registered nurses and nursing assistants are employed for junior positions, such as assisting at clinics and with records and providing other aids to the qualified public health nurse.

In some of the provinces public health programs are determined and carried out by the provincial departments of health. In others, particularly in the early-settled provinces with a population of predominantly British Isles descent, there is local autonomy, within certain regulations and with consultative services provided by the provincial department. Quebec, which is chiefly French in population and has retained the Napoleonic Code of Law and other French influences, has the problem of a population with two official languages. It was one of the first provinces to develop rural health units. Health units are now established in other provinces although there are still areas, gradually decreasing in number, in which no public health nursing service is yet available. The developing trend in the rural health unit is to supply bedside nursing as well as the more traditional services of the official agency. Newfoundland has particular geographical problems and has developed its out-port services and its cottage hospitals as well as the usual public health services in its larger centers.

The official agency in Canada has given leadership in the development of public health nursing from the early years.

OCCUPATIONAL HEALTH NURSING

The first known record of an industrial nurse in Canada was dated 1908. Growth of industrial nursing was stimulated to a large degree by the passing of Workmen's Compensation Acts and by World War I. Increasing industrialization following the war, particularly in the provinces of Ontario and Quebec, aroused governmental interest. Divisions of industrial hygiene were formed within the provincial departments of health, the first being established in 1920 in Ontario. Within these divisions it has been found desirable to have nursing consultants; the first full-time appointment was in 1943 in Ontario. A strong factor influencing the growth of industrial nursing during World War II was a federal government *order-in-council* requiring companies with certain war contracts to establish health services. Although this requirement was rescinded at the end of the war, a steady development of health services in industry has continued. Nursing consultants have been appointed in the Federal Department of Health and Welfare and in Ontario, Quebec, and Saskatchewan. Occupational health nursing, which was at first chiefly concerned with first-aid in factories, has since developed a broad public health program. It is now present in all types of industrial and commercial establishments and is increasing rapidly within hospitals.

CANADIAN RED CROSS SOCIETY

The Canadian Red Cross Society and its provincial divisions have aided greatly in the health programs of the country. Some of its stated projects have been: to fill gaps in public health services; to plan and to conduct well-balanced programs that could be continued within the framework of existing public health services; to experiment with new ideas and methods; to initiate pilot programs, demonstrate their values, and turn them over to official health services if and when this is appropriate; and to ensure that all of its programs are conduced at such a professional and technical level that they will serve as models. Some examples of the fulfillment of these projects are: the Out-Post Service of the Red Cross in the various provinces; financial support to universities for public health nursing courses as in 1920 to 1923; the provision of bursaries, scholarships, and loans for students enrolled in university basic and post-baccalaureate courses until such aids become available elsewhere; and most recently, the provision for the first Canadian fellowship for nurses to study at the doctoral level.

The financing of the independent Canadian Nurses' Association course in Windsor, Ontario, 1948 to 1952, was a major gift to nursing education. It resulted in the acceptance of an increase of independent schools throughout the country in the last decade.

THE UNITED STATES INFLUENCE

In other respects the development of Canadian nursing has closely resembled the development of nursing in the United States. It has appreciated the value of university affiliation, and in 1919 the University of British Columbia, in cooperation with the Vancouver General Hospital, established a department of nursing. This was soon followed by similar departments in other universities.

SIMILARITIES TO THE UNITED STATES

When the United States had its nursing situation surveyed by nursing organizations, and the Lancet Committee, largely sponsored by doctors, surveyed in England, Canada was surveyed by a joint medical-nursing committee under the direction of Professor G. M. Weir of the Department of Education of the University of British Columbia. The purpose of this survey was primarily to investigate the criticism that had been growing about Canadian nursing and training. The recommendations of the committee were not unlike those of the American survey. It recommended higher educational standards, higher requirements from the schools more graduate nurses on hospital staffs, general application of the eight-hour day, better-qualified instructors, and general introduction of tuition charges —in other words, less "working for your board" and more planned instruction. To meet the expense of such reforms, the report recommended increased government support. In line with this were recommendations for a stronger and expanded public health service; accordingly, a Proposed Curriculum for Schools of Nursing in Canada was prepared in 1936 by a committee of which several members were doctors and hospital administrators. A Supplement to a Proposed Curriculum for Schools of Nursing in Canada was prepared by The National Committee on Education of the Canadian Nurses Association and was Published in 1940. It amplified and further advanced the recommendations of the survey, endeavored to attract an increasingly finer type of young woman and to develop her initiative, and to provide cultural advantages offered by any form of higher education.

Unfortunately, much of this happened during the depth of an economic depression, and naturally so progressive a spirit would encounter much opposition, but in spite of all, Canadian nursing has been progressing toward the realization of its ideals.

The Canadian nurses were organized in many respects similarly to the American ones. In fact, the original Associated Alumnae and the Superintendents' Societies encompassed both Canadian and United States nurses. They separated only when the legal requirements of incorporation and other practical considerations rendered it necessary. The Canadian Associated Alumnae did not at first become incorporated in Canada, but in 1907 the Canadian Association of Superintendents of Training Schools for Nurses was formed. Miss Snively was its president. In 1917 it adopted the less cumbersome name of the Canadian Association of Nursing Education.

In 1924 the Associated Alumnae and the Association of Nursing Education were combined and called the Canadian Nurses' Association. It had three sections: nursing education, private duty, and public health nursing. Since 1930, membership in the national association has been limited to members of the provincial associations, each of which was similarly subdivided. Altogether this streamlined organization made for increased efficiency and flexibility.

The first *Canadian Nurse* journal was published in 1905. The journal was incorporated in 1910; it is owned and controlled by the Canadian Nurses' Association. In 1958 the French edition was first published.

In 1945 the journal had only seven thousand subscribers; in 1967 the figure had increased to over eighty thousand.

CANADIAN NURSING IN WORLD WARS I AND II

At the end of World War I many nurses who had been in service with the army transferred to Veterans' Service. A permanent corps of Nursing Sisters was established by the Royal Canadian Medical Corps, and a registry of graduate nurses was set up within the Department of National Defense so that in an emergency a nucleus of military nurses may be readily available. During World War II, Canada became a great training field particularly for the air forces of different allied groups. Many Canadian nurses served in the air force hospitals. Many others went overseas, either with the army, the navy, or the air force. A serious shortage in the nursing staffs of hospitals in Canada during the war resulted in the freezing of some nurses in the home positions. This was done to stabilize the nursing services. As in the United States, the government in Canada helped financially in the recruitment of students, in providing scholarships to graduates, and in training faculty members to meet the demands of increased enrollment. This grant was made through the former Department of Pensions and National Health. The student enrollment increased markedly. The need for subsidiary workers and volunteers in the health and hospital fields was recognized early in the war. They were used extensively, and since the war they have contributed a great deal to meet the nursing shortage.

DEVELOPMENTS IN PROFESSIONAL NURSING SINCE WORLD WAR II

The Canadian Nurses' Association is an affiliation of the ten provincial registered nurses' associations. The year 1958 marked the fiftieth anniversary of the founding of the Canadian Nurses Association. From a membership of a few hundred in 1908, the Association has grown to eighty thousand members in 1967. The Canadian Nurses' Association, a member of the International Council of Nurses since 1909, is the second largest Association affiliated with it. Miss Alice Gerard, Dean of the School of Nursing, University of Montreal, is president and will preside at the Council meeting in Montreal in 1969.

Changes in the Canadian Nurses' Association since World War II

In 1950 the Executive Committee of the Canadian Nurses' Association decided that the time had come for an impartial evaluation of the objectives, functions, machinery, and relationships of the Association as a whole. Accordingly, in January, 1951, "A Structure Study of the Canadian Nurses' Association" was begun under the directorship of Pauline Jewett, M.A., Ph.D. It was decided that the study should reexamine the purposes and functions of the Association, study the relations of these to the nurses and to society, and consider the interrelationship of the Canadian Nurses' Association to other health and welfare organizations. This study resulted in a reorganization of the structure of the Association, but the objectives and functions remained essentially the same. The membership of the executive committee was reduced. The national committees were reorganized and reduced, and the specialized sections were eliminated. Minor changes were implemented in 1967. In 1954, the Canadian Nurses' Association moved its headquarters to the national capital, Ottawa. In 1967 C.N.A. House was completed and opened, and became headquarters for the Association and the *Canadian Nurse* journal.

In November, 1957, the Canadian Nurses' Association sponsored the first national conference on nursing. More than one hundred nationally recognized representatives from federal and provincial governments, medicine, hospitals, public health, welfare, education, business, women's organizations, and the public, as well as from the nursing profession, participated in the conference.

The conference was organized to provide an opportunity for the Canadian public to consider with nurses the future demand for nursing service in Canada and how best it could be met.

Recommendations were presented to the executive committee of the Canadian Nurses' Association for consideration.

Research projects undertaken or assisted by the Canadian Nurses' Association

An experiment in a two-year program was conducted in the Metropolitan School of Nursing, Windsor, Ontario, under the joint sponsorship of the Canadian Red Cross and the Canadian Nurses' Association from 1948 to 1952. The course was designed to show that this school of nursing, independent of the service demands of a hospital, could prepare a nurse in less than the traditional three years. An evaluation of the experiment by Dr. A. R. Lord, a Canadian educator, showed that it had been a success.

In 1953, a "Study of the Functions and Activities of Head Nurses in a General Hospital" was carried out in the Ottawa Civic Hospital by the Research Division of the Department of National Health and Welfare at the request of the Canadian Nurses' Association. The study was an endeavor to find ways of conserving the time of the head nurse in the best interest of patient care. The report provided factual data that may be used in determining which duties of the head nurse can be assigned to other persons, to which persons these duties may be assigned, and in planning safeguards in the delegation of such duties.

In 1945 the Canadian Nurses' Association approved the principle of accreditation of schools of nursing in Canada. The general membership voted to proceed with a pilot project of evaluation of a few schools of nursing in Canada, at the 1956 biennial meeting. The purpose of the study was to determine what is involved in an accreditation program—the personnel, technics, cost, and so forth. In September, 1957, Miss Helen K. Mussallem, now the Executive Director of the Canadian Nurses' Association, was appointed Director of the Pilot Project for the Evaluation of Schools of Nursing. The report of the project was published in 1960.

PROVINCIAL NURSES' ASSOCIATION

There is a Registered Nurses' Association in each province, in nine of the provinces the association is the registering body, with registration and membership being synonymous. Ontario is the exception to this general pattern. In 1962 legislation was passed to permit the formation of a College of Nurses of Ontario, similar to the Ontario College of Physicians and Surgeons. This college has a council elected by the registered nurses of the province, plus two representatives of the Registered Nurses' Association, one from the Registered Nursing Assistants' Association and the Minister of Health, ex officio. The council has the authority to set minimum standards for nursing education, to approve schools of nursing, and to conduct registration examinations and subsequent registration of both the professional nurse and the nursing assistant. Membership in the Registered Nurses' Association of Ontario is voluntary; a majority of the 54,513 registered nurses were members in 1967.

Each province uses either the Canadian Nurses' Association's or its own minimum curricula; recently two-year curricula have been approved in several provinces. The majority of the provinces use the State Board Test Pool Examinations of the National League for Nursing as examinations for registration. Ontario, which conducts examinations in both English and French, has developed its own test pool in both languages (more adapted to the Canadian situation); it was first used in 1964. This is the basis for a Canadian Test Pool examination to be implemented by 1970.

Each association has conducted studies, surveys, and pilot projects (too numerous to list here) alone or in conjunction with the Canadian Nurses' Association or other professional groups to deal with its particular problems. Many of the ideas have been implemented, more are being considered, and further research is under way or projected. These studies have included clinical nursing, nursing service, nursing education, recruitment of male and married and older women students, and the use and training of auxiliary personnel and of home nursing projects.

TRENDS AND DEVELOPMENTS IN NURSING EDUCATION AND SERVICE SINCE WORLD WAR II (1945)

The most significant developments in nursing education since the end of World War II have been stimulated by the changes in health demands of the community. Even though there has been a considerable expansion of nurse power, the number of professional nurses does not meet the demands for nursing service today. As a result, auxiliary nursing personnel have been prepared in increasing numbers to assist in fulfilling the need.

As the staffing pattern has changed so has the pattern of nursing education in order to prepare the student for the responsibilities she must assume as a practitioner. Because of the increase in numbers of nonprofessional workers, the student has needed more preparation in the "team nursing" approach to patient care. Newer concepts in nursing care have modified the pattern of nursing education. There appears to be a trend toward inclusion in the basic program of more study of social sciences, communication skills, and the humanities.

Following the report of the Metropolitan

School of Nursing in 1952, a school to follow this pattern was organized in 1960. It was the Nightingale School in Toronto, financed by the Ontario Hospital Services Commission but with a separate board and an independent Nursing Advisory Committee. Since that time, other centers throughout Canada have organized or are organizing schools on this pattern. In Ontario alone, 25 schools have been thus organized. One, a unique experiment, is limited to applicants aged thirty to fifty years; two classes have successfully completed their course with high standing in the registration examinations. In the meantime, until sufficient finances can be obtained to support more of these schools, an increasing number of schools of nursing have changed their program from the traditional three-year program to an education-oriented two-year program plus one-year internship. There has been a small increase in the number of university degree programs and a small decrease in the number of hospital diploma programs. Increasing numbers of bursaries and scholarships have been made available to nurses through government sources and private agencies.

The international problem of increased demand for nursing service is one that has been accentuated in Canada by the introduction, in recent years, of government-sponsored provincial hospital insurance plans. (It is interesting that the ratio of graduate nurses employed in hospitals to beds has increased as follows: 1932, one nurse to 32 beds; 1962, one nurse to 2.7 beds.) Activities in the Province of Ontario will be cited as an example since this province has the largest population and contains some 300 hospitals.

The Ontario Hospital Services Commission Act provides that insured patients (99% of the population of Ontario) are entitled to "necessary nursing services." This does not include private-duty nursing but, rather, the cost of nurses engaged and paid by the hospital to the extent of its patients' medical needs. A staff of nursing consultants is maintained to study existing service and to report upon ways and means of developing greater efficiency in the use of professional nurses. Encouragement is given to the employment of registered nursing assistants, thereby permitting greater professional scope for registered nurses. Since 1960, the net cost of operating hospital schools has been charged as part of the cost of patient care. This has indirectly benefited nursing education. One outstanding project of the commission was the establishment of the Nightingale School of Nursing.

The realization that some patients recover better in their own homes and the greater demand for hospital beds made by the provision of hospital insurance have highlighted the value of home care. Several home-care projects under various auspices have been undertaken. These projects have been financed through the Ontario Hospital Services Commission; the Visiting Nurses have shared greatly in them.

THE UNIVERSITIES
AND NURSING EDUCATION

Twenty-one universities located in most of the provinces are providing some form of nursing education. As indicated earlier, the University of British Columbia was the first in Canada to undertake nursing education. In 1920, five universities with grants from the Canadian Red Cross Society began certificate or diploma courses of one year in preparation for public health nursing. The University of Toronto, realizing that this one-year course was not adequate, organized a four-year course in conjunction with Toronto General Hospital and its affiliating hospitals. The pattern of this course was similar to that adopted by the other universities. In 1933, the Rockefeller Foundation, impressed with the leadership in education demonstrated by the Director of the School, provided a five-year grant for

the purpose of the establishment of a school that in thirty-eight months undertook to prepare a student for all types of nursing service. This in turn, in 1942, led to a degree course, extending over a four-year period. The outstanding feature of the new course was an integration throughout of general and professional education as well as a clearly defined emphasis upon both the preventive and curative aspects of nursing. Throughout the entire life of the school a spirit of research has continued to dominate its work.

This program was shortly followed by McMaster University and more recently by other universities in Ontario and other provinces. In these programs, whether in the classroom, the hospital clinical field, or in the public health nursing service, the teaching is the responsibility of the university school staff. Most of these basic integrated courses are four years in length.

Most of the schools providing basic degree courses also provide a degree course for graduate nurses. It is increasingly the opinion of nurse educators, that the one-year diploma courses for graduate nurses are most inadequate and that as soon as expedient these should be replaced by courses leading to a degree for the graduate nurse.

The University of Alberta, besides the usual courses, provides a program in Advanced Practical Obstetrics, which is considered equal to Part I Mid-wifery of Great Britain.

Most universities require three years for the courses leading to a degree for the graduate nurse; the others are usually two years in length. Five years of high school is the entrance requirement of some universities, and in others preference is given to applicants with this qualification.

The importance of a broad university education in the preparation of the nurse who may become a leader in nursing education or nursing service is becoming more apparent. The enrollment indicates that this fact is appreciated by the nurses and employing agencies. Additional financial assistance in the form of scholarships, fellowships, and bursaries and loans has become available. The Canadian Nurses' Association has recently developed a Canadian Nurses' Foundation to assist in providing scholarships for post-baccalaureate study. The universities are attempting to develop a master's degree that is truly a nursing degree and also of the same high caliber as the other graduate degrees. Three universities are offering master's degrees, and others are expecting to do so shortly.

The need for research is great, and Canada needs nurses prepared to conduct research in many phases of nursing. One of the encouraging features has been the increasing cooperation between nurses of hospitals and public health agencies and nurses of other professional groups.

SIGNIFICANT ACTIVITIES

One of the most significant activities in 1962 was the presentation of briefs to the Royal Commission on Health; these briefs were prepared by: all Canadian nursing associations, national and provincial, provincial departments of health; university schools of nursing; Victorian Order of Nurses; the Red Cross Society; and other nursing groups. Most of their recommendations included the concept of bringing basic nursing education diploma programs within the general frame of education. This evidence resulted in a request from the commission to the Registered Nurses' Association of Ontario to develop a plan to implement such a program at the post-secondary school level. To fulfill this request, a specific research project was organized in 1964 in order that the feasibility of such a concept could be demonstrated. The Ontario Department of Education approved the project and an Institute of Technology and Applied Arts was authorized to conduct this experimental course. A report on the project will be available shortly. In the meantime, plans are going ahead to place schools of nursing in the various newly established community colleges. These briefs also emphasized the importance of not merely registering the professional nurse and the assistant group, but insisting upon licensing. Other recommendations from the briefs were considered by the Commission, which made its report and recommendations to the government. All recommendations are being studied by the nurses' associations.

The provincial associations throughout Canada are actively engaged in developing programs for collective bargaining to assure economic status and favorable working conditions for the nurse. After many efforts of the Canadian Nurses' Association, male nurses are being given officers' rank in the Armed Services, a status the female nurse has had for years.

In Canada's Centennial Year (1967), the Federal Government showed its appreciation of nursing education and service by awarding medals to a gratifying number of nurses. It has appointed nurses to many Royal Commissions, Federal and Provincial, and has thoughfully studied briefs submitted by various nursing associations. In December, 1967, two significant events occurred: a nurse was appointed as adviser to the Federal Deputy Minister of Health, and for the first time a national conference of doctors, nurses, and hospital administrators was held to discuss hospital-medical staff relationships.

CONCLUSION

This chapter has attempted to provide a brief history of nursing in Canada as well as a closer look at recent and current problems of nursing education and service and at the ways in which the Canadian profession is attempting to meet them.

To the reader from the United States, Canada may seem a country of small population, but the health care of its people has always been of great interest. Nursing has been accepted since the 90's as one of the preferred professions for young women of education and culture. If the progress in the rising standards of nursing education and service of the past ten years can be maintained during the next decade, many of today's hopes and dreams will be fulfilled.

Questions and study projects for unit ten

1. What are the three main influences in the development of Canadian nursing?
2. What were the contributions of the Ursuline Sisters to Canadian nursing?
3. What are some of the recent developments in nursing education in Canada?
4. Describe the contributions of the following to nursing: Jeanne Mance, Agnes Snively, and Professor G. M. Weir.
5. Show how the developments in nursing education in Canada have paralleled those in the United States.
6. Describe the development of public health nursing in Canada.
7. Make an annotated bibliography of recent articles appearing in *The American Journal of Nursing, Nursing Outlook, Nursing Research,* and any other journals available in your library relating to the discussion in this chapter.
8. What contributions has the Canadian Red Cross made to the development of Canadian nursing?
9. What influences have the following developments had on Canadian nursing:
   (a) Hospital insurance plans
   (b) Home care
   (c) Public demand for increased nursing service

References for unit ten*

Cadwallader, Marian F.: Nursing problems in the Labrador, American Journal of Nursing **40**:861-864, August 1940.

Canadian Nurses' Association, American Journal of Nursing **29**:135, 1929.

Carpenter, Helen M.: Nursing education in Canada, International Nursing Review **13**(5):29, 1966.

Gibbon, J. M., and Mathewson, Mary: Three centuries of Canadian nursing, Toronto, 1947, The Macmillan Company.

Historical overview of approaches to staffing the hospital nursing service department, Ottawa, Canada, the Canadian Nurses' Association, 1966.

Judson, Helen: Edith Cavell, New York, 1941, The Macmillan Company.

Kivimaki, Anna: Nursing with the Grenfell Mission, American Journal of Nursing **37**:593-598, June, 1937.

MacLaggan, Katherine: Portrait of nursing, New Brunswick Nurses' Association, Fredericton, N.B., 1967.

Report of Royal Commission on Health Services, 1967, Toronto, Ontario Department of Health.

Seymer, Lucy Ridgely: A general history of nursing, New York, 1933, The Macmillan Company.

Sloan, Raymond P.: Through faith we serve, Modern Hospitals **64**:43-45, March, 1945.

Status of Nursing among French Canadians of Quebec, American Journal of Nursing **29**:283-286, March, 1929.

Weir, G. M.: Survey of nursing education in Canada, Toronto, Canada, 1932, University of Toronto Press.

*For current comments on Canadian nursing consult the monthly issues of The Canadian Nurse.

Unit eleven

Nursing in other countries

Nursing, a vital function in every culture, is always influenced in its development by differences in national patterns. The customs and mores, particularly in regard to the family, the position of women, and education, are always evident in the way nursing develops in any country.

The reports of nursing in other countries were compiled with the cooperation of the official organizations in these lands. America's history, trends, progress, and advancements should be more meaningful when compared to happenings in our profession in other countries. We have chosen one to explore in some depth. Our discussion of nursing in other selected areas presents an international flavor and dimension to our study. In discussing nursing in the British Isles, we try to show only the relationship to our own development in the beginning years. Therefore the history ends with the Lancet Commission report in 1932. There are many definitive histories of British nursing for those who wish to pursue the study further.

Chapter 41

Nursing in the British Isles

The British Isles have always been more closely related to the United States than has the European Continent. This is easy to understand, because our development has been extensively dominated by men of Anglo-Saxon (and Irish) extraction. A common language has given the two countries a common heritage of traditions and ideals. It is, therefore, not surprising that the beginnings of many of the reforms in nursing may be found across the ocean. If this book were a chronological record of past events, this chapter may well have preceded the section on American nursing. However, our aim is to give the nurse an understanding of the evolution of the nursing profession. Having understood the development of its various elements in this country it is profitable for the nurse to learn how many of them had their origins or parallels in England.

We concluded our discussion about England with the death of Florence Nightingale in 1910. Her life span had encompassed many nursing reforms that she had directed or in which she had been actively interested. We have repeatedly considered the principles of the "Nightingale School" upon which the great nursing reform was based. We have seen that emissaries from the United States studied it and that the early American schools were more or less based upon its principles.

SCHOOLS OF NURSING

England, in the early days, perhaps placed greater emphasis than did America upon the importance of ward teaching and endowment for the school. In addition, British schools maintained two classes of students —privileged ones who came from the upper class, and average ones who came from the middle class. The privileged ones paid tuition and were prepared for higher, executive positions. They constituted roughly 10% of the classes. The average pupil nurse—all but the exceptional ones—could only hope for promotion to the top.

The school at St. Thomas' Hospital maintained a high standard. Its primary purpose was to produce pioneers who would organize and work in similar schools elsewhere, at home and abroad. Most of those who left England went to the Colonies. Best known, however, is the small group of "Nightingales" who, under the direction of Miss Lucy Osborn, went to Sidney, Australia. Her undertaking flourished and soon other nurses followed. Miss Alice Fisher, another Nightingale nurse, came to the Blockley Hospital in Philadelphia, where she did outstanding work. And so it was in England; the nursing service throughout the general hospitals underwent sweeping reforms during the thirty years following the opening of the school at St. Thomas. When the reforms were not actually carried out by nurses trained under Miss Nightingale's auspices, they were conducted on lines markedly influenced by the Nightingale reforms. Ultimately the nursing had been reorganized in all the leading English hospitals.

THE LIVERPOOL EXPERIMENT

In 1860, the year in which the school at St. Thomas' Hospital was established, another event occurred that indirectly was destined to have the most profound effect on nursing in Britain and far beyond its borders. Mrs. Rathbone, the wife of a Liverpool philanthropist, died. The tragedy of her illness and death made her husband appreciate the value of good and devoted nursing. He decided to devote his wealth to the relief of the indigent sick. He employed Mrs. Rathbone's nurse, Mary Robinson, full time to visit the poor sick people and saw that her requirements in the way of supplies and diets were met. Although Mary Robinson had no particular training, she was a faithful soul and, as may be expected, the undertaking was eminently successful. The work expanded so that Mr. Rathbone was interested in getting assistants for Miss Robinson. He was well acquainted with Miss Nightingale's work and turned to her for help; but she had no nurses available and besides, the Nightingales were not being trained for this kind of work. Miss Nightingale suggested that he start his own school, offering training especially in district work. Mr. Rathbone accepted the idea, and in cooperation with the Liverpool Royal Infirmary, a school building was constructed in connection with that institution. Miss Nightingale supplied the superintendent, Miss Merryweather. The pupil nurses were to receive the regular nurses' training, but, in addition, they were to be given special instruction in district work. Eighteen such visiting nurses were each allotted her own district, supervised by "lady visitors" and by Mr. Rathbone who followed the work closely.

This was the start of organized visiting nursing.

A corollary to this work was one of the most beautiful and, in its way, romantic chapters in nursing. While carrying on this work, Mr. Rathbone found that when the poor became very sick they objected as long as they could to going to the City Workhouse and House of Correction where the incurable and chronically sick were supposed to receive care. Investigating the conditions in this institution, he found them horrible beyond all description: crowding, filth, vice, drunkenness, and violence abounded. Medical care, kindness, adequate food, and cleanliness were unknown and impossible to obtain under the circumstances. Again Mr. Rathbone dipped into his pockets and offered to staff the place with nurses if Miss Nightingale could find him a superintendent for them.

Miss Nightingale's choice fell upon Miss Agnes Jones, who has gone down in history as one of the matyrs of nursing, for her life was truly sacrificed unnecessarily although not in vain. She was apparently a most attractive young woman when she, at the head of twelve certified nurses, moved into this hell on earth. Mr. Rathbone did everything he could to enable her to carry on; still, at first the job seemed entirely beyond her, for not only were the physical difficulties appalling but the very human material with which she had to work seemed beyond recall to decency and clean living. When she thought back to the clean wards of Kaiserswerth or St. Thomas', where she had been trained, the contrast was too great to bear, and in her despair she turned to Miss Nightingale. The answer she received was just the kind that would challenge a young worthwhile nurse: "It was Scutari all over again." With the example of the great leader before her she went to work with her little staff, and in three years she had the place organized. Her staff increased and the hospital was no longer a chamber of horrors but a place in which the indigent sick could receive kind and sympathetic care. Her task thus barely accomplished, Miss Jones became ill with an infection contracted in the line of duty. The strain of the many months of hard work had lowered her resistance, and she succumbed, deeply mourned by all who knew her, not least by Miss Nightingale, who had expected much from her in the future. But her work had not been in vain: it had shown the world how bad workhouses were and what could be done to clean them up. A reform swept England, and in ten years these were changed places.

MRS. BEDFORD-FENWICK

Another nursing leader is a woman to whom was given not only the gift of leadership but also a long life devoted to the cause. She was Ethel Gordon Manson, better known under her married name of Mrs. Bedford-Fenwick. She was a contemporary of Mrs. Hampton Robb, whom she knew well. The lives of the two women were similar in many respects; in fact, Mrs. Fenwick initiated in England many of the reforms that Mrs. Hampton Robb was later to carry out in America. Through her activities at the World's Fair in Chicago in 1893, she was indirectly responsible for the organization of the American Society of Superintendents of Training Schools.

She was born in 1856 and trained in Manchester. She was a ward Sister at the London Hospital when she was called upon to take charge of and reorganize the nursing at St. Bartholomew's Hospital, where a previous attempt to begin a modern school of nursing had been unsuccessful. She accomplished the task in the six years she was there. She resigned to marry Dr. Bedford-Fenwick. As in the case of Mrs. Robb her marriage did not terminate her interest in nursing. On the contrary, it placed her in a position in which she could advantageously work for the profession. Again like Mrs. Robb, she was involved in most of the nursing reforms in her country during the next generation. Her first great task was

the organization of the British Nurses' Association, which became the prototype for similar American organizations. She was in charge of the British Nurses' Exhibit at the Chicago World's Fair in 1893, and the same year she founded the *Nursing Times*. She became very interested in international work among nurses and became the first president of the International Council of Nurses, retaining that position until 1912. In 1926 she founded the British College of Nurses.

VISITING NURSING IN BRITAIN

Visiting nursing originated with the apostolic deaconesses who visited the sick; it was the guiding principle of the early nursing orders and reached its highest early development with the Sisters of Charity who were organized for the very reason that the increasing severity of the Church prevented extramural nursing activities of the holy orders. For centuries, until the full development of the modern municipal hospitals, home visiting remained the mainstay of nursing of the sick; consequently, it was also a prominent feature of nursing during its early renaissance; Mrs. Fry's Protestant Sisters of Charity, St. John's Home, the Order of St. Margaret, and other such organizations were all organized primarily for this purpose. Dr. Fliedner's Deaconesses received a considerable part of their training in the field.

However, as a secular profession, comparable to the "Nightingale Nurse," the visiting nurse did not emerge until 1860 in Liverpool when Mr. Rathbone employed Miss Robinson to visit the needy sick. The whole undertaking developed into a powerful organization; a leader in its field, the Liverpool experiment soon influenced the organization of other visiting nurses' societies in both town and country. The need for this kind of nursing was obvious. It was inaugurated during a period of philanthropy, and its demands far exceeded the possible supply of nurses. During the next few years visiting nursing suffered from the uneven, often poor quality of its votaries, a fact that to some degree accounted for its early difficulties. In some cases the "nurses" employed were entirely without preparation.

The best of the societies of visiting nursing was the East London Nursing Society. It was founded in 1861 and guided by definite regulations that became important in the formation of later organizations when in 1874 the whole visiting nurses' movement came under the scrutiny of a committee. Mr. Rathbone was chairman of this committee; a Nightingale nurse, Miss Florence Lees, assumed the heavy load of the investigation. Miss Nightingale's genius appeared also in this undertaking.

The outcome of the work of the committee was the formation of the Metropolitan and National Nursing Association in 1875 under the leadership of Miss Lees. This was a great step forward, for not only was the new organization better organized than its predecessors but it also appealed to educated women as a career. It was believed that this work, to be successful, must be carried out by people who could exert the necessary authority by example as well as by knowledge. The responsibility of independent action, often under adverse and trying circumstances, could best rest on socially superior women who, by their very presence, could elevate the character of the undertaking. Many, including Miss Nightingale, were skeptical as to the success of this new departure, but, as we said, the spirit of philanthropy was prevalent and the general movement of emancipation of women had by now reached a stage at which it was possible to recruit such a service from among the daughters of the well-to-do. In this manner visiting nursing prospered as best it could with the limited resources of private enterprise until it received great help in 1887 when Queen Victoria celebrated her fifty years' jubilee. One action of hers in this memorable year was to donate 70,000 pounds, a very large sum in those days, out of the women's jubilee offering, to the cause of visiting nursing. Augmented from other sources, this sum constituted a foundation, "The Queen Victoria's Jubilee Institute for Nurses." The institute received its Royal charter in 1889. Now visiting nursing could be organized upon a financial sound basis. Branches were established throughout the country and the Empire.

Not only was the "Jubilee Nurses" a splendid organization in itself, but throughout the Empire it set an example that was followed by the organization of similar foundations, of which the Victorian Order of Nurses in Canada, the King Edward VII Order in South Africa, the "Bush" Nursing Association in South Africa, and the Plunkett Nurses in New Zealand are outstanding examples.

The Queen's Nurses are all registered nurses who in addition to their basic nursing course have received six months' special instruction in visiting nursing. The organization also makes its influence felt where it cannot carry the whole load, for in out-of-the-way districts it helps finance what we would call practical nurses, there known as "village nurses." Considerable stress is also placed on midwifery. Before World War I, the general extension of such an organization tended to provide Great Britain with an adequate nursing service for the sick who had not been admitted to hospitals.

So far, few had thought that the interest of society extended beyond the care of the indigent sick, but the war brought a terrible revelation. The recruiting services discovered an incidence of physical defects far in excess of what had been expected, and at once great agitation was begun to remedy the situation. There were not enough nurses to look after the health as well as the illnesses of the people, nor was the elaborate technical training of a nurse considered necessary for this purpose, but it was essential to see that the population was enabled to live up to certain standards of hygiene. The task of supervising this project was placed in the hands of a newly created group of people—the "health visitors." These were not trained nurses, but they did have some training enabling them to acquire the necessary facts, discipline, and knowledge to deal with situations that they encountered. However, as time passed on, it was found desirable that "health visitors" should possess more and more information found in the nurses' courses; it seemed that other educational advantages could never quite substitute for the knowledge of midwifery, infectious diseases, and preventive medicine, which seemed necessary for this career. So gradually, as nurses became available after the war, an increasing number of health visitors were graduate nurses, until now they are almost all nurses. The result in England has been that what is called public health nursing, but what may better be termed nursing in preventive medicine, is largely in the hands of "health visitors," while the care of the sick is a matter for the visiting nurses.

BRITISH AND AMERICAN NURSING COMPARED

It will now be necessary briefly to investigate some of the British nursing reforms and establish their relation to American advances; in doing so it will be noted that the professions in the two countries have advanced much along parallel lines, as shown by Table 41-1.

At the same time there are some important differences between nursing in the two countries: The British have stressed nurses' training in midwifery, a subject largely neglected by American nurses (except for their basic experience in obstetrical services, but that does not make them midwives). The British were much more profoundly affected by World War I, and they have been more active in establishing insurance schemes, funds, and associations that further the cause of nursing. Outstanding among them are the Royal College of Nursing and the British College of Nurses. In spite of that, the profession has not flourished in Britain as it has in America, for the Lancet Committee was not appointed so much to improve nurses' education as to inquire into the scarcity of nurses and into remedies for the situation. Public health nursing, which originated in England, has reached a high degree of development there.

After this brief comparative survey we shall now examine some of these points more in detail.

BRITISH NURSES' ASSOCIATIONS

Mrs. Bedford-Fenwick's first important activity was to organize the British nurses into a professional group. The British Nurses' Association did not develop out of local alumnae associations as did the American Nurses' Association. It was actually conceived and planned by Mrs. Fenwick as

Table 41-1. Comparison of early professional developments in Britain and the United States

	Britain	United States
Nurses' association	British Nurses' Association (1887)	Associated Alumnae (1897)
Teachers' association	Matrons' Council of Great Britain (1894)	American Society of Superintendents of Training Schools (1896)
Journal	*Nursing Times* (1893)	*The American Journal of Nursing* (1900)
Registration	State registration (1919)	State registration (1899)
Commissions	Lancet Commission (1930)	Goldmark Committee (1920) Committee on Grading Schools of Nursing (1925)
Preliminary courses	1893	1899
Leader	Mrs. Ethel Bedford-Fenwick	Mrs. Isable Hampton Robb

a means of obtaining a professional standing for British nurses, comparable to that obtained by British doctors and other professional groups that had gained strength through organization. Consequently, it met much more resistance than did its American sister organization; doctors and hospital administrators were afraid of losing the control that they exerted over the nurses. However, Mrs. Fenwick saw to it that it had the proper backing of Royalty, which was so important in those days. It has a Royal Charter and is presided over by Royalty. After Miss Nightingale's opposition to this scheme had subsided, it expanded to include most certified nurses. It has been responsible for the further advances of the profession, including the state registration of nurses.

In 1894, the year the American Society of Superintendents of Training Schools was organized, the Matrons' Council of Great Britain was also formed. It, too, became a powerful organization that is largely concerned with improvements in nurses' education and organization. It was this council (not the British Nurses' Association) that in turn sponsored local associations corresponding to our alumnae associations. In 1904 it became affiliated with the National Council of Nurses of Great Britain, with Mrs. Fenwick as its first president. So, although the British nurses obtained organizations similar to ours, the interrelationship of these organizations is different.

COLLEGES OF NURSING

The colleges, to which we have no exact equivalents, were more or less outgrowths of World War I. The first, the Royal College of Nursing, was formed in 1916 with an endowment of $500,000 for the purpose of nursing education, scholarship, relief, and so forth. It sponsored the registration of nurses and developed special sections for various branches of nursing such as; head nurses, student nurses, and public health nurses. It also has a fine library and imme-

diately adjoins the Cowdrey Club. The Cowdrey Club was formed by Viscount and Viscountess Cowdrey for the rest and recreation of nurses. It is housed in a very fine building in London. Its membership now encompasses over half the British registered nurses. After World War I it particularly sponsored international cooperation. "British College of Nurses" was founded in 1926 under the sponsorship of Mrs. Bedford-Fenwick with another $500,000 foundation. It, too, has for its purpose "the advancement of the educational and social status of nurses" and has a large membership, about one-third of all registered nurses. In addition, there are numerous special nursing societies in Britain, for example, the Mental Hospital Matrons' Association and the Infectious Hospitals Association. To the American student the advantage of so many separate associations with approximately the same aims and scope would seem dubious. In unity there is strength.

NURSING JOURNALS

As may be expected, until recently the principle of strength in unity applied to nursing journals. The entire American Nursing Organization united in using *The American Journal of Nursing* for an outlet until 1952. (The *Pacific Coast Journal of Nursing* is of more local interest; consequently, this journal is very strong). In England Mrs. Bedford-Fenwick, in 1893, founded the *Nursing Times,* which later became the *British Journal of Nursing* and which officially represents the British Nurses' Association, the Matrons' Council, and the British College of Nurses. The title *Nursing Times* was resurrected in 1905. This journal has since become the official organ for the Royal College of Nursing. In addition, there are several other nursing journals in Great Britain.

PUBLIC HEALTH NURSING

The evolution of nursing that followed the reorganization of the schools followed essentially practical lines in keeping with the national temperament. It was considered more important that British nurses be able to shift for themselves if stranded in the wilderness than to obtain academic standing. As a result, the stress was placed upon public health nursing, district nursing, and midwifery. In fact, nearly all British nurses are also midwives registered by the Central Midwives Board. The advantage of this training for nurses working in poor districts or in regions in which doctors are scarce cannot be exaggerated. Seeing the advantage of such training, many American nurses have gone to England to obtain it, for work where a thorough knowledge of obstetrics is needed. In the big hospitals student nurses are sent into the district to deliver babies, a type of training similar to that which is offered to the medical students.

UNIVERSITY AFFILIATIONS

Britain has had much less agitation than America for university affiliation. To understand this difference from the American development, it must be remembered that British university degrees are considerably more august than American degrees. Most general medical practitioners do not possess university degrees but are licensed by examining boards. The Lancet Committee, therefore, although it encouraged better professional and social status for nurses in every way, it did not express any enthusiasm for better university affiliations. To the English mind a university degree is something that should be reserved for those in the highest administrative positions. However, in order to give to nurses the advantage of university education, two universities, Leeds and London, have established courses for them, leading to diplomas but not to degrees.

PRELIMINARY COURSES

The British were the first to recognize the advantage of the preliminary course. This course was originally introduced by Mrs. Rebecca Strong of the Glasgow Royal Infirmary when she sent her students to St. Mungo's College for three months' preliminary work before they were admitted to the wards. This was the scheme that was later to be so successfully adopted in the United States.

WORLD WAR I

World War I affected Britain much more profoundly than it affected us. The nursing resources were drained to beyond the minimum requirements of civilian hospitals. The British army enrolled 10,000 nurses, there were 6,000 territorial nurses and 13,000 in the reserves, the British Red Cross had 6,400 trained nurses, and beyond that Britain had to draw upon the colonies, dominions, and the United States for more nurses to care for her wounded soldiers; yet all of these proved insufficient. So the Voluntary Aid Detachment (V.A.D.) was organized. It eventually included some 60,000 men and women. This corps consisted of lay persons who received a short course of three to six months in the elements of nursing and then gave their time and labors wherever they could do the most good. They did not restrict their work to nursing but undertook maid's work, cleaning, and all tasks for the benefit of the service. Many wealthy persons organized private hospitals in their homes and staffed them with voluntary aids. Altogether it may be said that the war accelerated the development of nursing in Britain as it did in the United States. British nurses went wherever the Union Jack flew during the war, and often beyond, for in the reconstruction period that followed hostilites, the British Red Cross was active in many foreign lands.

REGISTRATION

One of the most important developments immediately following World War I was the final passing of the registration bill. It had been hotly contested by Miss Nightingale on the grounds that registration was the wrong way to maintain the high standards of nursing because the personal qualities that are essential in the formation of a good nurse were ignored. However, Miss Nightingale was now dead, and the nurses as a group had grown so strong that they could enforce the legislation that was necessary to protect them. Finally, in 1919, the register was established. From an American viewpoint it lacks the uniformity that would be the strength of the ideal American national register, for in England there are several registers: for general nurses, for mental nurses, for nurses of infectious diseases, and so forth. The English, however, seem to like it, for the Lancet report recommends that the system be continued.

THE LANCET COMMISSION

British nursing advanced in the years following World War I to higher standards and greater professional freedom; but in spite of this growth British nursing suffered from one vital defect: lack of recruits. There were not enough nurses to fill vacancies. In 1930, the medical journal, the *Lancet,* appointed a commission consisting of educators, physicians, hospital administrators, and nurses to look into the situation. Their report, published in the *Lancet* in 1932, presented a most interesting view of the English attitude toward nursing, both inside and outside of the profession. The report was practically unanimous, indicating that the facts it brings to light are generally acceptable. The material was not collected under the auspices of a nurses' association, but there were nurses on the commission, and what the report lost by not being issued strictly from a nurse's point of view, it may have gained from the wider perspective resulting from its being the product of teamwork by leaders in many different professions concerned with women's careers.

The committee first established the existence of a real shortage of nurses that seriously threatened the efficiency of the nursing service of the hospitals. In some cases the efficiency had already been affected. It was acknowledged that the discipline of

nursing schools was unnecessarily severe and regulations often annoying. These policies had been carried down from early days of the nursing school when nursing was the only career open to women who entered it from the protecting walls and the severe discipline of a Victorian home, unfitted to shift for themselves and to face the realities of life alone. This outlook was so thoroughly ingrained into many of those women, who by 1930 were in responsible positions, that they could see no other way of handling nursing students.

Another difficulty was the conflict between the educational and the practical aspects of the training. Many head nurses were still insisting that the attention to patients must come before classes, and not that provisions must be made for seeing that students appear fresh, receptive, and on time in their classrooms. Not only were these attitudes found to be too prevalent in nursing schools but the realization that they did exist was so widespread in circles that were influential in shaping young nurses' careers that they acted as deterrents even from schools that had adopted up-to-date methods. Since the opening of nursing schools established careers for young women, many other professions developed real competition to nursing, offering more convenient or shorter working hours and often better remuneration.

The committee believed that the number of nurses could be increased without thoroughgoing reforms if the couse in nursing and subsequent prospects could be made more attractive to young women. They recommended that appeals be made to the right type of girls and that, if necessary, scholarships be established to occupy these girls between leaving school and reaching the age when they could enter nursing schools. The salaries of graduate nurses should be generally elevated to an attractive level (even then they were considerably below American standards). Arrangements should be made to enable all registered nurses to join superannuity and pension plans (a point at which American nurses are as yet far behind those of Great Britain). The hours on duty should be definitely limited, (the proposed standards still far exceed the eight-hour working day adopted by most American schools). They also recommended better conditions of admission and service, offering certain conveniences (such as telephone facilities) which young ladies may reasonably expect and doing away with unnecessary restrictions such as rules against smoking in quarters or lights out at 10:30 P.M., and so forth.

They recommended (1) that courses for nurses be limited to schools approved by the General Nursing Council, (2) that proper preliminary terms be generally established, (3) that examinations in anatomy, physiology, and hygiene precede admittance to work on the wards, and (4) that the number of instructors bear a reasonable proportion to the number of students. The committee was hopeful that by such reforms, many of which had even then been widely adopted, the crisis could be overcome and the supply of nurses again be made to equal the demand. There had hardly been time to learn the effects of these reforms when England became involved in another great and horrible war.

Chapter 42

Nursing in South America

The development of professional nursing has been slow in South America. Educationally, economically, and socially the countries in this vast continent have been backward or at least have not become industrialized as rapidly as their northern neighbors in the United States. Education until the middle 1920's was only for the few in the privileged classes. Until the end of the nineteenth century women had few educational opportunities and no political right. By 1937 women were being admitted to all universities and professional schools in the Spanish-American countries.

In Catholic countries most nursing was done under the supervision of the Church, and hospitals were developed under its supervision. Different national groups built and staffed hospitals for their own people. It was not until after World War I, however, that the various republics in South America really became interested in establishing schools for the preparation of professional nurses. In many instances, educational requirements are still low.

In all of Latin America, Spanish and Portuguese religious orders have been responsible for nursing. In fact, nuns are found in the majority of hospitals there today. In some of the South American countries, modern nursing is about sixty years old. About the turn of the century some

British nurses were brought to Argentina, Chile, Uruguay, and Cuba to organize schools of nursing similar to the St. Thomas' pattern. Because of the position of women in the Spanish and Portuguese cultures, young women did not usually leave the home to enter the professions. They were expected to remain at home until they married. Girls did not mix with society outside the home. As long as foreign nurses, that is, British and American, were in charge of the schools in these countries, a certain amount of prestige was given to them; but when these schools were given to the South Americans, a certain amount of family disapproval existed.

Before World War I, most of the physicians in Latin America had gone to Europe, particularly France, Germany, Italy, and Spain, for study. During and immediately after World War I, however, they tended to go to the United States where they came in contact with the modern professional nurse. Some of these doctors approached the Rockefeller Foundation between World Wars I and II for help in organizing the modern schools of nursing. Assistance was given through consultation service, fellowship programs, and financial aid for the construction and equipment of nursing schools in some of the countries.

This move to modernize nursing service

and nursing education was accelerated during and after World War II. The Rockefeller Foundation, the Kellogg Foundation, the Institute of Inter-American Affairs, and the Pan-American Sanitary Bureau, later the Regional Office for the World Health Organization have been active in helping in the establishment of schools of nursing. At the same time, slowly changing conditions have stimulated young women to seek work and professional training outside the home. As is to be expected with such developments, there is great variation in the standards of schools in South America. It is similar to the great differences found in schools of nursing in this country prior to and immediately following World War I. A few of the schools compare very favorably with good schools in the United States. In a few of the countries, there are still no national nurses' organizations. In over twelve of the remaining countries in Central and South America, nursing leaders are working hard and hope in time to be admitted to the International Council of Nurses. The minimum standards set by the International Council of Nurses for membership are that the associations must be directed by nurses and must represent all graduate nurses in the country, and it is recommended that membership be restricted to graduates of three-year schools of nursing whose entrance requirements include complete secondary education. Only in a few countries has much been accomplished toward legislation regarding the practice of nursing, including state board examinations and registration. In some countries any nurse who

graduates from a state-recognized school is allowed to register. In other words, it is the school that is inspected and not the individual. If the state recognizes the school from which the nurse graduates, this nurse automatically is allowed to register. The interest in nursing in Central and South America is at present very high and in line with the interest in modern health and medical developments.

Through the Institute of Inter-American Affairs, cooperative health programs of the United States and Latin America have developed throughout health and sanitation divisions since 1942. These programs are comprehensive, and doctors, sanitary engineers, nurses, and other health workers are employed in carrying out their activities. Experts from the United States in all of these fields have usually gone there to start the program. When the program is advanced and well established, it is taken over by the individual country. Prevention of disease through health teaching, early and better diagnoses, and effective treatment are some of the aims of these programs. Many Latin Americans have been trained as auxiliary workers, and many professional workers, including several hundred chief engineers and nurses, have been given study grants for postgraduate work in this country. This is all part of what is often referred to as a "good neighbor policy." It is interesting to note that American nurses have been very much in demand to start the program in these South American countries and to help in the early supervision.

Chapter 43

Nursing in Europe

We have now followed the evolution of nursing in Europe before 1850, in England, the United States, and Canada; this study includes most of the factors that have been important in modeling modern nursing. We shall now briefly note their effects in the rest of the world. Since this study is not a catalogue of nursing conditions but rather a study of its principles, our discussion will be general.

CATHOLIC ORDERS

The original Catholic nursing orders, badly handicapped in Protestant countries, have dominated in Catholic ones; in some places, such as France and Catholic Germany and wherever these influences reached, nursing was good. In orders, notably the Mediterranean and Balkan countries, nursing was exceedingly backward; in Spain it is still so. It would be interesting to study how this state has been determined by the factors (or rather their absence) that we noted as the principal determinants of modern nursing, such as the Industrial Revolution, modern medicine, modern hospitals, and the emancipation of women. As these movements have penetrated into our sister republics of the western hemisphere, standards of nursing have risen rapidly, often under the tutelage of British and American nurses. As the various govern-

ments awakened to the need for professional nurses and, especially, for public health nurses, the Rockefeller Foundation stepped in and rendered valuable assistance. At the present time Rockefeller support is active in almost all the Central and South American Republics.

INFLUENCE OF KAISERSWERTH

The other great pre-Nightingale factors in nursing were the Kaiserswerth deaconesses. Except for the United States their influence has not been considerable beyond the European Continent, but there it has made itself felt throughout the Protestant countries, notably Scandinavia. The deaconesses were important in elevating nursing standards throughout Germany and the countries that were medically close to it, but they did not go far enough. Their educational standards were not so high as those achieved in England, and they were too much controlled by the medical profession, which emphasized proficiency for a given task rather than the all-around education of a professional woman. The rules of the various deaconess orders varied greatly; some were nearly as strict as the Catholic ones. The nursing training that had been established in Kaiserswerth gradually became accepted in purely secular hospitals, such as the Red Cross and the many government hospitals, but the nurses did not achieve the degree of independence that they had in England under the guidance of Miss Nightingale, nor were they recruited in the same extent from the upper middle class. As a protest against this state, the Free Sisters (also called the "Wild Sisters") appeared at the beginning of this century. They requested complete freedom for nurses with consequent improvement of their general status. This movement resulted in five different nurses' organizations, which eventually have become coordinated through a central committee. These developments are now of only historical interest. Following the depression of the postwar years, nursing shared in the general improvement of Germany in the 1930's. The effects of World War II cannot yet be conjectured.

The smaller countries surrounding Germany all underwent similar changes tempered by English, and later American, influences and by national traditions. In Austria the development was even slower than in Germany; such progress as there was was largely initiated by doctors. Catholic orders were strong but generally maintained low standards. The working conditions of Austrian nurses were admittedly poor and their social standing low. Not until quite recent times has there been an attempt at improvement, and this has been greatly hampered by the unfortunate political and economic fate of Austria. Even recently there were only eight acceptable schools of nursing in the whole country. Conditions in Switzerland were somewhat better, largely because of the stimulus produced by La Source in Lausanne. The government took active interest in the training of nurses, and all the important factors of the surrounding countries, Catholic orders, the Red Cross, and the deaconesses, also operate in Switzerland. The result is that Switzerland has very satisfactory nursing. In Holland nursing was largely done by deaconesses, but until the turn of the century their status was poor. Then the unsatisfactory conditions were ac-

knowledged as a result of an inquiry by the Dutch Association for Sick Nursing. Since then Dutch nursing has steadily advanced, largely under government auspices.

INFLUENCE OF ENGLISH AND AMERICAN NURSING

One cannot study the development of nursing in foreign countries without being impressed with the tremendous influence, first of English, and later of American nursing. Almost in every country nursing reforms have been initiated either by native nurses who have gone to study in London or America or by English or American nurses who have been called in to start modern nursing education. In general, it may be stated (1) that English nursing gave the impetus to nursing in France, Italy, and a few other European countries, (2) that after World War I this work was continued and expanded to other European countries mostly by Americans, (3) that nursing in the British Empire has advanced largely on English lines, almost according to a set pattern, and (4) that American nursing has dominated the modernization of nursing in the Far East, in the United States dependencies, and in South America.

AFTER WORLD WAR I

Although the early developments in many European countries had emanated from St. Thomas and other London hospitals, England has had relatively little influence on European nursing after World War I. This event brought American nurses to almost all parts of the Continent, and many remained after the war to participate in the relief work. Also the Rockefeller Foundation sponsored projects in various countries as it became increasingly interested in European public health activities. American nurses became attached to many of these, and thus American nursing began to have an important bearing on postwar nursing in Europe and, especially, throughout the Near East.

Following the war Dr. Hamilton of France came to visit the United States, and through the American Nurses' Association a fund was established for a nurses' home for her school at Bordeaux. It was erected as a memorial to the American nurses who died in the war. Another example of the American influence is that Miss Charlotte Munck, the outstanding leader in Danish nursing, was a graduate of the Presbyterian Hospital in New York.

Several of the countries in Eastern Europe turned to the United States for guidance of their nursing reforms. When in 1922 the state school of nursing in Czechoslovakia was reorganized under the Red Cross, three American nurses were asked to head this reorganization. They completed their job in a year and then turned the school over to Czechoslovakians.

Greek nurses had come to the United States for education even before the war. At one time there were seven Greek girls studying nursing under Greek royal patronage in this country. In 1922-1923 occurred the great disaster in Asia Minor when one and a half million Greeks were literally thrown out of their homes and suddenly repatriated with resulting great suffering and deprivation. The Near East Relief was organized under American auspices to cope with this situation, and American nurses came in and immediately did much to relieve the situation. Later they laid the foundation for modern schools and public health projects throughout Greece and Asia Minor.

From 1923 to 1926 they ran the school of nursing at Athens Polyclinic Hospital, and, also in 1923, a training school for nurses was established at the American Women's Hospital in Salonika; it was later (1927) transferred to Athens. Miss Alice Carr did outstanding work at this time in malaria control around Corinth and Marathon. American nursing played an important part in relieving the disaster in Asia Minor. Miss Emma Cushman had been in Asia Minor and the Balkans since 1899 and took a prominent part in the organization of hospitals and in extending aid to refugees and orphans. She received high official recognition for her work. Ann Slack is another American nurse who, under the Near East Foundation, worked for several years to promote public health measures in the Near East. Since 1866 there has been an American university in Beirut. In 1905 a school of nursing was established there under Miss Jane Van Zendt; although the students are somewhat cosmopolitan in nature, the school is conducted on American principles and has educated leaders and administrators in nursing throughout the Near East, England, and South America.

Nursing enterprises under leadership of American nurses are scattered throughout Turkey, Iran, Iraq, and Armenia. Some of them are sponsored by the Near East Relief, but many more are mission hospitals. Some are strictly private undertakings, as, for instance, the American Hospital in Istanbul. It is natural that with the later influx of British and American armies into this region, these efforts should receive further stimulus.

In Scandinavia nursing development was advanced by the high general educational standards. Good nursing material was more readily available, and when nursing reforms started, partly under the impulse of the deaconess movements and partly through the influences from England, directly through the Nightingale schools and indirectly through the Red Cross, they advanced rapidly. Systematic training of nurses began in 1876 in Denmark, in 1884 in Sweden, and in 1894 in Norway. Great emphasis has been placed upon public health and district nursing. This has been further favored by the progressive social legislation in those countries. Because nursing in Denmark early came under the auspices of educated women, nurses in Denmark also produced the first national nurses' organization on the Continent (the Danish Council of

Nurses, 1899); Norway and Sweden followed a few years later. Stimulated by their generally international outlook, these countries have taken an active part in efforts at international cooperation between nurses.

ITALY

Italy underwent a development similar to that of France, but because the social restrictions surrounding young girls were even more confining in Italy than in France any attempt at establishing a women's profession was bound to meet with marked resistance. Even the nuns had no professional freedom but worked entirely under the control of the priests. Again the first attempts at improvement were made under British auspices but with American influence. Miss Grace Baxter was born in Florence of English parents and was trained at Johns Hopkins Hospital in Baltimore. She was induced by Miss Turton, a Scotch woman living in Italy, to return to Italy and there to establish a school of nursing. This she did in Naples in 1896. In spite of hard work her school developed very slowly, especially because of the prejudice among the upper class Italians against nursing as a profession. In 1910 Miss Turton founded another school, this time in Rome, again under the direction of an English nurse, Miss Dorothy Snell. These early schools had a hard time until the social structure of Italy changed. The value of trained nurses had been demonstrated during the war and when the Fascist revolution won, many conditions were changed by decree. Although we may not agree with the dictator's way of doing things, it was generally conceded that in its early days Fascism effected many desirable reforms in Italy. It put its weight behind the training of nurses and gave to Italian girls a freedom which has resulted in a change in the type of girl who now enters the profession. The Catholic organizations have cooperated and Italy is now rapidly achieving an influential place in nursing, largely under their auspices.

BELGIUM

A similar development to that in Italy occurred in Belgium; here the pioneer work was done by the City of Brussels, under whose auspices Miss Edith Cavell from the London Hospital organized the first modern school of nursing. She later obtained world fame because she was executed by the Germans during World War I for helping wounded British prisoners to escape. The improvement in education here also led to the establishment of government examinations and registration and to the formation of an official nurses' society with its own periodical.

FRANCE

In France nursing remained in the hands of religious orders up until quite modern times. Their work, originally good, had gradually deteriorated and did not advance with the nursing reforms elsewhere in the nineteenth century in spite of several efforts, notably by Dr. Bourneville. The reform in French nursing is largely the work of Dr. Anna Hamilton, who was a French physician of British-French parentage. In her thesis, written about 1900 after a study of the English system, she insisted that schools of nursing must have some educational standards for entrance requirement, that qualified nurses should give the practical instruction, that the theoretical teaching should be simplified, and that schools of nursing should be directed and controlled by qualified nurses. These requirements, modest enough, caused considerable controversy, but finally Dr. Hamilton obtained the support of the Protestant Hospital at Bordeaux. A school was organized there under the direction of a qualified nurse. It became a pioneer institution in nursing education in France. In 1930 Dr. Hamilton received the cross of the Legion of Honor in appreciation of her nursing reforms.

The social structure of France was not favorable to a high development of nursing. French girls were on the whole, not well educated, the higher education that they did receive was often in Catholic private schools, and they tended to marry early. Thus it was difficult to obtain educated girls for nursing, and candidates were therefore recruited from the lower strata of society. The war changed much of that, for it led many girls of the better classes into nursing and with the great loss of men many women had to find careers for themselves. Under the leadership of prominent Frenchwomen, the work started by Dr. Hamilton soon became more widely adapted. Minimum standards for nursing education have been established in accredited schools. The nurses are licensed by the state after examinations by the state; they have their official society and journal. These improvements in nursing education extend also into the schools of the religious orders, which consequently have become greatly improved.

SPAIN

Spain was never able to make a proper start. By the time the country had reached a point at which nursing reforms that had been started may have been successful she became embroiled in internal disturbances, which up to the present, have seriously interfered with social progress.

British nurses influenced the early development of nursing. Nurses from St. Thomas' Hospital were called to Spain, and a Swedish nurse trained there founded an excellent Red Cross training school.

RUSSIA

Before the Bolshevik Revolution of 1917 nursing was done by women of the lower classes. They were deeply devoted to their work, which was considered "semi-religious" in character; the Sisters of Mercy, organized by the Grand Duchess Helena, rendered good services during the Crimean War. Until the Russian Revolution nursing was, not advancing fast; many nurses were quite illiterate. Nursing reforms were included, however, in the Five-Year Plan, and every effort has been made to create an efficient and up-to-date nursing profession. How far it has succeeded is not fully known, but such information as was available regarding nursing during World War II indicated that Russian nursing, like the Russian war machine, had been greatly underrated.

CONCLUSION

It has been pointed out that between World War I and World War II the influence of American nurses increased greatly in Europe. This has been accelerated since World War II and in most countries has not been prevented by political conditions. Graduate nurses look to America for leadership; an increasing number of nurses are coming to the United States for graduate study. In all European countries, the improvement of the educational program for students and the improvement of personnel policies for graduate nurses have been strong items in recruitment programs. In several countries, postgraduate courses are being established.

Chapter 44

Nursing in Greece*

The first hospitals in Greece appeared early in the seventh century B.C. and were named "Asculapea" after the ancient god of medicine, Aesculapius. Nurses are mentioned in the old texts, but there is no evidence that these nurses were women. Later in the Christian era, we find women working in the hospitals, the "nosokomea" of the Byzantine Empire as deaconesses or as lay nurses, "nosokomos." During the four centuries of Turkish occupation, hospitals did not exist in Greece, and very few women are mentioned as nurses accompanying the rebels in their struggle for freedom during the Greek Revolution early in the nineteenth century.

FIRST EFFORTS

The first efforts for nursing education in Greece were made by Queen Olga who, in 1875, established a two-year training school for nurses. This school subsequently, in 1885, was attached to the "Evanghelismos" Hospital when this hospital was founded for the training of nurses. The school continued to function until 1930 when it was reorganized for a three-year program. This school is successfully functioning and is still attached to the same hospital, which has now

*Contribution by Miss Sophia Ledakis.

become the largest general hospital in Greece; it has 1,200 beds.

In 1914 Queen Sophia established a two-year training school on a voluntary basis under the administration of the Red Cross. The school was directed by a Greek nurse trained in England. The graduates of the school worked very successfully during the period of war from 1914 to 1921. The Red Cross continues to give six- to eight-month courses for volunteer nurses. There are about 9,000 volunteer nurses who work in Red Cross institutions and are ready to help the graduate nurses in times of need, such as war, epidemics, and catastrophies caused by the elements of nature. Graduate nurse instructors in Greece provide courses for the volunteer nurses. These courses consist of about 150 hours of theory and sixty working days of practice. In order to keep them up to date with new techniques, each year the nurses are invited to a thirty-day practice period in Red Cross institutions.

It was a group of these nurses from the first class (1914-1916) who, in the light of their experience from the difficult years of World War I, sensed the need for up-to-date professional nursing education. They contributed greatly toward the establishment of the Greek Red Cross School of Nursing and public health nursing in Athens in

1924. This school was the first in Greece to be operated on a three-year program based upon the internationally accepted curriculum of that time.

This school was directed during the first two years of its existence by the Helen Vassilopoulou, a Red Cross nurse with a "diploma d'Etat Francais." From 1926 to 1954 the director of the school was Miss Athena Messolora, a Red Cross nurse of the class 1912-1916. She had worked as a volunteer in military hospitals and missions catering to displaced persons in Constantinople and Asia Minor. She had taken a postgraduate course in public health nursing at the King's College, London University, in 1921. The course was sponsored by the League of the Red Cross Societies. During her long professional career Miss Messolora's devoted services and wise leadership greatly contributed to the development of nursing in Greece.

In 1927 a three-year nursing school was founded by the American Women's Association. This school was placed under the administration of an American-trained nurse but had to close in 1933 because of lack of facilities. Only twenty-seven graduated from that school.

STATE SCHOOL

In 1938 the third three-year school for nurses and public health nurses was established by the state; it was placed under the administration of a Greek nurse. Four other three-year schools of nursing have been founded since World War II: the Military School of Nursing in 1946, the State School of Nursing in Salonika in 1954, the Princess Irene School of Nurses at the Children's Hospital (the Aghia Sophia) in 1940, and the Pikpa School for Nurses and Public Health Nurses in 1963.

Along with these three-year training schools for professional nurses, a number of one-year training schools for assistant nurses were established. In 1930 a one-year school for assistant public health nurses

was founded; it functioned until 1932. Another one-year temporary school was established in 1939; but it closed down in 1940. In 1946 a one-year school for assistant public health nurses was established but was not recognized and closed down within a few years. In 1949 the School for Assistant Nurses of Soteria Hospital was founded; it continues to operate. In 1954 two similar schools were established and continue to operate, one at King Paul's State Hospital and one at the Patriotikon Foundation of Social Welfare and Hygiene. In 1962 a school for assistant nurses was started in Agrinion.

In 1947 the nursing section of the Ministry of Health was first established, and Miss Helen Petralia was appointed as Chief Nurse. Foreign nurses working for United Nations Relief and Rehabilitation Administration at that time caused the establishment of this bureau at the Ministry of Social Welfare.

FIRST LEGISLATION

In 1948 the first nursing legislation was enacted and Law 683/48 was passed by the parliament. The Nursing Bureau of the Ministry of Social Welfare, Hygiene Division, was legally recognized, and nursing education and registration were put under its supervision. Entrance requirements to schools of nursing were considerably raised. For the three-year schools of nursing a gymnasium (high school) diploma is required, that is, twelve years of studies. In order that these schools of nursing be recognized by the state and their graduates granted state registration, they must meet the minimum requirements set by the decree mentioned above.

A unified educational program is set by this bureau, and schools are supervised so that the schedules are carried out. The register is also kept by the Nursing Bureau of the Ministry of Social Welfare. Registration of graduates of the state-approved schools of nursing is effected as soon as their diplomas are confirmed by the Minister of Social Welfare. All graduate nurses in Greece are required to work successfully for three years in an institution or service defined by the Ministry of Social Welfare. After this period, they are granted their license, which is life-long.

Conditions of service, rank, promotion, and so forth, as defined by Law 683/48 have been improved by subsequent Law 3097 of 1954.

NURSING ORGANIZATION

The Hellenic National Graduate Nurses Association was founded in 1923 by eleven Greek nurses who had been trained abroad. In 1927 the first graduates of the Hellenic Red Cross School of Nursing joined the Association. In 1929 the Association was accepted in full membership by the International Council of Nurses of Montreal, Canada. The Association had been inactive during the years of war but renewed international contact soon after the liberation of Greece from German occupation in 1947. The Association is now very active and has a total of 1980 members. In 1965 the Association organized the first postgraduate study week. The Association circulates a nursing bulletin four times a year.

SOCIAL AND ECONOMIC CONDITIONS OF NURSES IN GREECE

Since 1948 when the 683 Law for nurses and public health nurses was passed by the parliament, the social and economic status of the nurses improved remarkably. The standards of entrance requirements and training have been raised, and the recruitment conditions of candidates have been greatly improved. There are more than five applications for every one admission to the various schools. This enables the schools to give a strict entrance examination and select the best candidates.

The grading of graduate nurses is similar to that of the state employees; their salaries compare very favorably to those of school

teachers and social workers. Nursing is accepted as an honorable profession for a girl, and many applicants seek entrance each year. Nursing education is given free in all schools, and students are not paid. Nursing education is comprehensive in Greece; the program in all schools covers all branches of nursing, including public health. Students must spend eight weeks in the public health field. Three of the schools have an extended course in public health nursing, thus specializing their graduates for public health work.

Most of the schools are independent educational institutions and have their own administration and management. Only two of the schools are attached to hospitals. Postgraduate education does not exist in Greece. Plans are being made for the establishment of a postgraduate school in Athens, but this has not been accomplished because of financial difficulties. Specialization in nursing administration is acquired abroad. Scholarships are offered by the State Scholarship Foundation and the World Health Organization. In the postwar years many scholarships were offered by other organizations, such as the Rockefeller Foundation, the American Mission to Greece, the Florence Nightingale International Foundation, and others. About 200 nurses have had the opportunity of postgraduate studies and specialization abroad.

Nurses of many nationalities worked in Greece under the United Nations Relief and Rehabilitation Administration. They greatly helped in improving the conditions. Today, the picture of nursing in Greece is that of development and expansion, following the progress of technology and always keeping upmost the high traditions that have been the source of inspiration for nurses in the past years.

Greek nurses have learned that recognition and esteem for their work is not offered by society, but it is earned by hard work and sacrifice. About 4,000 graduate and volunteer nurses worked hard during the war years and the German occupation, as well as the Civil War. Thirteen nurses lost their lives on active service, and sixteen Florence Nightingale medals were awarded to Greek nurses for excellent services. Young students today must face the problem of continuing and maintaining the heritage that the passing generation of nurses is entrusting to them.

There are over 3,000 graduates of the three-year schools and over 2,000 from the one-year schools of training. About 250 nurses graduate every year from the seven schools. The three schools of assistant nurses have an enrollment of about 200 students per year; in addition, there are about 3,000 professional midwives who have graduated from the three-year schools of midwifery.

About 3,000 practical nurses are working in the various institutions. These practical nurses are not registered or licensed by the state. A short, two month course of in-service training is given to practical nurses by graduate nurses, according to a program prescribed by the Nursing Bureau of the Ministry of Social Welfare.

Chapter 45

Nursing in Asia

THE AMERICAN INFLUENCE

We still should discuss how modern nursing has been brought to the Far East. Although many nations have had a share in this movement, it has predominantly been an American undertaking, except for India, partly by foreign missions and partly by great foundations like the Rockefeller. The tendency has been, insofar as possible, to train native nurses for administrative positions. This most essential part of the program has often been very difficult to attain because of the social position of Oriental women. The opposition has been overcome, slowly and gradually at first but at an ever-increasing tempo.

JAPAN

In Japan the first attempt to train native nurses was made in 1885 in Kyoto. Miss Linda Richards was placed in charge. She remained for five years. Her school was successful and passed eventually into Japanese hands. About the same time (1887) a Japanese Red Cross was established, and soon it began to establish hospitals and train nurses. Japanese Red Cross hospitals have continued to operate nurses' training schools. The standards of these schools are high. The graduates are available for military service.

The other official Japanese schools are run by the government; their standards are not so high, but they give extensive postgraduate training. Several have university affiliations.

The outstanding American nursing institution in Japan is the school of nursing of St. Luke's Hospital at Tokyo. Its standards are as high as are found anywhere in the world. It belongs to the Protestant Episcopal Church of America. With the support of the Rockefeller Foundation it has established a College of Nursing that gives a four-year course training nurses for leading positions. Thus, it is similar to Teachers College, Columbia University. Up to the outbreak of World War II nursing in Japan was aiming at the highest standards.

Professional nursing and schools of nursing suffered seriously during World War II. In 1945 the United States military government offered to help in the reorganization of nursing education in Japan. Under the Nursing Affairs Division of the Public Health and Welfare Section of the Supreme Command of Allied Powers, a study was made of the Japanese schools of nursing. In 1946 the Red Cross Demonstration School of Nursing was established in Tokyo. This school, set up as a demonstration unit, is now a center for refresher courses for nursing administrators, educators, and clinical specialists.

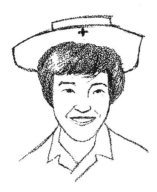

Japanese Red Cross College School

The National Nurses' Association, known as the Japanese Midwives, Clinical Nurses, and Public Health Nurses' Association, was registered by the Japanese government in 1947 with the aim of promoting education, both professional and general. This organization has applied for membership in the International Council of Nurses and is working hard to meet its standards.

CHINA

One of the most interesting developments in nursing is that which has occurred in China. Chinese health conditions were appallingly primitive in spite of the high culture of the country, and the first few mission hospitals that were established seemed pitifully inadequate. Although medical schools soon were established, nursing was long done by "dressers"—untrained men and women who had been taught to perform simple tasks but who were uneducated and of low social standing. About the turn of the century the education of women began; no longer were the feet of baby girls bound. Soon efforts were being made to train Chinese girls to become nurses. Because of social customs it became necessary also to train male nurses to nurse men—this trend is now waning. From the beginning the education of nurses was in the hands of English and American nurses of the mission hospitals. In 1909 Miss Cora Simpson united them into a Nurses' Association of China for the purpose of establishing standards and trends. She was eminently successful; by 1912 a standard curriculum had been established and a central registration committee had been empowered to accredit schools.

The nursing profession of China gained a distinct advantage by expanding from a central national organization, for it became much easier to enforce rules and regulations. The result was a tremendous development; it was favored by the support of both the Chinese government and the China Medical Missionary Association, as well as by the respect of the average Chinese for education.

The immediate task of the organization was to train Chinese for leading positions, and for this purpose valuable aid was received in two ways. The national organization achieved an enviable position: At first the president was a missionary nurse, but as soon as possible the presidency passed to a Chinese. European- and American-prepared nurses, many of them Chinese, continued to control the development. In fact, most promising Chinese nurses were sent to American or English institutions; many of them obtained advanced degrees. In 1937 the Association obtained a national headquarters in Nanking; a nursing journal had been established in 1920. A great many English and American nursing texts have been translated into the Chinese.

The second important development was the organization in 1921 of the Peiping Union Medical College by the Rockefeller Foundation. Five mission hospitals were united and received modern buildings and the finest possible organization. The Foundation provided visiting teachers from Europe. Although the College was organized to advance medicine as a whole in China, the fact that public health was especially emphasized helped the cause of nursing greatly. The school of nursing was organized on the highest standards; minimum requirements were two years of college and, as in the case of St. Luke's Hospital in Tokyo, the purpose was primarily to provide administrators and teachers for other schools.

Until China was crippled by the war, she, therefore, bid fair to become one of the leading nations in the world in nursing. China had launched a tremendous public health program that was expected to require 50,000 nurses; every encouragement was given to midwifery and child welfare. In 1937 the education of nurses was placed under the Ministry of Education; license was to be obtained after an examination by a national board. By 1937 over 200 nursing schools had been established and over 10,-000 nurses had been graduated. Since then, however, nursing activities in free China have been very much handicapped, first by the war with Japan and then by the Chinese Communists. Before the Communists took over most of China, the educational minimum for young women entering schools of nursing was graduation from a junior high school, which was followed by three years in a school of nursing. The Communists have reduced educational standards to primary school graduation and two years of nurses' training. At present free China has in Taiwan four nursing schools and over 600 students. Already, over 700 have graduated from these schools. This number is not nearly enough to meet the need but it is the nucleus.

INDIA

India presents a few points of special interest to nurses, for it, more than any country outside the British Isles, had Miss Nightingale's attention. For many years she was actively interested in improving public health conditions in this vast country. Although she never set foot on Indian soil, she was in close touch with every important official who went there from England. The high standards of ancient times had long since been abandoned; the whole social structure was averse to the progress of modern medicine. When we study the state of nursing in a country like India, we are impressed with the importance of those factors that we discussed in the introductory section, in the evolution of nursing. We see here a country with an age-old culture of the highest order, in which poetry and other literature ranked high, riches had been amassed almost beyond comprehension, and religious and ethical philosophy were highly developed as well as the social structure. Though this culture may seem strange to the Western mind, it certainly was not primitive or undeveloped as that in the Australian or African wilderness. Yet this great civilization remained for many years untouched by the Industrial Revolution and all that it implies, including medical advance and modern hygiene as expressed in hospital construction. Its women were confined by narrow social customs. Furthermore, their activities were restricted by castes and religious considerations, the dominating religions, Hinduism and Mohammedanism, being in sharp conflict.

This social structure offered a resistance to Western Civilization that is still strong. Although it may be argued that people with so high a culture should be allowed to live and die as they please, it is still hard for the Western mind to face so much unnecessary suffering without attempting to relieve it. This was the motivating force in Florence Nightingale's work for India. It was she who planned the public health reforms that have been carried out during the last two or three generations. Here, as in other colonies, nursing was greatly aided by the support given by the nobility. In 1885 when Miss Nightingale was still at her height, Queen Victoria instructed Lady Dufferin, wife of the Governor-General, to plan work to bring the advances of modern medicine to Indian women. Lady Dufferin lived up to the Queen's expectations; as the result of her work a large fund was created under the auspices of royalty and nobility for the purpose of supplying hospitals, dispensaries, and medical and nursing aid to the various parts of this vast country. As the fund increased, its activities became even more extensive; an increasing emphasis was placed upon the education of native doctors and nurses. The fund gradually became government administrated. Many Americans came out to aid in the work. This was difficult work, for not only was it necessary to train women doctors, as well as nurses, because of the social conditions, but the women to be trained were illiterate and had no elementary education. The social order was against their education. All this is now slowly changing, and it seems that the value of health and of the modern measures that are available to obtain it are being increasingly appreciated. These reforms are, therefore, likely to go on, whatever may be the outcome of the present struggle.

Some historical data may be of interest to American nurses who are likely some day to find themselves in India.

Training of nurses in India preceded even the Nightingale schools, for the Madras Hospital began it in 1854; several hospitals followed suit, especially after 1880 when the mission hospitals began to realize its importance. They have established a United Board of Training for Mission Nurses. Serious efforts are being made to extend nursing education to native girls; therefore, mission schools often instruct in the native languages while the government schools require English as the official language. There are now many accredited schools, and as can be expected, great emphasis is being placed upon the teaching of midwifery. Wherever English administration prevails, attention is paid to public health. Some of the most important health working is being done by the Red Cross Society of India. It finds the various shrines of India particularly favorable for dissemination of knowledge, for these are visited by great numbers of people from all over the country.

The official organization of nurses is similar to that of the English-speaking countries: After 1923 the various provinces rapidly adopted registration of nurses. There is an Association of Nursing Superintendents and a Trained Nurses' Association, as well as a *Nursing Journal of India*. All were established at the beginning of the century. Thus, India has the beginnings of organizations that may eventually bring modern health conditions to all its teeming millions.

Questions and study projects for unit eleven

Chapter 41

1. What was the effect of Mr. Rathbone's interest in public health nursing in Liverpool?
2. What are the main differences between British and American nursing?
3. How has the development of the registration of nurses in Great Britain differed from that in this country?
4. Describe the contributions of the following persons to nursing: Mrs. Bedford-Fenwick, Mr. Rathbone, and Agnes Jones.
5. Compare American and British nursing in their developments.
6. Describe findings of the Lancet Commission and its contribution to British nursing.

Chapter 42

1. What social and economic conditions influenced early nursing in these countries?
2. Discuss the great influence of America in the development of nursing in South America.
3. Discuss the cooperative plans in nursing education between the United States and South America.
4. Make an annotated bibliography of recent articles appearing in *The American Journal of Nursing, Nursing Outlook, Nursing Research,* and any other journals available in your library relating to the discussion in this chapter.

Chapter 43

1. What were some of the differences in the development of nursing in Catholic and in Protestant countries of Europe during the nineteenth century?
2. Show how the general social conditions, especially in the fields of education and those affecting the status of women, influenced the development of nursing in different European countries.
3. Write a short paper on, or be prepared to discuss, the influence abroad of English and American nursing:
   (a) Before World War I
   (b) Between World Wars I and II
4. Make an annotated bibliography of recent articles appearing in *The American Journal of Nursing, Nursing Outlook, Nursing Research,* and any other journals available in your library relating to the discussion in this chapter.

Chapter 44

1. Would you say Greek nursing was influenced more by British or American nursing? Why?
2. List at least six examples of the influence of modern war on nursing in Greece.
3. Can you explore or trace the influence of war upon nursing from the time of the crusades, through Florence Nightingale to modern times?

Chapter 45

1. What have been the main influences in the development of nursing in the British colonies and dominions?
2. Trace Miss Nightingale's influence on nursing in India.
3. Discuss the prewar activities of medical missionaries and the use of private funds from America in modern nursing in the Asiatic countries.
4. Show how the political conditions in these countries affect professional nursing. Give specific examples.
5. Make an annotated bibliography of recent articles appearing in *The American Journal of Nursing, Nursing Outlook, Nursing Research,* and any other journals available in your library relating to the discussion in this chapter.

References for unit eleven

Chapter 41

Dock, Lavinia L., editor and co-author: A history of nursing, vol. 3, New York, 1907, G. P. Putnam's Sons.

Edwards, Muriel M.: Nursing in Britain, 1937-1943, American Journal of Nursing **44**:125-133, February, 1944.

Goodall, Frances G.: The college of nursing, American Journal of Nursing **31**:1245-1250, November, 1931.

Lancet Commission on Nursing: Final report, London, 1932, The Lancet, Ltd.

Nursing in Britain, American Journal of Nursing **37**:281-284, May, 1947.

Pavey, Agnes: The story of the growth of nursing, London, 1938, Faber & Faber, Ltd.

Seymer, Lucy Ridgely: A general history of nursing, New York, 1933, The Macmillan Co.

Seymer, Lucy Ridgely: Agnes Jones, 1832-1932, International Nursing Review **8**:43-51, 1933.

Sidley, Irene: No. 15 Manchester Square, American Journal of Nursing **37**:590-592, June, 1937.

Some impressions of British nursing, American Journal of Nursing **37**:589, June, 1937.

Wheelock, Ruth V.: In Miss Nightingale's London, American Journal of Nursing **38**:978-981, September, 1938.

Chapter 42

Adams, Sara E.: A school for nurses in Chile, American Journal of Nursing **27**:1029-1030, December, 1927.

Control of nursing in Brazil, American Journal of Nursing **31**:1034, September, 1931.

Larrabure, Sister Rosa: The National School of Nursing in Peru, International Nursing Review **7**:63-68, 1932.

Mackie, Janet W.: Nursing in the other American republics, American Journal of Nursing **45**:355-357, May, 1945.

North and South American nurses consider legislation and advanced education, American Journal of Nursing **53**:1462, December, 1953.

Our South American colleagues, American Journal of Nursing **40**:47-51, January, 1940; **40**:153-160, February, 1940.

Parsons, Ethel: Development of nursing in Brazil, International Nursing Review **10**:54-60, 1936.

Pioneers in Argentina, American Journal of Nursing **48**:578-579, September, 1948.

Pullen, Bertha: Modern nursing in Brazil, American Journal of Nursing **35**:345-350, April, 1935.

Storgerer, Beatrice: A good neighbor fellowship program, American Journal of Nursing **48**:440-443, July, 1948.

Chapter 43

Andrell, Majsa: Nursing in Sweden, American Journal of Nursing **40**:1336-1341, December, 1940.

Cantor, Shulamith L.: Nursing in Israel, American Journal of Nursing **51**:162, March, 1951.

Ernsberger, Rose G.: Nursing in Russia, Nursing Outlook **2**:883, December, 1963.

Hallsten-Kallia, Armi: International influences on nursing in Finland, American Journal of Nursing **46**:154-156, March, 1946.

Kroeger, Gertrud: Nursing in Germany, American Journal of Nursing **39**:483-485, May, 1939.

Larsson, Sister Bergljot: Norway's nurses carry on, American Journal of Nursing **46**:308-309, May, 1946.

Nordendahl, Kerstin: Nursing in Sweden, American Journal of Nursing **48**:694-696, November, 1948.

Report from Czechoslovakia (editorial), American Journal of Nursing **46**:226, April, 1946.

Schroeder, Ellen Margrethe: Nursing in Denmark, American Journal of Nursing **37**:355-360, April, 1937.

Setzler, Lorraine: Nursing and nursing education in Germany, American Journal of Nursing **45**:993, December, 1945.

Setzler, Lorraine: Stockholm diary, American Journal of Nursing **46**:46-47, January, 1946.

Stevens, Wilma F.: Off duty in Syria, American Journal of Nursing **39**:1323-1327, December, 1939.

Witt, Elizabeth: Existing conditions amongst nurses (in Denmark), International Nursing Review **12**:5156, 1938.

Chapter 44

Messolora, Athina J.: A brief history of the evolution of nursing in Greece, Athens, 1956, Hellenic National Graduate Nurses' Association.

Chapter 45

Burnett, D. Lois: Nursing in the Orient, Nursing World **125**:298-300, July, 1951.

Kaneko, Mitsu: Public health nursing in Japan, Public Health Nursing **50**:97, January, 1950.

Korean assignment, American Journal of Nursing **53**:678-679, June, 1953.

Larson, Blenda: Report from Japan and Korea, American Journal of Nursing **48**:630-632, October, 1948.

Lin, Evelyn: Nursing in China, American Journal of Nursing **38**:1-8, January, 1938.

Sister M. Clare and Sister M. Laetitia: Nursing in India and Pakistan, American Journal of Nursing **49**:359-361, June, 1949.

Index

Sternberg, George M., 90
Stewart, Isabel Maitland, 105, 106, 108-109, 125
Stimson, Julia C., 159
Stokes, William, 34
Stone, Lucy, 39
Strong, Mrs. Rebecca, 305
Structure Study, 200, 201
Studies
   between World War I and World War II, 149-150
   contemporary, in nursing, 212-217
"Study of the Functions and Activities of Head Nurses in a General Hospital," 291
Subjection of Women, 39
Sultan of Egypt, 11
Superintendents' Society, 116
Surgery, first course of lectures on, 30
Sutherland, John, 37, 67, 74
Sydenham, Thomas, 22
Syme, James, 46
Syphilis, 83

T

Taylor, Effie J., 276
Teachers College, Columbia University, nursing education at, 124-125
Teams, health, 174
Technical nurse, functions of, 185-186
Temple of Cos, 9
Temple of Hygeia, 8
Terry, Luther, 184
Testimony, 264-265
Testing services, 215
Teutonic Knights, 13-14
Textbook of Nursing, 132
Third Order of St. Francis, 16-17
Todd, A. J., 43
Toronto University, School of Nursing at, 142
Tort(s), 243-253
   definition of, 243
Town and Country Nursing Service, 96, 107
Transylvania University School, 84
Tuberculosis, 83
Tuke, William, 32
Tulane University, women students at, 41
Turton, Miss, 313
Twenty Thousand Nurses Tell Their Story, 216

U

Un Souvenir de Solferino, 92-93
Undue influence and legal capacity, 239
Unfitness, actionable per se, 253
United States; *see* U.S.
University(ies)
   affiliations in British nursing, 305
   Canadian, nursing education at, 293-294
   schools of nursing, 125
University College Hospital, 53

University College Hospital in London, 99
University of Alberta, 293
University of British Columbia, 293
University of Chicago, women students at, 41
University of Minnesota, 142
University of Montpellier, 20
University of Padua, 20
University of Pennsylvania, 84
University of Toronto, 293
Ursuline Sisters, 54-55
   in Canada, 283
U.S. Cadet Nurse Corps, 157, 160
U.S. Indian Service, nursing in, 147
U.S. nursing; *see* American nursing
U.S. Public Health Service, 96, 119, 191
   insignia, 191
U.S.S. Higbee, 164
U.S.S. Relief, 146

V

Valerian, Emperor, 10
Van Buren, John, 58
van Leeuwenhoek, Anton, 33
Van Zendt, Jane, 312
Vasilopoulou, Helen, 316
Vassar, 40
   Training Camp, 135-136
      Program, 108
Venereal disease, 83
Vesalius, 21
Veterans Administration, nursing service in, 146-147, 195-196
Victorian Order of Nurses, 286
"Village nurses," 302
Vindication of the Rights of Women, 37
Virchow, Rudolf, 34, 47
Visiting nurse, 143
   British, 301-303
Visiting Nurse Quarterly, 131
Voltaire, 29
Voluntary Aid Detachment, 305

W

Wald, Lillian D., 96, 105, 106-107, 117, 121, 147
Ward Sister, 78
Wardell, William, 95
Warrington, Joseph, 86
Wasserman reaction, 83
Wellesley, 41
Western Reserve, 126
   School of Nursing of, 142
   women students at, 41
Westminster Hospital, 53
Wheaton College, 40
Whitfield, R. G., 76
WHO, 172, 277, 278
"Wild Sisters," 311